JUSTICE IN GLOBAL HEALTH

Rather than making another attempt at proposing a single and unifying theory of global health justice, this timely collection brings together, instead, scholars from a range of traditions to frame the issue more broadly, highlighting not only different perspectives but also key topics and debates.

The volume features chapters that offer both new theoretical approaches to global health justice, as well as fresh takes on existing frameworks. Others adopt a bottom-up approach to tackle specific problems, including the sexual rights of children and adolescents, artificial intelligence (AI) in medicine, framing of neglected tropical diseases, securitisation of health, and trademarks in global health. Brought together within one volume, the breadth of these chapters provides a unique and enlightening contribution to the wider Global Health field.

This important volume will be a fascinating read for students and researchers across Global Health, Bioethics, Political Philosophy, and Global Development.

Himani Bhakuni is a Lecturer at York Law School, United Kingdom. Before that, she was the Assistant Professor of Justice in Global Health Research at the University Medical Center, Utrecht University. She primarily works on issues within global health and human rights, particularly on questions surrounding justice, reparations, and global health law.

Lucas Miotto is a Senior Lecturer in Law at the University of Surrey and a core member of the Surrey Centre for Law and Philosophy. He works at the intersection between legal, moral, and political philosophy, dealing with questions about coercion, manipulation, wrongful interference, and forms of just governance.

JUSTICE IN GLOBAL HEALTH

New Perspectives and Current Issues

Edited by Himani Bhakuni and Lucas Miotto

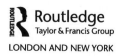

Routledge
Taylor & Francis Group

LONDON AND NEW YORK

Designed cover image: Getty Images

First published 2024
by Routledge
4 Park Square, Milton Park, Abingdon, Oxon OX14 4RN

and by Routledge
605 Third Avenue, New York, NY 10158

Routledge is an imprint of the Taylor & Francis Group, an informa business

British Library Cataloguing-in-Publication Data
A catalogue record for this book is available from the British Library

Library of Congress Cataloguing-in-Publication Data
Names: Bhakuni, Himani, editor. | Miotto, Lucas, editor.
Title: Justice in global health : new perspectives and current issues / edited by Himani Bhakuni, and Lucas Miotto. Description: Abingdon, Oxon [UK] ; New York, NY : Routledge, 2023. | Includes bibliographical references and index. |
Identifiers: LCCN 2023020046 | ISBN 9781032508474 (hardback) | ISBN 9781032508450 (paperback) | ISBN 9781003399933 (ebook)
Subjects: LCSH: Right to health. | Human rights. | Public health laws. | Bioethics.
Classification: LCC K3260.3 .J87 2023 | DDC 344.03/21--dc23/eng/20230802
LC record available at https://lccn.loc.gov/2023020046

ISBN: 978-1-032-50847-4 (hbk)
ISBN: 978-1-032-50845-0 (pbk)
ISBN: 978-1-003-39993-3 (ebk)

DOI: 10.4324/9781003399933

Typeset in Sabon
by MPS Limited, Dehradun

CONTENTS

PART V
Global Health Justice: New Frames,
New Approaches **239**

CONTRIBUTORS

Alice Trotter is a PhD candidate at the Centre for Applied Human Rights at the University of York, United Kingdom. Alice has been involved in the pluridisciplinary project 'Noma, The Neglected Disease. An Interdisciplinary Exploration of Its Realities, Burden, and Framing'. Her other research focuses on human rights in cities.

Alvaro Fernandez-Mora is a Lecturer at York Law School, United Kingdom. He holds a DPhil from the University of Oxford (DPhil) and an LLM from Harvard Law School (LLM). Dr Fernandez-Mora's research interests lie at the intersection between intellectual property law and other fields – notably human rights and competition law and economics. Dr Fernandez-Mora's work has been published in the *Berkeley Journal of International Law* (*BJIL*), the *International Review of Intellectual Property and Competition Law* (*IIC*), and the *Intellectual Property Quarterly* (*IPQ*), among others.

Daniel Elliot Weissglass is an Assistant Professor of Philosophy at Duke Kunshan University. His chief research interests with respect to health include models for improving the moral and political adequacy of global health governance, models of decision making for persons with compromised and/or variable cognitive capacities, assessing the values implicit in the tools used to measure and report health outcomes, and the risks and benefits of medical AI – especially in LMICs.

Erika Blacksher is the John B. Francis Chair at the Center for Practical Bioethics and Research Professor in the Department of History and

Philosophy of Medicine at the University of Kansas School of Medicine. Dr. Blacksher studies questions of responsibility and justice raised by U.S. health inequalities and the potential for democratic deliberation to build shared purpose across race, class, and geography and to make health a shared value. Her current work focuses on intersectional health inequalities, with a focus on class, poverty, and race, and the methodology of democratic deliberation.

Gottfried Schweiger is a Senior Scientist at the Centre for Ethics and Poverty Research (CEPR) and a member of the Philosophy Department (KTH) of the University of Salzburg, Austria. His research revolves around social and political philosophy with a focus on poverty, social and global justice, migration, childhood and youth, social work, sports, and critical theory.

Hendrik Kempt works mostly in applied ethics, with a focus on the ethics of medical AI, natural language processing, and human–machine relationships. He has published several books and articles, his latest being on "Synthetic Friends". He is a research associate at the Applied Ethics Group at RWTH Aachen.

Himani Bhakuni is a Lecturer at York Law School, United Kingdom. Before that, she was the Assistant Professor of Justice in Global Health Research at the University Medical Center, Utrecht University. She primarily works on issues within global health and human rights, particularly on questions surrounding justice, reparations, and global health law.

Ioana Cismas is a Reader and the Co-Director of the Centre for Applied Human Rights at the University of York, United Kingdom. Dr Cismas' interests span the broad discipline of public international law, the specialist branches of international human rights law and international humanitarian law, and related fields, such as law and religion and transitional justice. Her work has attracted substantial research grants from the UK Economic and Social Research Council (ESRC), the Swiss National Science Foundation, the Swiss Network of International Studies (SNIS), and several non-governmental organisations and charities. Currently, Dr Cismas co-coordinates the SNIS-funded project Noma, The Neglected Disease. An Interdisciplinary Exploration of Its Realities, Burden, and Framing.

Joanne Liu is an Associate Professor of Medicine at the University of Montreal, a Professor of Clinical Medicine at McGill University, and the former International President of *Médecins sans Frontières*. She is also a paediatric emergency medicine physician in Montreal.

Keerty Nakray is a Professor at Jindal Global Law School, NCR Delhi and Adjunct Faculty at the Centre for Ethics, Yenepoya University, Mangalore. She holds a PhD in Sociology and Social Policy from Queen's University Belfast, Northern Ireland. Her research deals with topics such as gender-based violence, social policy, child poverty, and social exclusion.

Lucas Miotto is a Senior Lecturer in Law at the University of Surrey and a core member of the Surrey Centre for Law and Philosophy. He works at the intersection between legal, moral, and political philosophy, dealing with questions about coercion, manipulation, wrongful interference, and forms of just governance.

Luciano Bottini Filho is a Lecturer in Human Rights Advocacy at Sheffield Hallam University and an affiliated researcher at the Petrie-Flom Center for Health Law Policy, Biotechnology, and Bioethics at Harvard University. His research studies resource allocation, global health, and the right to health. He has been both a Modern Law Review Scholar for his PhD studies at Bristol and a Chevening Scholar by nomination of the UK Foreign, Commonwealth and Development Office (FCDO).

Man-to Tang is a Visiting Fellow at the Department of Public and International Affairs, City University of Hong Kong. His research interests are in phenomenology, classical and contemporary Confucianism, and political philosophy.

Nils Freyer works in the field of machine learning, especially active learning and natural language processing. His research interests also include questions of AI ethics, with a focus on medical AI. He is currently a research assistant at FH Aachen – University of Applied Sciences.

Ryoa Chung is a Full Professor in the Department of Philosophy of the University of Montreal and Co-Director of the Center for Research in Ethics. She works in the field of international ethics, feminist philosophy, political philosophy, and health inequality. She also teaches medical ethics/bioethics at the Faculty of Medicine of the University of Montreal. Her works have appeared in edited volumes published by Oxford University Press, Presses universitaires de France, and in journals such as *Journal of Social Philosophy, Journal of Medical Ethics, Public Health Ethics, The Lancet,* and *Hastings Center Report.*

Sridhar Venkatapuram is an Associate Professor of Global Health and Philosophy at King's College London in the United Kingdom. He is based at the Global Health Institute, where he is Deputy Director, and Director of Global Health Education. He is the author of *Health Justice: An Argument from the Capabilities Approach* (2011), co-editor of *Vulnerable: The Law, Policy and Ethics of Covid-19* (2020) and *The Routledge Handbook of Philosophy of Public Health (2022)*. He can be found at @sridhartweet.

Xuanpu Zhuang is a PhD candidate at Bowling Green State University, Department of Philosophy. Xuanpu works on issues within political and practical philosophy, particularly on issues pertaining to equality, citizenship, and justice.

INTRODUCTION

Justice in Global Health

Himani Bhakuni and Lucas Miotto

As we write this introduction in early 2023, we are fortunate to have survived one of the most daunting global health emergencies of our time, but the world lost many to COVID-19. Health emergencies tend to refocus our attention not only on the value of life, but also on the centrality of health in preserving life. In the early days of the pandemic, COVID-19 was called "a great equaliser", that it would affect everyone the same. But soon enough, that thought went out the window quite like almost everything else that has been called a great equaliser before. It is not news that our world is riddled with staggering inequalities. Everything that threatens humankind tends to threaten some bits of humankind more than others. But that we continue to bear these inequalities despite there being other ways to think, reason, and act is even more staggering.

This book is about that – not about continuing to bear the different forms of health inequalities – but about challenging them. Our contributors, from varied disciplines, have thought of some problems in global health and have given reasons for why we would all be better off in thinking of a given problem in a particular way. Some have provided legal solutions; others have questioned the way we frame issues. Some have proposed newer frameworks that could be used to tackle injustices in global health, while others have used pre-existing theories of justice and applied them to modern-day health issues. But the goal of each chapter in this edited volume is the same – to provide some guidance on what would aid the field of global health in achieving its lofty aspiration of improving health for *all* people worldwide. We choose the overarching language of justice to do so.

Up until a few decades ago the notion of justice (in academic circles at least) was predominantly territory bound. There was international justice,

DOI: 10.4324/9781003399933-1

but it was largely about justice amongst nations. Lately, factors including globalisation, digitalisation, increasing climate change, economic interdependence, and enduring global effects of colonial histories, have all led to the expansion of the scope of justice. Today, we talk about *global* justice not only when we consider duties that we have towards others beyond nation-states, but also when we talk about worldwide inequalities as moral problems which are embedded in local contexts and shared norms. Global health justice then becomes an area of research that focuses on proposing, creating, and maintaining conditions that would enable *everyone*, not just a privileged few, to experience and achieve good health and life.

Philosophers and political theorists have attempted to provide an overarching theory of global health justice, wherein they have been particularly inspired by the capabilities approach.[1] Some have extended pre-existing theories of global justice and the rights-based approach to health.[2] Despite all these commendable efforts, it is quite likely that, given the multitude of global health problems, a single overarching theory of justice would still at best be a partial explanation of the duties and obligations of various stakeholders involved in the debate. Which is why this edited volume adopts a mix of approaches to look at justice in global health, it provides some new philosophical frames and fresher takes on existing frames, but it also tackles some more specific problems that we believe that any successful overarching theory of global health justice must address. While general frameworks of justice help to provide a better understanding of our world and our responsibilities within it, more specific incursions on specific issues allow us to see solutions to problems that might not be immediately available or salient to those who attempt to provide unifying frameworks.

We are aware that this book is releasing at a time when people might be going through a health-topic fatigue. A lot has been written (and is being written) about health, daily. But we nonetheless believe that this volume adds much more than just noise to the conversation. The volume contains 13 original contributions, most of which were first presented online at the *Justice in Global Health Workshop Series* in October 2022. The contributions address a wide range of issues and topics within global health justice: from specific challenges associated with an overlooked disease, future injustices caused by the development of new technologies, role of law in addressing commercial determinants of health, and institutional reforms, to new theoretical frameworks for global health justice. As editors, we are proud of the volume's thematic breadth. But we are also proud of the interdisciplinary dialogue that took place amongst contributors from different backgrounds and corners of the world. Such dialogue allowed us to identify some common threads and insights running across contributions, which we think would be valuable to anyone interested in global health and global health justice. To make the threads clearer to our readers, we have divided the volume into five parts. This division, however, should not be seen as an attempt to draw hard boundaries; some themes, arguments, and concepts recur through the volume. In what follows we provide an overview of the volume's contributions.

Part I. Citizenship, Power, and Relational Justice

The first part illustrates a pervasive theme in the book. Justice in global health requires more than a fair distribution of resources – it requires a fair distribution of the burdens necessary to maintain our health systems globally. It also requires addressing morally problematic relations of power and, more specifically, that we relate to one another as equals and respectfully in health-related contexts. Relational justice is, therefore, integral to global health justice. However, promoting relational justice in global health may require radical shifts in our current institutional and political architecture, as is argued by the two chapters in this part.

In *World Citizenship and Global Health* (Chapter 1), Xuanpu Zhuang argues for one of those shifts by favouring the introduction of the cosmopolitan ideal of world citizenship. "People are not just abstract moral beings"; their identity, rights, and obligations are shaped by their social and political arrangements. Citizenship marks an important form of membership in a social and political arrangement. It typically determines the political rights, liberties, and obligations that individuals have towards the state and towards other individuals living in the same territory. Often, however, social and political relations outgrow the confines of a state or territory: individuals interact as a global community on global matters. This raises a question about the need for a form of world citizenship which, Zhuang argues, is not simply national citizenship writ large. It is, instead, an extra layer of social and political association significant enough to ground certain entitlements to social goods, welfare, and capabilities.

Global health enters the scene because the capability of being healthy is, according to Zhuang, a necessary condition of functioning as a world citizen. To justify this claim, Zhuang introduces the four "Problematic Hierarchies"; four ways in which the absence of health undermines the sort of egalitarian relations which are constitutive of world citizenship. From the discussion, it becomes apparent that strengthening global health is necessary for maintaining the relational egalitarian ideal of world citizenship. But – the chapter also seems to entail – the relationship goes both ways: not only is the capability of being healthy a necessary condition of world citizenship, but some demands to promote global health justice also flow from and are (at least partly) constituted by broader demands of relational equality and respect enshrined in world citizenship.

A good illustration of the relationship between global health justice and relational egalitarianism is found in *AI-DSS in Healthcare and Their Power over Health Insecure Collectives* (Chapter 2). In this chapter, Nils Freyer and Hendrik Kempt discuss a dilemma that arises from the introduction of artificial intelligence-led decision support systems (AI-DSS) in expert-scarce areas – for example, a system that diagnoses and recommends treatment for a disease without the interference of a medical expert. These systems require what is known as "explainability standards": standards that allow humans to understand and assess the reliability of the conclusions and recommendations reached by an automated system. For optimal reliability, these standards must be stringent. But the costs, technology, and qualified personnel required to maintain stringent explainability standards cannot often be met by expert-scarce communities – or "collectives", as the authors believe we should call them. Hence the dilemma: either expert-scarce collectives do not introduce automated systems and abandon their hopes to reap the health benefits that these systems bring, or these collectives settle for a cheaper alternative and accept whatever explainability standards are offered to them by the relevant corporations. Because the second horn of this dilemma is often the more tempting one, the emergence of a "colonial mindset" and the introduction of a relation of domination between collectives and corporations are obvious risks.

The main difficulty, then, is whether this relation of domination can be avoided without abdicating the potential health benefits introduced by AI-DSS. The authors propose a way to negotiate explainability standards that do not require eschewing relational justice. The solution explored in the chapter is instructive, as it can be extended to contexts where a similar clash between health benefits and relational justice arises. For example, in contexts of clinical research where some researchers and participants are tempted to relax research regulations in the name of efficiency or short-term health benefits.

Part II. Responsibility for Justice: Law, Civil Society, and the Private Sector

The second part of the volume focuses on the role and responsibilities of courts, advocacy groups, and the private sector in the promotion of global health justice. The opening chapter, *Everything Is Unconstitutional – Contesting Structural Violence in Health Systems with Legal Mobilisation* (Chapter 3), highlights the use of constitutional remedies as a tool for the elimination of structural violence and inequality in global health. The author, Luciano Bottini Filho, centres the discussion on a case from 2021 where the Brazilian Supreme Court relied on the "state of unconstitutional affairs" doctrine to declare the entirety of the Brazilian public health system unconstitutional in light of its systematic and enduring violation of transgender people's right to health, life, and dignity.

The Court's decision helps to highlight the importance of relational justice in the context of global health justice. As we can infer from the chapter, not only was the declaration of unconstitutionality grounded on the denial of health resources, but it was also (and perhaps primarily) based on the systematic discrimination and exclusion of transgender people in the context of healthcare. The chapter also illustrates the vital role that courts can play in the broader transformation of health systems and society more generally. In so doing, it also aligns with the discussion about the just transformation of health systems that appears later in the volume (Chapter 10).

In *Framing Noma: Human Rights and Neglected Tropical Diseases as Paths for Advocacy* (Chapter 4), Alice Trotter and Ioana Cismas discuss the strategic importance of framing to strengthen the efforts of advocacy groups and campaigns and to bring about changes in global health. Roughly, to "frame" a given issue is to choose the way in which the issue is communicated to a selected audience; thus, a "frame" can be seen as a rhetorical device. In the chapter, the authors discuss the findings from their own empirical research on the uses of alternative frames for tackling noma, a relatively unknown disease that, despite being preventable and treatable, has an estimated mortality rate of around 90% in children. Noma primarily affects those living in extreme poverty, and its effects were initially framed as a medical or humanitarian emergency which, despite the relative success in attracting aid from charities and doctors from the Global North, also brought with it relations of dependency and "signalled a 'white saviour' trope". Here the chapter brings us back to the importance of relational justice to global health: the alternative framings considered by the authors – framing noma as a neglected tropical disease and as a human rights issue – were used precisely to make both material progress in combating the disease and relational progress, as it were, in avoiding the emergence of problematic social relations in the context of health. The chapter, therefore, illustrates how civil society and advocacy groups can play an effective role in tackling global health injustices by carefully choosing how to frame these injustices.

In this part's last chapter, *Trade Marks and the Right to Health: A Growing Tension* (Chapter 5), Alvaro Fernandez-Mora discusses policymakers' use of trade mark-restrictive policies to protect health and health rights. Such policies range from advertisement bans to more aggressive restrictions on packaging and aim at making harmful products less attractive to consumers. These policies stem from the assumption that manufacturers of such harmful products – most notably the tobacco industry – cannot be exempted from a responsibility to promote health. Hence, the sacrifice of their rights to intellectual property and freedom of expression in the name of health seems justified. Be this as it may, Fernandez-Mora identifies a rapid expansion of such health-oriented restrictions into the control of alcoholic products and foods high in fat, sugar, and salt. There, the justification of implementing such restrictions may not be straightforward, and the risk of undesirable spillover effects is higher. Courts, being key to the success of health-promoting policies, must be mindful of these hurdles when deciding on the adequacy and legality of such expansionist policies. Though tempting, the "protect health by any means" approach can sometimes cause more harm than the prospective harms from which health-oriented policies seek to protect us. Doing justice in global health – and this is a lesson that we can draw from the chapter – sometimes requires that we take a counter-intuitive step away from the short-term protection of the right to health and focus our efforts on other rights which can sometimes be more important to societal well-being in the long run.

Part III. Sexual Rights and Reproductive Justice

The third part of the volume considers some significant issues within a specific branch of global health justice: sexual and reproductive justice. Sexual health and rights are often subsumed under reproductive health and rights, but both are conceptually distinct, albeit related, areas. WHO's working definition of sexual health states that it "requires a positive and respectful approach to sexuality and sexual relationships, as well as the possibility of having pleasurable and safe sexual experiences, free of coercion, discrimination and violence".[3] While much has been written about sexual rights of adults and able-bodied persons, two groups stand out as understudied and undertheorized in this area: children and adolescents and persons with disabilities (PWDs). The chapters included in this part address these two groups.

In *The Capability Approach and the Sexual Rights of Children and Adolescents* (Chapter 6), Gottfried Schweiger considers how sexual rights reflect the developmental dynamics of child and adolescent autonomy and what aspects of well-being, or what capabilities, these rights protect and enable. Schweiger uses the capability approach to enumerate the sexual rights of children and adolescents, while also focusing on the differences between children and adolescents. His argument is that while sexual rights of children largely deal with defence against dangers and attacks, they must not be limited to that. By relying on the capabilities approach, he proposes a conceptual expansion of sexual rights for children and adolescents: sexual rights should also empower and enable children and adolescents to develop in a sexually healthy way so that they can express their agency according to their level of maturity. This conceptual expansion places sexual education policies as well as measures to raise awareness of contraceptives and sexually transmitted diseases amongst teenagers at the forefront of children and adolescent health. The capabilities approach assists in clarifying that sexual development is part of healthy development and that there are good reasons to break some of the taboos associated with the talk about sexual health of children and adolescents if we want to make progress in global health.

In *Reproductive Justice and Ethics of Consent in Assisted Living Facilities for Disabled People: A Critical Reflection for Socio-Legal Policies on Long-Term Care in India* (Chapter 7), Keerty Nakray claims that people suffering from severe intellectual disability are subjected to what is known as "erotic segregation": the conception according to which disabled people are asexual and not supposed to engage in sexual activities. She uses the framework of critical disability studies to diagnose the cause for this as stigma and discrimination faced by not only the PWDs but also their carers. Her chapter summarises the Indian legal framework dealing with consent of PWDs and discusses leading precedents that demonstrate that despite having a legally recognised right to consent over sexual and reproductive matters, this right for PWDs is barely upheld. Given this and other issues with long-term social care in India, Nakray proposes that some individuals might be able to achieve sexual decision-making capacity through the assistance of a decision-making support network. And that such "network consent" could create opportunities for new social justice paradigms and assure long-term *humane* care of PWDs.

Part IV. Health Governance, Security, and Transitions

Global health governance refers to the use of formal and informal institutions, processes, and rules created and employed by various stakeholders to effectively deal with challenges to global health that require collective action within and across borders. Since its inception, the World Health Organization (WHO) has been the primary institution dealing with health governance as it remains the only international health organisation that can promulgate treaties and regulations with the power to legally bind member states. But (sometimes) with great power, comes greater scrutiny. In the chapter *Justice in Global Health Governance: The Role of Enforcement* (Chapter 8), Daniel Elliot Weissglass scrutinises some key provisions of the WHOs legally binding International Health Regulations (IHR) and establishes a pattern of pervasive noncompliance with those provisions. He argues that noncompliance with IHR creates not only practical, but political problems, as it creates an environment for the continuation of both substantive and procedural injustices.

Weissglass regards noncompliance as a violation of the Rawlsian 'principle of fidelity', which in short means that promise keeping under appropriate circumstances is a fundamental principle of justice. When states fail to meet their obligations under IHR they violate this principle which leads to unfairness in the outcomes of the global health system and perpetuation of health disparities. He further argues that noncompliance leads to unfairness in the processes of global health governance as it erodes the very normative force of IHR and results in weaker perceived obligations by state parties, thereby feeding further noncompliance. But Weissglass does not stop at merely making a factual and philosophical case for the role of compliance in global health governance. As steps towards increasing compliance, he suggests that the WHO could name and shame noncompliant states, provide conditional support (for instance, by 'outcasting' or make access to funds and other cooperative enterprises contingent on compliance of member states), and deploy sanctions (beginning with least severe and coercive and escalating based on the situation).

Global health governance is not only suffering from a problem of noncompliance, but also reeling from some adverse consequences of the narrative of securitisation of health. In *The Ethical Issues Raised by the Securitization of Health* (Chapter 9), Ryoa Chung and Joanne Liu consider the moral conundrums associated with framing health issues as national and international security threats. The salience of framing established in Chapter 4 is also illustrated in this chapter. Framing and elevating matters as security threats provides governments a podium through which emergency and other non-standard measures can be hoisted upon people, and often these measures subordinate human rights of people both within and outside national borders.

The authors provide three illustrations of the clash between securitisation of health and human rights. The first being states' responses to SARS-Cov-2 which, among other human rights violations, disproportionately exacerbates health nationalism. The second example involves instrumentalisation of health issues in the context of armed conflict or violent political tensions (e.g., attacks on hospitals and health workers during armed conflicts or violent tensions). And the third example builds upon the perception of refugees, asylum seekers, and irregular migrants as security threats and a burden on the health system. Chung and Liu argue that securitisation of health can aggravate the perceived threat posed by migrant populations to the health systems and well-being of nationals. By combining topical illustrations and philosophical reflection on the ethical issues raised by the narrative of securitisation of health, the authors urge us to strengthen the human right to health, at least until other conceptual and practical alternative proves itself more successful.

The last chapter in this part is by the editors of this volume. In *Transitional Health Justice* (Chapter 10), we find important similarities between failing political systems in conflict-affected states and failing health systems post health emergencies, viz., pervasive structural inequality, normalised individual or collective wrongdoing, existential uncertainty, and uncertainty about authority. These similarities led us to borrow some theoretical insights from the traditional transitional justice framework and to derivatively name our account *"transitional health justice"* (THJ). If transitional justice aims at just transformation of a society, THJ demands just transformation of health systems. But transforming our health systems within a background of resource scarcity and inequality would not be easy. It would require the relevant actors to make important choices about how to deal with past failures and the wrongs perpetrated by their respective health systems. These choices would also require a balance between distributive and reparative demands, blame and forgiveness, truth and efficiency.

In proposing a structure of THJ, we look to improve the circumstances of transitional health justice. Essentially this would require institutional reforms; reforms which will aid in the rebuilding of social trust in health institutions, abating of existential uncertainty, and tackling the uncertainty regarding the authority of health experts and governments on questions of health. These reforms will also aid in reducing structural health inequalities and in reckoning with the truth of past wrongs. We offer some ways in which heath systems in transition could do all this and conclude the chapter by positing that THJ can have an important role in allowing for broader projects of societal transformation which are typical of transitional justice initiatives.

Part V. Global Health Justice: New Frames, New Approaches

The fifth, and last, part of the volume is where three authors present the foundations of three general frameworks – or *theories*, if you like – of global health justice. Erika Blacksher opens this part by extending Nancy Fraser's two-dimensional theory of justice to matters of global health. Her contribution, titled *"Redistribution and Recognition in the Pursuit of Health Justice: An Application of Nancy Fraser's Framework"* (Chapter 11), aptly distinguishes between distributive and relational injustices (i.e., "maldistribution" and "misrecognition") while acknowledging that these forms of injustice intersect and interact. Under Fraser's (and Blacksher's) framework, the legitimacy of claims of maldistribution and misrecognition – i.e., the measure of justice – is given by participatory parity: the requirement "that social and economic arrangements permit all (adult) members of society to interact with one another as peers". Health and health inequalities are relevant to justice (and questions about health injustices are genuine questions of justice) – Blacksher argues – because health is both instrumentally and intrinsically valuable to participatory parity. Health is, therefore, as relevant to participatory parity as the latter is to health justice.

Blacksher also considers in some detail the application of the proposed Fraser-inspired framework to population health studies. In so doing, she demonstrates the practical upshot of the framework, which grants it some plausibility points and, arguably, a comparative advantage over rival theoretical frameworks. It should be noted at this point that despite some of the examples of epidemiological and population health studies as well as some examples of social relations discussed in the chapter being from the United States, they are not confined to the United States. They illustrate much broader population trends and relations: relations of oppression, domination, and discrimination in the context of health which are unfortunately omnipresent. For that reason, these are important examples to think about in global health justice. Additionally, the United States has a particular history of class and race inequalities – and a particular approach to healthcare – that cannot be ignored by any theory of justice that strives to be global in character.

It is also worth mentioning that Blacksher closes her chapter with some initial thoughts on how the proposed framework could be further extended to address questions of children and young people's health. Interestingly, this brings us back to Gottfried Schweiger's contribution (Chapter 6) and to the importance accorded to the development of children's and adolescent's health capabilities. Perhaps the ability to explain the challenges associated with children's health is more important to a theory of global health justice than is acknowledged by previous theorists of health justice.

In *"Beyond Egalitarianism: A Confucian Approach to Justice in Global Health"* (Chapter 12), Man-to Tang proposes an alternative to theories of global health justice centred around health rights and egalitarian principles. Drawing from both contemporary and classical Confucian doctrine, Tang defends the primacy of sufficientarian principles of distribution and an agent centred, as opposed to institution-centred, approach to global health justice. The core sufficientarian idea in global health justice entails the provision of sufficient health resources and conditions. The measure of sufficiency is a flourishing life, a life where one can cultivate harmony of social relations and expand one's cardinal virtues. Harmony of social relations may require the introduction of hierarchies, and this may raise some questions about whether Tang's account can meet the demands of relational justice in the context of global health. Tang, however, emphasises that the virtue of *Ren* – the motivation and desire to care for oneself and for others – is a necessary condition of harmonious social relations, which suggests that the proposed account may have the theoretical resources to explain some forms of relational injustice.

Despite rejecting egalitarian principles, Confucian justice – Tang argues – is sensitive to egalitarian considerations in a specific context: in extreme circumstances where "resources are insufficient to maintain basic human needs". In such contexts, all must bear the burdens equally. This idea also illustrates another core aspect of Confucian justice: that it is agent centred. The responsibility to promote global health justice lies, according to Tang's account, on all individuals – and not exclusively (or primarily) on institutions. Health justice arises from the gradual expansion of our virtues: we first show concern for our own health, and then expand this concern to our relatives, neighbours, friends, and ultimately to the global community. Tang's account is not intentioned to simply lay down some ideals for global health justice; he sees it as belonging to the realm of non-ideal theory. Tang illustrates the feasibility of his Confucian approach to health justice by describing how a similar approach was implemented in Hong Kong during the early stages of the COVID-19 pandemic.

The concern for a theory of global health justice to be feasible and apply to real-world situations is shared by both Blacksher and Tang – despite both endorsing largely distinct approaches to global health justice. In the final chapter of this volume – *What do We Want from a Theory of Global Health Justice?* (Chapter 13) – Sridhar Ventakapuram takes a step back and proposes three criteria for a successful theory of global health justice. Not surprisingly, the concern for feasibility and real-world application is the first among them. This is what he calls the criterion of "relevance", and it involves both a theory's ability to explain and identify real-world injustices (theoretical relevance) as well as its ability to guide the elimination of such injustices (practical relevance). Ventakapuram proposes two further criteria: perseverance and inter-theoretical coherence. The former is a requirement to avoid parochialism: theories of global health justice must not be solely concerned with a specific health problem of the here and now; they must have enough generality to deal with a broad spectrum of health injustices over time. This may suggest that the criteria of perseverance and relevance are mutually reinforcing. To guide the elimination of a broad spectrum of health injustices over time, a theory of health justice must persevere. And to persevere, the theory must remain relevant.

The final criterion, inter-theoretical coherence, works as a justificatory standard: the more a theory of global health justice coheres and integrates insights from other disciplines – such as economics, epidemiology, medical and social sciences, anthropology, and so on – the more robust it is. Hence, Ventakapuram invites global health justice theorists to get out of the confines of their own disciplines and actively engage in cross-disciplinary work. He briefly shows that some global health justice theorists have tried to do so, but to a limited extent. He highlights the need to integrate a theory of global health justice with history, something that he is trying to do in his ongoing work. Towards the end, Ventakapuram offers a brief argument – couched in some recent examples – in defence of a capabilities approach to global health justice. According to him, the capabilities approach can not only meet all the proposed criteria, but also offer a more refined and capacious understanding of health which allows us to see a theory of global health justice "as an argument for not only more justice in global health but for more global justice".

Notes

1 Venkatapuram S, *Health Justice: An Argument from the Capabilities Approach* (Polity Press 2011); Ruger JP, *Global Health Justice and Governance* (Oxford University Press 2018).
2 Pogge TW, 'Human Rights and Global Health: A Research Program' (2005) 36 Metaphilosophy 182; Segall S, *Health, Luck, and Justice* (Princeton University Press 2009); Shue H, *Basic Rights: Subsistence, Affluence, and U.S. Foreign Policy* (Second, Princeton University Press 1996); Daniels N, *Just Health: Meeting Health Needs Fairly* (Cambridge University Press 2007); Ruger JP, *Global Health Justice and Governance* (Oxford University Press 2018).
3 World Health Organization (WHO), Definition of Sexual Health, 2006a.

PART I

Citizenship, Power, and Relational Justice

1

WORLD CITIZENSHIP AND GLOBAL HEALTH

Xuanpu Zhuang

1.1 Introduction

Although contemporary theorists usually endorse the ideal of moral equality as one of the fundamental premises in social and political life, people do not agree on what the ideal of moral equality requires.[1] Egalitarians usually assert some stronger claims on social life, *e.g.*, certain egalitarian policies and arrangements. There are two main groups of egalitarians in the discussions: distributive egalitarians and relational egalitarians. To put it simply, distributive egalitarians pursue the distribution of certain social goods in a way that reflects the ideal of equality.[2] Differently, relational egalitarians believe the point of equality is to live as equals.[3] For relational egalitarians, justice requires that people relate to one another as equals. And as the standard question of justice focuses on a single society, an intuitive and direct claim for relational egalitarians is that everyone ought to relate to one another as equal *citizens*.[4] But the claim based on the notion of national citizenship meets some difficulties when we consider global justice. It is not hard to recognise huge global distributional inequalities.[5] In 2019, for example, around a tenth of the world's population lived on less than $1.90 a day and more than 40% of the world's population (almost 3.3 billion people) lived below the $5.50 line, while individuals in high-income economies made $12,696 or more.[6,7] But what would the claim on the ideal of living as equals demand from us regarding global inequalities? And what does relational egalitarianism require for people who are not co-citizens in the usual sense?

In this chapter, I argue for a weak notion of equal world citizenship, which implies that individuals in the world ought to live as equal world citizens in a significant sense, and then discuss its implications in global health. In

DOI: 10.4324/9781003399933-3

Section 1.2, I present a relational egalitarian version of cosmopolitanism, which requires people to relate to one another as equal and full participants in global political and social activities. To support this conception of equal world citizenship, I follow the capabilities approach, which requires sufficient social goods for everyone to function as an equal world citizen in Section 1.3. Among those social goods, medical support is crucial, as people who lack health support are vulnerable and thus live as inferiors in different aspects. Specifically, the lack of medical support *causes*, *follows*, and *strengthens* some problematic social hierarchies in which some people do not live as equal world citizens, which are exemplified in various ways. I examine several cases to show why medical support is crucial in sustaining equal world citizenship in Section 1.4. Finally, Section 1.5 discusses the importance of certain egalitarian arrangements in the international order to sustain equal world citizenship.

1.2 World Citizenship and Relational Egalitarianism

Equality is not always incompatible with differences in treatment. For example, assume that Alf is a member of a dance club and Betty is a member of a music club. As such, Alf, but not Betty, is allowed to enter the dance club's locker room. Alf and Betty are treated differently: they have different rights and benefits associated with their identities (specifically, the club memberships). But this case of inequality seems neither unjust nor unreasonable; Betty does not become inferior to Alf even without the right to enter the locker room, as long as other conditions associated with her equal memberships (*e.g.*, being an equal fellow student on campus) are fulfilled.

Things become more difficult when we consider the inequalities between citizens and foreigners (non-citizens) living in the same country. In this context, it is unclear which inequalities, if any, would be justified. This problem follows two seemingly conflicting intuitions. On the one hand, it seems wrong if a foreigner is treated as inferior. On the other hand, there are at least a few defensible differences between citizens and foreigners concerning their statuses. For example, in some circumstances, it seems impermissible for foreigners to have a say in a country's long-lasting political decisions. So, a country may be justified in depriving foreigners from the right to vote or participating politically. But this is not devoid of problems, after all political equality is usually the main indicator of the ideal of equality today.[8] For instance, suppose that a certain policy may harm the interests of foreigners, *e.g.*, some rules that may deprive them of opportunities to get a better education in their country of residence.[9] It is usually disallowed for foreigners to donate money to a political candidate who argues against this. But foreigners could choose to demonstrate or sign a petition. The latter kind of action seems to be a reasonable claim on one's interests, while the former may be seen as a case of an unjustified foreign intervention in the political institutions of a country.

If the asymmetry between citizens and aliens, *i.e.*, the two levels of social and political status, is intuitive, and we usually appeal to the conception of national citizenship to explain the higher level, then what explains the lower level for foreigners?[10] A possible reply, as one could imagine, is that any human being ought to have some basic rights, which are associated with one's status as a person. In other words, people share the same status as equal moral beings. For example, if one owns a book, *i.e.*, one has the right to keep, use, sell, lend, and even destroy this book, then it seems that no one else is allowed to violate her right by, for example, burning the book without her permission. Such rights ought to be respected no matter where one comes from, which country one lives in, or which national citizenship one has. Similarly, some believe that each person has certain basic human rights that cannot be violated regardless of one's national citizenship, which provides a minimum level of one's social and political status.[11] Call it the "Moral Equals View."

Despite capturing some basic human rights on a fundamental level, the Moral Equals View fails to explain the universal level of social and political status that everyone has for two reasons. First and foremost, the Moral Equals View does not capture positive rights and claims easily. Understandably, one has the right to use their book no matter which country one belongs to. But it is unclear why one would have a stake in certain policies made in a country one does not belong to, if one is nothing more than a moral equal. Second, the Moral Equals View does not view human beings from a perspective of social relations. People are not just abstract moral beings. Rather, people live in social relationships, which provide them access to different organisations and unions, in which they gain different types and levels of memberships. If national citizenship is a kind of important social and political membership in one's social identity, then we may need a concept for the membership of living in the world as well.

I believe that the cosmopolitan tradition, which claims certain forms of world citizenship, works better here. Let us begin with national citizenship. As usual, citizenship is fundamentally a kind of membership that entails certain civil rights, obligations, and benefits.[12] A member of a certain union differs from a person outside the union even when both are deeply affected by the union. Assume that a dance club is located near a music club on campus. The members of the dance club may have legitimate and reasonable rights to demand the music club to control the volume when they are disturbed by the music, but it is unreasonable for them to choose a leader for the music club's meetings. If this is true, then we could distinguish between two claims here, both of which are based on the ideal of equality without sharing the same content. That is, we believe that the members of the music club and the members of the dance club are equals – after all, they all do the activities on campus, while they do not have the same legitimate claims in choosing the leadership for the music club. Similarly, in the case of citizens and foreigners, we view citizens and foreigners as equals though they have different levels of legitimate claims. We may say foreigners have the right to claim their interests and thus act against some policies, especially the ones that may harm them.[13] But engaging in the election of a political candidate, which is usually seen as one of the key elements in political institutions of a country, is not open to foreigners. Strictly speaking, it is not directly relevant to their basic status as equals.[14]

Then what does basic status mean? I argue that a weak version of citizenship at the global level, *i.e.*, world citizenship, holds for every individual whichever country the individual lives in. That is, citizens have both world citizenship and national citizenship in their own country, while foreigners only have world citizenship, which provides them with equal status as they relate to one another as world citizens.[15] The notion of world citizenship may provide an intuitive explanation for why foreigners could have a legitimate claim in certain political affairs no matter where they live.[16]

A direct problem, however, is that given that world citizenship does not depend on the territorial state, it may be thought that this form of citizenship lacks the institutional framework that provides meaning and support for citizenship.[17] In other words, we may wonder whether there are good reasons to support the notion of world citizenship when it is divorced from, and does not require engagement with, a democratic institution. After all, the notion of citizenship originates from the historical tradition including Athenian democracy, Republican Rome, and the Italian city-states and workers' councils, and from the philosophical traditions of Aristotle, Cicero, Machiavelli, and Rousseau. It seems to contain at least both civic self-rule and equal legal status, which strongly presupposes some political institutions which citizens live with.

To pursue a plausible version of world citizenship, I believe that a global version of relational egalitarianism could help. Egalitarians usually hold that the intuitive requirement of moral equality implies some stronger claims on social life, *e.g.*, certain egalitarian policies, arrangements, or norms, though the criterion for "stronger claims" is inaccurate. Relational egalitarians believe that we ought to understand the requirement of moral equality as the ideal of living as equals. Thus, relational egalitarianism, as a theory of justice, usually holds that a situation is just only if everyone it involves relates to each other as equals, *i.e.*, justice commits to the ideal of living as equals. An inclusive conception of relational egalitarianism is as follows:

Relational Egalitarianism: A situation is just only if everyone it involves relates to each other as equals.

When pursuing justice as the ideal of "living as equals," relational egalitarians usually are opposed to the problematic hierarchies of domination, esteem, standing, etc., which are understood in a broad sense.[18] As the discussions on justice are usually focused on a single society, relational egalitarians also focus on the ideal of "living as equals" inside a single society. So, relational egalitarians usually claim that everyone ought to relate to one another as equal *citizens*.

The notion of "relations," which is defined as the "process of interactions" by Elizabeth Anderson, however, seems to require less than what a national citizenship needs.[19] Although Anderson and Samuel Scheffler appeal to democratic institutions in their relational egalitarian theories, it does not mean that they have strong presumptions on an institutional framework in the problem of *global justice*. Or to put it in another way, different processes of interactions imply different relations. We may suppose that the interactions occur in different dimensions such as political institutions, markets, and social activities. If we view the world as a global union based on the close interactions in the time of globalisation, then we need a notion for its membership.[20] Different from national citizenship based on the birthplace and residential address, world citizenship is based on the link with social and political activities: citizens participate in certain institutions and practices as social and political agents, which constructs significant interactions and mutual awareness as a global union. Relational egalitarians typically argue for a sufficiency proviso, *i.e.*, every individual gets sufficient social goods for living as a free, equal, and full *participant* in a social and political cooperative system.[21] This participating membership is usually understood as (national) "citizenship" inside a nation. But a weaker, and arguably more plausible, version would take world citizenship, and its substantial claims, as not dependent on the existence of a global community.

1.3 A Relational Egalitarian Version of Equal World Citizenship

Given the weaker version of "relations," we may acknowledge that the lack of a strong democratic institution does not necessarily exclude the possibility of world citizenship.[22] For many people, boundaries and nationality do not define their engagement with political institutions. For example, a foreigner may be much more engaged and linked with the country where they live than with their homeland.[23] On the other hand, sometimes we may feel a connection with every corner of this world. Assume that John – who never attends political manifestations or votes – only focuses on his own business of selling bananas. He does not have a clear political view and does not have a sense of political policies. However, any political decisions made in a faraway country responsible for a large share of banana's global consumption are significant to John. In this sense, John has much more significant interactions with that far-away country than with his country of residence. Of course, this in and of itself does not provide John with citizenship in that country. But the close connection John has with that far-away country illustrates how our world is a system of social cooperation to a degree that was before unimaginable. And because our world currently works as a social cooperation system, it inevitably implies a substantial kind of social relation amongst people. It is safe to say, therefore, that social changes such as globalisation have an impact on our current understanding of citizenship – as well as on the institutional and political frameworks surrounding it. Today, we have various international (and global) organisations that work in political, economic, and social domains, such as the United Nations and its agencies, the World Trade Organization, the International Criminal Court, the International Monetary Fund, and some regional organisations such as European Union and Association of Southeast Asian Nations. Even granted the limitations of different international organisations, it seems we have good reasons to see our world as a union to some extent.

If we have reason to view the world as a global union, then we need a notion for the membership of this big union. Different from national citizenship based on the difference of birthplace and residential address, world citizenship is based on some link with social and political activities: citizens participate in certain institutions and practices as political agents, which constructs significant interaction and mutual awareness as a global union.[24] The link is weaker than that in national citizenship, but it is still significant.[25] It does not mean that an individual must live in a country that is a member of the United Nations or other organisations to obtain this world citizenship. Instead, every individual ought to be recognised as an equal world citizen only because he or she is involved in global interactions directly or indirectly, which is usually unavoidable for human beings. In this sense, every individual is a world citizen, which implies that they ought to be viewed as equal world citizens in the fundamental aspects of social life, no matter who they are, where they live, what they do, and which views they hold.[26] To sum up, a conception of equal world citizenship could be stated as follows:

Equal World Citizenship: A world is just only if everyone it involves relates to each other as an equal social and political participant, *i.e.*, a *world citizen*.[27]

To put it in another way, it is wrong to view a person as inferior merely because they possess a different national citizenship, as every person holds equal world citizenship. More specifically, people ought to relate to each other as equals because we all engage in social practices of global affairs – climate, resources, economic growth, and cultural communications, which implies that we are at least in the same social union even without a common democratic institution. We have seen that different international organisations have constructed a net of international orders that is neither perfect nor sufficient yet. For instance, European Union citizens with their inter-state parliaments might be one example in the sense of transnational and regional citizenship.[28] Now we could have a picture of a relational egalitarian theory in global justice based on this understanding of world citizenship.

But what does it mean to function as an equal *world* citizen? It seems that every world citizen is entitled to certain social goods such as necessary rights and liberties (expression, communication, and so on), a basic level of welfare (food, housing, and so on), natural resources (water, electricity, and so on), and opportunities (education, job, and so on). Without sufficient resources (broadly understood), one cannot function as a full participant in global political and social activities. When relational egalitarians argue for a sufficiency proviso, many of them adopt a capabilities approach.[29] This approach calls the states of being and doing "functionings," *e.g.*, the opportunity to do or be the things such as being educated, working, travelling, and so on. One's capabilities consist of sets of functionings one can achieve. Relational egalitarians claim that each individual ought to have the capabilities necessary for functioning as an equal citizen in different situations. In what follows I will explore the capabilities that a relational egalitarian version of world citizenship would require.

1.4 Why Is Medical Support Required by Equal World Citizenship?

With the capabilities approach, the theory of equal world citizenship could shed light on the problem of global health. Among the social goods that are individually necessary and jointly sufficient for functioning as a world citizen, health conditions play a key role. This is because people (especially in developing countries) who lack health conditions are vulnerable and thus live as inferiors in various aspects. Just like relational egalitarians are opposed to problematic social hierarchies, medical support for individuals is crucial for world citizens because people lacking sufficient medical support will lose their equal world citizenship at least in the following five ways.

1.4.1 The Problematic Social Hierarchies of Esteem

First, people who lack medical support tend to be esteemed in a stigmatising way. One's social identity, *i.e.*, who one is, consists of various aspects, for example, one's birthplace, profession, and interests. People tend to accord esteem to different features of one's social identity including certain nationalities, races, achievements, and so on. People always esteem each other and esteeming does not seem wrong in and of itself.[30] For example, if someone lies we tend to criticise or reproach them, and if someone sacrifices oneself to help others, we usually praise them. But some ways of esteeming are problematic. We could call the problematic esteem hierarchies "stigmatising."[31] To put it simply, the esteem hierarchies are stigmatising when the inferiors are connected to some negative stereotypes, and thus separated into certain distinct categories. So, in the case of stigmatising, certain kinds of esteeming are so significant and pervasive that they deeply shape one's social identity, and thus lead to deep influences on various aspects and areas of one's social life. An ordinary example of stigmatising esteem hierarchies, as one can imagine, is the discrimination against people of colour, who are minorities regarding their racial identity. For instance, some people hold negative attitudes toward persons who are African or Asian. They may see people of colour as violent or stupid, disparage them, or even believe that people of colour are related to certain infectious diseases and avoid contacting them.

The lack of medical support plays an important role in constructing and sustaining the problematic social hierarchies of esteem. This is because people who lack medical support are typically more vulnerable to diseases, which makes it easier for those people to get weak and even viewed as dangerous in the case of infectious diseases. The problematic social hierarchy of esteem occurs frequently in the case of infectious diseases. For example, during the COVID-19 pandemic, the poor who could not get vaccinated were easily seen as dangerous and ostracised. Again, as many developing countries cannot provide sufficient vaccines and relevant medical resources for their people, people from those countries will typically be unvaccinated. In this process, people in the world are separated into two groups: vaccinated and unvaccinated. And it is easy for people from developing countries to be labelled as unhealthy and infectious. As we can see, the stigmatising esteem can be formed without any agents exercising or pursuing it on purpose, which forms an example of structural inequality.[32] To eliminate structural inequalities, positive actions are required, actions like providing medical resources to the people who cannot afford them.

1.4.2 The Problematic Social Hierarchies of Treatments

Second, people lacking medical support are not treated with equal respect because of the differences in their health conditions. Of course, one may see that it is counter-intuitive to treat everyone in the same way – we have also shown that there are differences between national citizenship and world citizenship above. But failing to treat one with equal *respect* makes one feel inferior in social status rather than being an equal world citizen.[33] Treating one with equal respect usually implies giving appropriate recognition to or treating one's significant interests appropriately. Different from the social hierarchies of esteem, which are problematic only when they are stigmatising, the hierarchies of respect are always problematic, as equal respect is required for living as equals.[34] Besides, one can be treated without equal respect even if there is no stigmatisation. An example of treating one's significant interests differently is the case of "redlining" in the United States, where certain institutions, such as banks, tend to hold housing mortgages and other services from potential customers who reside in neighbourhoods classified as "hazardous" to investment.[35] Those neighbourhoods usually consist of a number of racial and ethnic minority groups and other low-income residents. This treatment is bad because the institutions do not treat those groups' significant interests (housing needs in this case) as weighty as the interests of others. It is not easy to spell out what the significant interests are, but a better description here is to call it "treating one with equal respect."

The problematic social hierarchy of treatment is usually related to the differences in health resources and health standards. For example, top universities with international reputations typically require a health record when accepting foreign students. For example, they may require prospective students to prove that they have not been exposed to a certain epidemic in order to be accepted. However, it is sometimes difficult for people who are born in many developing countries to satisfy the requirements, as many cannot provide acceptable medical documents or avoid the epidemic at all. In this way, people from less developed countries miss important opportunities without violating the seemingly fair rules or by being esteemed in a stigmatised way.

1.4.3 The Problematic Social Hierarchies of Attitudes

Third, people who lack medical support may be regarded as inferiors in different situations. Following Lippert-Rasmussen, we could distinguish between cognitive and non-cognitive attitudes, implicit and explicit attitudes here.[36] A cognitive attitude of regarding one as an equal is believing that one is an equal, while non-cognitive attitudes include conative elements, e.g., believing that one is an equal but it is better if one is not.[37] An explicit belief is usually held by one consciously, while an implicit belief is not.[38]

The lack of medical support also frequently leads to different attitudes at the global level. A controversial example of different attitudes is the vaccination passport that was considered during the COVID-19 pandemic. Broadly speaking, the vaccination passport is an immunity passport recording one's vaccination status. For people with vaccination passports, the companies could be fully open for business, and the countries would have resumed international travel without requiring quarantines. The vaccination passport is supposed to help boost economies and make life convenient while limiting the spread of the disease, as fully vaccinated groups are seen as protected from lethal risks and safe for others. However, by providing vaccination passports for people who could get vaccinated, governments treat the group lacking vaccines in a different way. Without sufficient vaccines, people from less developed countries or certain regions are treated in a different way, which expresses problematic attitudes toward them. For example, assume that a ship is travelling across the Mediterranean and requires a vaccination passport for boarding. In this case, we may see that people from Europe (where vaccination rates are usually high) have the right to board, while people from Africa and Asia (where vaccination rates might be lower) are not allowed to board. Although there is no stigmatising esteem here, people who are denied access are not viewed as equal citizens merely because their countries do not have sufficient vaccines. In this way, vaccination passports in practice deny the basic rights of some people and thus regard them as second-class world citizens.

1.4.4 The Problematic Social Hierarchies of Power

Fourth, some developing countries and their people are dominated by other countries, organisations, and companies when rich countries and companies monopolise medical resources. Domination is a problematic social hierarchy of power. Intuitively, power is the capacity to influence how things go in the world. To have dominant power over one is to have the capacity to arbitrarily interfere in one's life.[39] For example, assume that a tenant with a low income could only afford a particular apartment provided by a property owner. In this case, as the tenant has no choice but to rent this apartment, the landlord gains domination power over the tenant. For example, the landlord may order the tenant to take care of the children of the landlord. This is an arbitrary use of power, as the tenant has no obligation to do childcare for the landlord. But it will be hard for the tenant to reject the demand if he or she does not want to risk being kicked out. Domination power could appear in other domains as well. Sometimes powers may be exercised without agents. In other words, power may be a "net-like" organisation, in which people may feel dominated without a particular dominant agent.[40] For example, in the previous case, if the landlord does not demand the tenant to do childcare but every other tenant in the building does it for the landlord, then the new tenant may feel pressurised to do it.

The problematic social hierarchy of power is especially displayed in cases where governments in poor countries have to enter unfair treaties with rich countries and companies. For example, assume that a poor country P, lacking in medical technology, can neither produce vaccines nor purchase them from the international market during a pandemic.[41] An international medical company C promises to provide the vaccines for P on the condition of permitting C to perform a series of low-risk medical experiments on the people of P for ten years. In this case, P cannot refuse the condition because P has little medical support to deal with the pandemic save for the vaccines provided by C, and thus P must accept the demands made by C. So, C has domination power over P given the advantages it provides to the country's public health. Intuitively, the people of P are dominated by C and lose the status of being equal world citizens.

1.4.5 The Problematic Social Hierarchies of Deliberation

Finally, we do not count people in developing countries as equal world citizens when international organisations tend to focus on rich countries (and their economic growth and death rates) while evaluating a health crisis and considering its measurements. This is a problematic social hierarchy of deliberation. Scheffler puts forward a so-called "deliberative constraint" for egalitarian decision making: in an egalitarian relationship, people are disposed to treat one another's interests as significantly as theirs.[42] As a device for egalitarian decision making, the "deliberative constraint" also distinguishes between procedural justice and substantial justice in terms of the ideal of equals. This is because egalitarian decision making does not necessarily lead to an equal level.[43] Broadly understood, failing to obey the egalitarian deliberative constraint shows that there is a disposition to treat one's interests not as weighty as the interests of others.

The problematic social hierarchy of deliberation is related to the medical support that can be provided by international organisations. For example, the WHO (World Health Organization) plays an important role in the global plan for dealing with the COVID-19 pandemic. However, the pandemic does not have the same effect in all countries due to various factors. For example, some countries may have much higher vaccination rates than others, and the spread of different variants of COVID-19 differs from country to country. Given the various conditions of countries, it is controversial how the WHO evaluates the danger of a pandemic. If the WHO suggests fewer measurements on the spread of the disease, it may be good for the powerful economies and companies, while posing higher risks to the countries that do not have high vaccination rates and medical support. In this sense, we may claim that the WHO does not consider the significant interests of the less developed countries as weighty as the interests of others.

1.5 Global Health and the International Order

As I have shown above, individuals cannot relate to one another as equal world citizens without sufficient health conditions and relevant considerations. In this section, I argue that a better international order based on equal world citizenship is required for dealing with the problem of global health.

During a pandemic, companies and countries with strengths in medical technology and resources have the duty to provide some service for the countries and people who cannot prevent or treat a disease. In the long term, viewing individuals as equal world citizens requires that we provide those basic medical goods and construct a better international order in global health.

Like the problem of global poverty, it is well-known that many people live without even a minimum level of health conditions, especially in Africa and Asia. No doubt it would be better if we could do something for them. But is the action of helping them morally required or just supererogatory? Peter Singer, as a consequentialist, famously argues for our duty of donating to and helping the poor far away from us. His argument rests on the following thought experiment: imagine that you find a child drowning in a shallow pond and the only cost of saving the child for you is getting your clothes muddy.[44] As this cost is insignificant compared to life, it is morally wrong if you decide not to save the child. In the meantime, so many poor people subsist in this world and the only cost of saving one of them is to donate some money. If the case of poor people is analogous to the case of the drowning child, then it is also morally wrong if you decide not to donate. Thomas Pogge argues that globalisation harms the poor countries and their people because the international institutions are governed by rich countries and some international companies that take the advantage of poor countries.[45] As the rich countries are responsible for the harms and oppression brought to the poor countries and their people, rich countries have to take the responsibility for helping the poor and eliminating poverty. Although both Singer and Pogge provide some good reasons for helping the poor, and I do share some intuitions with them (especially Pogge's claims), they still see it as a project of effective altruism or a distribution plan.[46] I argue that the responsibility of promoting global health is grounded on equal world citizenship. It would be wrong if we do not view individuals in the world as equals. And for an individual to live as a free and equal world citizen, some substantial requirements regarding health conditions must be met.

As I have discussed above, world citizenship could be understood with the capabilities approach. World citizenship is supposed to promote a degree of equity and reciprocity among citizens. It seems that every world citizen is entitled to certain social goods such as necessary rights and liberties (expression, communication, and so on), a basic level of welfare (food, house, medical support, and so on), natural resources (air, water, electricity, and so on), and opportunities (education, job, and so on).[47] Basic rights and liberties are associated with civil membership and are necessary for citizens to participate in the world's political and social processes. A basic level of welfare, natural resources, and opportunities are implied by the benefits associated with the membership. Some education opportunities are needed to support equal participation in the political, economic, and social processes. Some basic social status and social relations are also necessary, such as membership in some communities and certain associations, certain obligations, and social benefits. If these social goods are necessary for sustaining world citizenship, then we have a strong reason for promoting global health as our responsibility. This is not something that is done out of goodwill; it is a claim grounded on a global egalitarian ideal of citizenship of the sort that I have argued for in the chapter. A just institution based on relational egalitarian claims can also work on other issues such as justice in climate change, health policy, and war. For example, during the pandemic, companies and countries with strengths in medical technology and resources have the duty to provide some service for the countries and people who cannot treat, prevent, or control the disease alone. Furthermore, a just institution is also required to deal with some cases in which the basic liberties, rights, or status of individuals are violated if we treat equal world citizenship seriously.

I am, however, not simply arguing for the extension of national citizenship or rejecting the notion of national citizenship altogether. Rather, what I propose is that there are different levels of citizenship, the global one of which implies that we ought to live as equal world citizens. It might be helpful to consider two potential objections here. First, given the current situation (including the extreme inequalities, limited resources, and weak international agencies), it seems difficult to support world citizenship and extend it to everyone at this moment. To this, I have two replies. On the one hand, this is not a problem particularly for world citizenship. In other words, we face similar problems in the case of national citizenship as well. On the other hand, even though we cannot achieve the ideal of sustaining equal world citizenship now, it is still *pro tanto* wrong to disadvantage one in terms of one's world citizenship by causing, following, or strengthening the problematic social hierarchies discussed earlier. The other problem is about the bearers of the responsibility in pursuing equal world citizenship. As some may think that since the claim of justice focuses on wrongdoings, which are usually subject to coercive power, it seems hard to define the bearers of responsibility – after all, we have no world government and probably do not need one at all. I believe that the claim of equal world citizenship may work for different kinds of agents. As I argued above, people can be wronged not only by governments but by other institutions, agencies, companies, and even individuals. So, it might be necessary to emphasise that in these cases not only governments but also other institutions, agencies, companies, and even individuals are responsible for taking certain actions against world citizens.[48]

1.6 Conclusion

In this chapter, I argue that a notion of world citizenship is worth pursuing, and it provides us with the possibility of a relational egalitarian version of cosmopolitanism, which sheds light on the issues of global health. I argue for a weak notion of equal world citizenship, which requires that people relate to one another as equals and full participants in global political and social activities. With this notion, we can see that universal medical support is crucial, as people who lack such support are vulnerable and thus live as inferiors in various aspects. And this requires certain egalitarian arrangements in a new international order.

Notes

1 For example, Will Kymlica seems to believe that all contemporary political theories share the premise of moral equality. See Kymlicka W, *Contemporary Political Philosophy* (Clarendon Press, 1990) 5.
2 Some philosophers who are usually seen as distributive egalitarians include G. A. Cohen, Richard Arneson, and Ronald Dworkin. But people may not agree with the label. See Cohen GA, 'On the Currency of Egalitarian Justice' [1989] Ethics 906; Cohen, 'Equality of What? On Welfare, Goods, and Capabilities' in Martha Nussbaum and Amartya Sen (eds.), *The Quality of Life* (Oxford University Press 1993); Cohen, *Self-Ownership, Freedom, and Equality* (Cambridge University Press 1995); Cohen, *If You're an Egalitarian, How Come You're So Rich?* (Harvard University Press 2000); Arneson R, 'Equality and Equal Opportunity for Welfare' [1989] Philosophical Studies 77; Arneson, 'Equality of Opportunity for Welfare Defended and Recanted' [1999] Journal of Political Philosophy 488; Arneson, 'Luck Egalitarianism and Prioritarianism' [2000] Ethics 339; Arneson, 'Luck and Equality: Richard J. Arneson' [2001] Aristotelian Society Supplementary Volume 73; Dworkin R, *Taking Rights Seriously* (Harvard University Press 1977); Dworkin, *Sovereign Virtue: Equality in Theory and Practice* (Harvard University Press 2000); Dworkin, 'Equality, Luck, and Hierarchy' [2003] Philosophy and Public Affairs 190.
3 Some philosophers who are usually seen as relational egalitarians include David Miller, Iris Marion Young (1990), Elizabeth Anderson, Joshua Cohen, T. M. Scanlon, and Samuel Scheffler. But people use different terms for their positive views—the terms at least include "social equality," "democratic equality," "relational equality," and "equality of status." See Miller D, *On Nationality* (Clarendon Press 1995); Miller, 'Equality and Justice' [1997] Ratio 222; Young IM, *Justice and the Politics of Difference* (Princeton University Press 1990); Anderson E, 'What Is the Point of Equality?' [1999] Ethics 287; Anderson, 'Expanding the Egalitarian Toolbox: Equality and Bureaucracy' [2008] Aristotelian Society Supplementary 139; Anderson, 'The Fundamental Disagreement between Luck Egalitarians and Relational Egalitarians' [2010] Canadian Journal of Philosophy 1; Anderson, *The Imperative of Integration* (Princeton University Press 2010); Anderson, 'Equality' in David Estlund (Ed.), *The Oxford Handbook of Political Philosophy* (Oxford University Press 2012); Anderson, 'Durable Social Hierarchies: How Egalitarian Movements Imagine Inequality' (Items, 19 July 2016) <https://items.ssrc.org/what-is-inequality/durable-social-hierarchies-how-egalitarian-movements-imagine-inequality> accessed 15 December 2022; Anderson, *Private Government: How Employers Rule*

Our Lives (Princeton University Press 2017); Cohen J, 'Democratic Equality' [1989] Ethics 727; Scanlon TM, 'The Diversity of Objections to Inequality' in Matthew Clayton and Andrew Williams (Eds.), *The Ideal of Equality*. (Palgrave Macmillan 2002); Scanlon, *Why Does Inequality Matter?* (Oxford University Press 2018); Scheffler S, 'What is Egalitarianism?' [2003] Philosophy and Public Affairs 5; Scheffler, 'Choice, Circumstances and the value of Equality' [2005] Politics, Philosophy & Economics 5; Scheffler, *Equality and Tradition: Questions of Value in Moral and Political Theory* (Oxford University Press 2010); Scheffler, 'The Practice of Equality' in C. Fourie, F. Schuppert, and I. Wallimann-Helmer (eds.), *Social Equality: Essays on What it Means to be Equals* (Oxford University Press 2015).

4 For example, in the groundbreaking paper *"What Is the Point of Equality,"* Anderson claims that egalitarian principles ought to "express equal respect and concern for all *citizens."* (Emphasis added) See Anderson, 'What Is the Point of Equality?' [1999] Ethics 289.

5 For example, Pogge develops a Rawlsian framework of global justice. See Pogge T, 'Rawls and Global Justice' [1988] Canadian Journal of Philosophy 227; Pogge, *World Poverty and Human Rights* (Polity Press 2002)

6 "PovcalNet". 'Investment Climate', <iresearch.worldbank.org> Accessed 15 December 2022.

7 "World Bank Country and Lending Groups – World Bank Data Help Desk", World Bank, <https://datahelpdesk.worldbank.org/knowledgebase/articles/906519-world-bank-country-and-lending-groups> Accessed 15 December 2022.

8 For example, Thomas Christiano believes that the principle of equality is fundamentally related to justice in a *political* society and thus constitutes the basis of democratic and liberal rights. See Christiano T, *The Constitution of Equality: Democratic Authority and its Limits* (Oxford University Press 2008) 12.

9 A policy that treats some persons badly is not necessarily illegal. It only needs to favour other groups to constitute bad treatment.

10 There may be other types of social and political status, e.g., permanent residents, who usually are not citizens but still have some benefits that foreigners do not have. But I do not consider them for now.

11 This view is similar to certain forms of "moral cosmopolitanism," i.e., the view focused on respecting and promoting basic rights for every human being. For example, see Singer P, *One World: The Ethics of Globalization* (Yale University Press 2002); Unger P, *Living High and Letting Die: Our Illusion of Innocence* (Oxford University Press 1996).

12 See Bellamy R, *Citizenship: A Very Short Introduction* (Oxford University Press 2008) 12–17.

13 For example, Arash Abizadeh argues that coercive power is legitimate only if it is justified by and to the very people over whom it is exercised, which implies that foreigners do have claims if a policy influences them. See Abizadeh A, 'Democratic Theory and Border Coercion' [2008] Political Theory 37; Abizadeh, 'Democratic Legitimacy and State Coercion: A Reply to David Miller' [2010] Political Theory 121.

14 The division of the world into states is usually both intuitive and defensible, and we may have strong reasons to hold at least a distinction between national citizens and foreigners. For example, see Coleman JL, and Harding SK, 'Citizenship, the Demands of Justice, and the Moral Relevance of Political Borders' in W. F. Schwartz (ed.), *Justice in Immigration* (Cambridge University Press 1995); Habermas J, 'Citizenship and National Identity' in *Between Facts and Norms* (MIT Press 1996); Kolodny N, 'Rule Over None II: Social Equality and the Justification of Democracy' [2014] Philosophy & Public Affairs 287;

Kymlicka, 'Territorial Boundaries: A Liberal-Egalitarian Perspective' in D. Miller, S. H. Hashmi (eds.), *Boundaries and Justice. Diverse Ethical Perspectives* (Princeton University Press 2001); Song S, 'Democracy and Noncitizen Voting Rights' [2009] Citizenship Studies 607.

15 Some also point out that we could understand citizenship rights as full rights while seeing extra-territorial citizenship rights as less than full rights, as the latter ones do not include voting rights. For example, see Lenard P, 'Residence and the Right to Vote' [2015] International Migration and Integration 131. Some countries do allow certain voting rights for non-citizen residents, but it seems controversial. See Lopez-Guerra C, 'Should Expatriates Vote?' [2005] *Journal of Political Philosophy* 216; Pogonyi S, 'Four Patterns of Non-resident Voting Rights' [2014] Ethnopolitics 122.

16 So, my proposal is a version of cosmopolitanism based on the conception of relational equality. For citizenship and multiculturalism, see Barry B, *Culture and Equality. An Egalitarian Critique of Multiculturalism* (Harvard University Press 2001); Benhabib S, *The Claims of Culture: Equality and Diversity in the Global Era* (Princeton University Press 2002); Benhabib, *The Rights of Others. Aliens, Residents and Citizens* (Cambridge University Press 2004); Kymlicka, *Multicultural Citizenship: A Liberal Theory of Minority Rights* (Clarendon Press 1995); Kymlicka, 'Citizenship in an Era of Globalization: A Commentary on Held', in I. Shapiro and C. Hacker-Cordon (eds.), *Democracy's Edges* (Cambridge University Press 1999); Kymlicka, 'New Forms of Citizenship' in T. J. Courchesne and D. J. Savoie (eds.), *The Art of the State: Governance in a World Without Frontiers* (Institute for Research in Public Policy 2003); Kymlicka, 'The Multicultural Welfare State?' in Peter A. Hall and Michele Lamont (eds.), *Successful Societies: How Institutions and Culture Affect Health* (Cambridge University Press 2009); Miller, *Citizenship and National Identity* (Polity Press 2000); *National Responsibility and Global Justice* (Oxford University Press 2007); *Strangers in our Midst* (Harvard University Press 2016); Scheffler *Boundaries and Allegiances: Problems of Justice and Responsibility in Liberal Thought* (Oxford University Press 2003); Scheffler, *Equality and Tradition: Questions of Value in Moral and Political Theory* (Oxford University Press 2010); Young IM, 'Polity and Group Difference: A Critique of the Ideal of Universal Citizenship' [1989] *Ethics* 250. For cosmopolitanism, see Scheffler S, 'Conceptions of Cosmopolitanism' [1999] Utilitas 255; Bohman J, 'Cosmopolitan Republicanism: Citizenship, Freedom and Global Political Authority' [2001] The Monist 3; Bohman, 'Republican Cosmopolitanism' [2004] Journal of Political Philosophy 336; Caney S, *Justice Beyond Borders: A Global Political Theory* (Oxford University Press 2005); Laborde C, 'Republicanism and Global Justice' [2010] European Journal of Political Theory 48; Pettit P, 'A Republican Law of Peoples' [2010] European Journal of Political Theory 70; 'The Globalized Republican Ideal' [2016] Global Justice: Theory Practice Rhetoric 47.

17 See Cohen, 'Changing Paradigms of Citizenship and the Exclusiveness of the Demos' [1999] International Sociology 245; Kymlicka and Norman W, 'Return of the Citizen: A Survey of Recent Work on Citizenship Theory' [1994] *Ethics* 352.

18 As one could imagine, it is not problematic if someone is an epistemic superior in a certain domain, *e.g.*, one medical expert is epistemically superior to ordinary people when diagnosing a certain disease. So, relational egalitarians are usually opposed to the problematic social hierarchies. For example, see Anderson, 'Equality' in David Estlund (Ed.), *The Oxford Handbook of Political Philosophy* (Oxford University Press 2012); Nath R, 'Relational Egalitarianism' [2020] Philosophy Compass 1.

19 See Anderson, 'The Fundamental Disagreement between Luck Egalitarians and Relational Egalitarians' [2010] Canadian Journal of Philosophy 16–17.

20 Another possibility is to see democratic institutions, which usually imply a collective decision-making process, from another perspective. For example, according to John Keane, we are experiencing a new form of democracy—monitory democracy, which refers to a form of democracy defined by the rapid growth of many kinds of extra-parliamentary, power-scrutinising mechanisms. For Keane, "[... ...] the era of representative democracy is passing away, that a new historical form of 'post-representative' democracy has been born, and is spreading throughout the world of democracy," and now the word "democracy" itself comes to have a new meaning: the public scrutiny and public control of decision-makers. See Keane J, *The Life and Death of Democracy* (Simon and Schuster 2009) xxvi. When democratic consciousness and basic human rights are accepted by more and more nations and people, more and more fields of social and political life are included in democratic ideals. But I do not assume that we must accept this new conception of democracy in this chapter.

21 For some background on sufficientarianism and the sufficiency proviso, see Shields L, 'Sufficientarianism' [2020] Philosophy Compass 1. Sufficientarianism usually claims that the point of (in)justice is whether individuals have secured enough of certain goods.

22 The thought of seeing the nation as the proper and dominant form of political organisation, on the contrary, could be seen as a cognitive bias called methodological nationalism. See Sager A, 'Political Philosophy Beyond Methodological Nationalism' [2021] *Philosophy Compass* e12726.

23 See Bosniak L, *The Citizen and the Alien. Dilemmas of Contemporary Membership* (Princeton University Press 2006).

24 There are controversies about birthright citizenship. See Bauböck R, 'Stakeholder Citizenship: An Idea Whose Time Has Come?' in Bertelsmann Stiftung, European Policy Centre, and Migration Policy Institute, *Delivering Citizenship: The Transatlantic Council on Migration* (Brookings Inst Press 2008) 35; Shachar A, *The Birthright Lottery. Citizenship and Global Inequality* (Harvard University Press 2009) 165.

25 Some believe that we could understand citizenship at different levels of governance: local, national, regional, and global. For example, see Pogge, 'Cosmopolitanism and Sovereignty' [1992] Ethics 58; Young *Inclusion and Democracy* (Oxford University Press 2000) 266.

26 For another proposal of world citizenship on individual engagement in political activities, see Kuper A, *Democracy Beyond Borders. Justice and Representation in Global Institutions* (Oxford University Press 2004). For another proposal of global relational egalitarianism, see Heilinger JC, *Cosmopolitan Responsibility: Global Injustice, Relational Equality, and Individual Agency* (De Gruyter 2019) Chap. 4.

27 The notion of world citizenship provides some substantial requirements for living as equals. In this sense, different from what Temkin claims, the concept of equality pursued by relational egalitarians is not merely comparative but at least implies certain sufficiency provisos. See Temkin LS, *Inequality* (Oxford University Press 1993).

28 For example, see Kollar E, 'From Surplus Fairness to Prospect Fairness: Why a Deeply Egalitarian Social Union Is Indispensable for a Free Europe' [2022] European Journal of Philosophy 503.

29 For the capabilities approach, see Sen A, *Inequality Re-examined* (Clarendon Press 1992). Martha Nussbaum also provides a detailed account of the capabilities approach. See Nussbaum M, *Women and Human Development: The Capabilities*

Approach (Cambridge University Press 2000); Nussbaum, *Frontiers of Justice* (Harvard University Press 2006); Nussbaum, *Creating Capabilities* (Harvard University Press 2011). For an example of the capabilities approach in the relational egalitarian theory, see Anderson, 'What Is the Point of Equality?' [1999] Ethics 316–321.

30 As Fourie puts it, "… advocating *equality of esteem* seems absurd on a number of levels. Esteeming is unavoidable, and at least many individual acts of esteeming and disesteeming appear to be perfectly morally permissible, probably even the "correct" moral response to admired or disliked characteristics, respectively." See Fourie C, 'To Praise and to Scorn: The Problem of Inequalities of Esteem for Social Egalitarianism' In Carina Fourie, Fabian Schuppert, and Ivo Wallimann-Helmer (Eds.), *Social Equality: Essays on What It Means to Be Equals* (Oxford University Press 2015) 89.

31 The concept of "stigma" is famously presented by the sociologist Erving Goffman to refer to a special discrepancy between virtual social identity (the category and attributes we impute to a person) and actual social identity (the category and attributes a person could in fact be proved to possess), where one is reduced "from a whole and usual person to a tainted, discounted one." See Goffman E, *Stigma: Notes on the Management of Spoiled Identity* (Prentice Hall 1963) 1–3. Link & Phelan argues that the concept of "stigma" has five components: labelling, stereotyping, separation, status loss (and discrimination), and power. See Link BG, and Phelan JC, 'Conceptualizing Stigma' [2011] Annual Review of Sociology 363.

32 I use "structural inequalities" to refer to certain cases of inequalities that cannot be attributable to individual actions of specific agents (individuals, states, or other institutions).

33 Stephen Darwall distinguishes two kinds of respect: recognition respect and appraisal respect. Broadly speaking, recognition respect consists in "giving appropriate consideration or recognition to some feature of its object," while appraisal respect consists in "a positive appraisal of a person, or his qualities." The notion of "(equal) respect" in this paper is used in the sense of recognition respect. See Darwall S, 'Two Kinds of Respect' [1977] Ethics 38–39.

34 For more discussions on the difference between esteem and respect, see Runciman WG, "Social' Equality' [1967] Philosophical Quarterly 221; Darwall, 'Two Kinds of Respect' [1977] Ethics 36; Fourie, 'To Praise and to Scorn: The Problem of Inequalities of Esteem for Social Egalitarianism' In Carina Fourie, Fabian Schuppert, and Ivo Wallimann-Helmer (Eds.), *Social Equality: Essays on What It Means to Be Equals* (Oxford University Press 2015).

35 For example, an investigation report by Bill Dedman demonstrated how Atlanta banks would often lend in lower-income white neighborhoods but not in middle-income or even upper-income Black neighborhoods in the report "The Color of Money," which wins the 1989 Pulitzer Prize. See Dedman B, 'The Color of Money' [1988] *The Atlanta Journal-Constitution* May 1–4.

36 See Lippert-Rasmussen K, *Relational Egalitarianism: Living as Equals* (Cambridge University Press 2018) 85–87

37 For example, some could believe that the black and the white are equals now but hope that the white could be superiors.

38 For example, some do not hold explicit discrimination beliefs but avoid communicating with any people of colour unconsciously.

39 The concept of domination is famously introduced by the theorists of republicanism such as Phillip Pettit, who understands the concept of political liberty as non-domination or independence from arbitrary power. According to Pettit, "someone has dominating power over another … to the extent that 1. they have

the capacity to interfere 2. on an arbitrary basis 3. in certain choices that the other is in a position to make." See Pettit P, *Republicanism: A Theory of Freedom and Government* (Oxford University Press 1997) 52

40 This term comes from Foucault M, *The History of Sexuality, Volume 1: An Introduction*, Robert Hurley (trans.) (Vintage 1979)

41 Also see Freyer N, and Kempt H, 'AI-DSS in Healthcare and Their Power over Health Insecure Collectives' In Himani Bhakuni and Lucas Miotto (Eds.), *Justice in Global Health: New Perspectives and Current Issues* (Routledge 2023)

42 Scheffler says, "each person accepts that the other person's equally important interests—understood broadly to include the person's needs, values, and preferences—should play an equally significant role in influencing decisions made within the context of the relationship. Moreover, each person has a normally effective disposition to treat the other's interests accordingly." See Scheffler, 'The Practice of Equality' in C. Fourie, F. Schuppert, and I. Wallimann-Helmer (eds.), *Social Equality: Essays on What it Means to be Equals* (Oxford University Press 2015) 25.

43 Scheffler says that "… in joint deliberations where the parties' values are at stake, what the egalitarian deliberative constraint requires cannot without distortion be described as achieving an equal level of interest-satisfaction. Instead, what the constraint requires is that the parties' decisions should be equally sensitive to the diverse implications of their actions for the values of each of them." See Scheffler, 'The Practice of Equality' in C. Fourie, F. Schuppert, and I. Wallimann-Helmer (eds.), *Social Equality: Essays on What it Means to be Equals* (Oxford University Press 2015) 28–29.

44 The thought experiment is a reconstruction from Singer P, 'Famine, Affluence, and Morality' [1972] Philosophy and Public Affairs 229.

45 Pogge, *World Poverty and Human Rights* (Polity Press 2002). Also, see Tan KC, *Justice Without Borders. Cosmopolitanism, Nationalism and Patriotism* (Cambridge University Press 2004).

46 In other words, it is still a kind of mutual aid instead of an obligation to give equal weight to the interests of foreigners. See Walzer M, *Spheres of Justice: A Defense of Pluralism and Equality* (Basic Books 1983) 48.

47 For more possible descriptions in the *Universal Declaration of Human Rights*, see Assembly UNationsG, *The Universal Declaration of Human Rights*, 1948. https://www.un.org/en/about-us/universal-declaration-of-human-rights accessed 15 December 2022.

48 For some discussions on how individual actions work in social justice, see Pourvand K, 'Must Egalitarians Rely on the State to Attain Distributive Justice?' [forthcoming] Social Philosophy and Policy. Deveaux also argues the social movements of alleviating global poverty ought to be led by the poor in the Global South. See Deveaux M, 'Poor-Led Social Movements and Global Justice' [2018] Political Theory 698.

Bibliography

Abizadeh A, 'Democratic Theory and Border Coercion' [2008] *Political Theory* 37.

Abizadeh A, 'Democratic Legitimacy and State Coercion: A Reply to David Miller' [2010] *Political Theory* 121.

Anderson E, 'What Is the Point of Equality?' [1999] Ethics 287.

Anderson E, 'Expanding the Egalitarian Toolbox: Equality and Bureaucracy' [2008] *Aristotelian Society Supplementary* 139.

Anderson E, 'The Fundamental Disagreement between Luck Egalitarians and Relational Egalitarians' [2010] *Canadian Journal of Philosophy* 1.

Anderson E, *The Imperative of Integration* (Princeton University Press 2010).

Anderson E, 'Equality' in David Estlund (Ed.), *The Oxford Handbook of Political Philosophy* (Oxford University Press 2012).

Anderson E, 'Durable Social Hierarchies: How Egalitarian Movements Imagine Inequality' (Items, 19 July 2016) <https://items.ssrc.org/what-is-inequality/durable-social-hierarchies-how-egalitarian-movements-imagine-inequality> accessed 15 December 2022.

Anderson E, *Private Government: How Employers Rule Our Lives* (Princeton University Press 2017).

Anderson E, 'Equality of Opportunity for Welfare Defended and Recanted' [1999] *Journal of Political Philosophy* 488.

Anderson E, 'Luck Egalitarianism and Prioritarianism' [2000] *Ethics* 339.

Anderson E, 'Luck and Equality: Richard J. Arneson' [2001] *Aristotelian Society Supplementary* 73.

Arneson R, 'Equality and Equal Opportunity for Welfare' [1989] *Philosophical Studies* 77.

Barry B, *Culture and Equality. An Egalitarian Critique of Multiculturalism* (Harvard University Press 2001).

Bauböck R, 'Stakeholder Citizenship: An Idea Whose Time Has Come?' in Bertelsmann Stiftung, European Policy Centre, and Migration Policy Institute, *Delivering Citizenship: The Transatlantic Council on Migration* (Brookings Inst Press 2008).

Bellamy R, *Citizenship: A Very Short Introduction* (Oxford University Press 2008).

Benhabib S, *The Claims of Culture: Equality and Diversity in the Global Era* (Princeton University Press 2002).

Benhabib S, *The Rights of Others. Aliens, Residents and Citizens* (Cambridge University Press 2004).

Bohman J, 'Cosmopolitan Republicanism: Citizenship, Freedom and Global Political Authority' [2001] *The Monist* 3.

Bohman J, 'Republican Cosmopolitanism' [2004] Journal of Political Philosophy 336.

Bosniak L, *The Citizen and the Alien. Dilemmas of Contemporary Membership* (Princeton University Press 2006).

Caney S, *Justice Beyond Borders: A Global Political Theory* (Oxford University Press 2005).

Christiano T, *The Constitution of Equality: Democratic Authority and its Limits* (Oxford University Press 2008).

Cohen GA, 'On the Currency of Egalitarian Justice' [1989] *Ethics* 906.

Cohen GA, 'Equality of What? On Welfare, Goods, and Capabilities' in M Nussbaum and A Sen (eds.), *The Quality of Life* (Oxford University Press 1993).

Cohen GA, *Self-Ownership, Freedom, and Equality* (Cambridge University Press 1995).

Cohen GA, *If You're an Egalitarian, How Come You're So Rich?* (Harvard University Press 2000).

Cohen J, 'Democratic Equality' [1989] *Ethics* 727.

Cohen J, 'Changing Paradigms of Citizenship and the Exclusiveness of the Demos' [1999] *International Sociology* 245.

Coleman JL, and Harding SK, 'Citizenship, the Demands of Justice, and the Moral Relevance of Political Borders' in W. F. Schwartz (ed.), *Justice in Immigration* (Cambridge University Press 1995).

Darwall S, 'Two Kinds of Respect' [1977] Ethics 36.

Dedman B, 'The Color of Money' [1988] *The Atlanta Journal-Constitution* May 1–4.

Deveaux M, 'Poor-Led Social Movements and Global Justice' [2018] *Political Theory* 698.

Dworkin R, *Taking Rights Seriously* (Harvard University Press 1977).

Dworkin R, *Sovereign Virtue: Equality in Theory and Practice* (Harvard University Press 2000).

Dworkin R, 'Equality, Luck, and Hierarchy' [2003] *Philosophy and Public Affairs* 190.

Foucault M, *The History of Sexuality, Volume 1: An Introduction*, R Hurley (trans.) (Vintage 1979).

Fourie C, 'To Praise and to Scorn: The Problem of Inequalities of Esteem for Social Egalitarianism' in C Fourie, F Schuppert, and I Wallimann-Helmer (eds.), *Social Equality: Essays on What It Means to Be Equals* (Oxford University Press 2015).

Freyer N, and Kempt H, 'AI-DSS in Healthcare and Their Power over Health Insecure Collectives' in H Bhakuni and L Miotto (Eds.), *Justice in Global Health: New Perspectives and Current Issues* (Routledge 2023).

Goffman E, *Stigma: Notes on the Management of Spoiled Identity* (Prentice Hall 1963).

Habermas J, 'Citizenship and National Identity' in *Between Facts and Norms* (MIT Press 1996).

Heilinger JC, *Cosmopolitan Responsibility: Global Injustice, Relational Equality, and Individual Agency* (De Gruyter 2019).

Keane J, *The Life and Death of Democracy* (Simon and Schuster 2009).

Kollar E, 'From Surplus Fairness to Prospect Fairness: Why a Deeply Egalitarian Social Union Is Indispensable for a Free Europe' [2022] *European Journal of Philosophy* 503

Kolodny N, 'Rule Over None II: Social Equality and the Justification of Democracy' [2014] *Philosophy & Public Affairs* 287.

Kuper A, *Democracy Beyond Borders. Justice and Representation in Global Institutions* (Oxford University Press 2004).

Kymlicka W, *Contemporary Political Philosophy* (Clarendon Press, 1990).

Kymlicka W, *Multicultural Citizenship: A Liberal Theory of Minority Rights* (Clarendon Press 1995).

Kymlicka W, 'Citizenship in an Era of Globalization: A Commentary on Held', in I. Shapiro and C. Hacker-Cordon (eds.), *Democracy's Edges* (Cambridge University Press 1999).

Kymlicka W, 'Territorial Boundaries: A Liberal-Egalitarian Perspective' in D. Miller, S. H. Hashmi (eds.), *Boundaries and Justice. Diverse Ethical Perspectives* (Princeton University Press 2001).

Kymlicka W, 'New Forms of Citizenship' in T. J. Courchesne and D. J. Savoie (eds.), *The Art of the State: Governance in a World Without Frontiers* (Institute for Research in Public Policy 2003).

Kymlicka W, 'The Multicultural Welfare State?' in Peter A. Hall and M. Lamont (eds.), *Successful Societies: How Institutions and Culture Affect Health* (Cambridge University Press 2009).

Kymlicka W and Norman W, 'Return of the Citizen: A Survey of Recent Work on Citizenship Theory' [1994] *Ethics* 352.

Laborde C, 'Republicanism and Global Justice' [2010] *European Journal of Political Theory* 48.

Lenard P, 'Residence and the Right to Vote' [2015] *International Migration and Integration* 119.

Link BG, and Phelan JC, 'Conceptualizing Stigma' [2011] *Annual Review of Sociology* 363.

Lippert-Rasmussen K, *Relational Egalitarianism: Living as Equals* (Cambridge University Press 2018).

Lopez-Guerra C, 'Should Expatriates Vote?' [2005] *Journal of Political Philosophy* 216.

Miller D, *On Nationality* (Clarendon Press 1995).

Miller D, 'Equality and Justice' [1997] *Ratio* 222.

Miller D, *Citizenship and National Identity* (Polity Press 2000).

Miller D, *National Responsibility and Global Justice* (Oxford University Press 2007).

Miller D, *Strangers in our Midst* (Harvard University Press 2016).

Nath R, 'Relational Egalitarianism' [2020] *Philosophy Compass* 1.

Nussbaum M, *Women and Human Development: The Capabilities Approach* (Cambridge University Press 2000).

Nussbaum M, *Frontiers of Justice* (Harvard University Press 2006).

Nussbaum M, *Creating Capabilities* (Harvard University Press 2011).

Pettit P, *Republicanism: A Theory of Freedom and Government* (Oxford University Press 1997).

Pettit P, 'A Republican Law of Peoples' [2010] *European Journal of Political Theory* 70.

Pettit P, 'The Globalized Republican Ideal' [2016] *Global Justice: Theory Practice Rhetoric* 47.

Pogge T, 'Rawls and Global Justice' [1988] *Canadian Journal of Philosophy* 227.

Pogge T, 'Cosmopolitanism and Sovereignty' [1992] *Ethics* 58.

Pogge T, *World Poverty and Human Rights* (Polity Press 2002).

Pogonyi S, 'Four Patterns of Non-resident Voting Rights' [2014] *Ethnopolitics* 122.

Pourvand K, 'Must Egalitarians Rely on the State to Attain Distributive Justice?' [forthcoming] *Social Philosophy and Policy*

Runciman WG, "Social' Equality' [1967] *Philosophical Quarterly* 221.

Sager A, 'Political Philosophy Beyond Methodological Nationalism' [2021] *Philosophy Compass* e12726.

Scanlon TM, 'The Diversity of Objections to Inequality' in M. Clayton and A. Williams (Eds.), *The Ideal of Equality*. (Palgrave Macmillan 2002).

Scanlon TM, *Why Does Inequality Matter?* (Oxford University Press 2018).

Scheffler S, 'Conceptions of Cosmopolitanism' [1999] *Utilitas* 255.

Scheffler S, *Boundaries and Allegiances: Problems of Justice and Responsibility in Liberal Thought* (Oxford University Press 2003).

Scheffler S, 'What is Egalitarianism?' [2003] *Philosophy and Public Affairs* 5.

Scheffler S, 'Choice, Circumstances and the value of Equality' [2005] *Politics, Philosophy & Economics* 5.

Scheffler S, *Equality and Tradition: Questions of Value in Moral and Political Theory* (Oxford University Press 2010).

Scheffler S, 'The Practice of Equality' in C. Fourie, F. Schuppert, and I. Wallimann-Helmer (eds.), *Social Equality: Essays on What it Means to be Equals* (Oxford University Press 2015).

Sen A, *Inequality Re-examined* (Clarendon Press 1992).

Shachar A, *The Birthright Lottery. Citizenship and Global Inequality* (Harvard University Press 2009).

Shields L, 'Sufficientarianism' [2020] *Philosophy Compass* 1

Singer P, 'Famine, Affluence, and Morality' [1972] *Philosophy and Public Affairs* 229.

Singer P, *One World: The Ethics of Globalization* (Yale University Press 2002).

Song S, 'Democracy and Noncitizen Voting Rights' [2009] *Citizenship Studies* 607.

Tan KC, *Justice Without Borders. Cosmopolitanism, Nationalism and Patriotism* (Cambridge University Press 2004).

Temkin LS, *Inequality* (Oxford University Press 1993).

Assembly UNationsG, The Universal Declaration of Human Rights, 1948. <https://www.un.org/en/about-us/universal-declaration-of-human-rights> accessed 15 December 2022.

Unger P, *Living High and Letting Die: Our Illusion of Innocence* (Oxford University Press 1996).

Walzer M, *Spheres of Justice: A Defense of Pluralism and Equality* (Basic Books 1983).

Young IM, 'Polity and Group Difference: A Critique of the Ideal of Universal Citizenship' [1989] *Ethics* 250.

Young IM, *Justice and the Politics of Difference* (Princeton University Press 1990).

Young IM, *Inclusion and Democracy* (Oxford University Press 2000).

2

AI-DSS IN HEALTHCARE AND THEIR POWER OVER HEALTH-INSECURE COLLECTIVES

Nils Freyer and Hendrik Kempt

2.1 Introduction

Given the continuous development and distribution of AI-based technologies in most areas of human activity, such as for medical diagnostics, transportation, communication, or marketing, their governance becomes increasingly important from an ethical, legal, and technical perspective. These perspectives become especially relevant in questions of how we relate to and interact with each other. To preserve and pursue justice in the way we interact and relate in times of AI, however, we require a theory from which we can assess these technological developments. Relational egalitarianism is a form of egalitarianism that understands a just society as one in which citizens claim one another's moral equality,[1] as moral equality demands equal standards for all, relational egalitarianism sits well with theories of global justice and helps expand the notion of citizenship.[2] Therefore, relational egalitarianism favours global standards of AI governance, possibly implemented by a system of global AI governance. Healthcare constitutes a concern to relational justice, as the ability to meet basic health needs is a necessary condition to function as an equal member of a society.[3] Global inequalities in the distribution of health resources and expertise violate the demands of relational justice. Thus, relational justice demands to equalise expertise by the distribution of knowledge and resources. However, redistribution demands time, and due to the acuteness of healthcare needs, time is not always available.

Sophisticated medical AI systems are promising in offering precise diagnoses and treatment recommendations for specific diseases such as breast cancer.[4] Especially in expert-scarce areas, in which medical expertise is not

DOI: 10.4324/9781003399933-4

accessible to everyone or only with hurdles, such automatic systems may lift the quality of healthcare in a significant manner and thus, diminish inequalities in health. For instance, advances in machine learning have led to AI-based decision support systems (AI-DSS) that may significantly improve the quality of radiology by diagnosing breast cancer, contributing to an advanced quality of healthcare.[5] AI-DSS could also help with the detection of diabetic retinopathy using eye scans.[6] However, the global deployment of medical AI systems can have some epistemological pitfalls, as their implementation demands global explainability standards, that is standardised degrees of explainability that must be met for the deployment of AI-DSS to be morally acceptable.[7] But often enough such standards are not – or cannot be – met in already disadvantaged areas, which impedes the use of such technology as a tool to diminish inequalities in these expert-scarce areas. And because the demand for such technologies is high (and because of them being a valuable tool), it becomes tempting for collectives in expert-scarce areas to accept the replacement of global explainability standards with less demanding ones. But setting for lower standards risks creating other, and sometimes more serious, wrongs, and injustices, in particular when considering historical and contemporary uneven power structures, economic influence, and healthcare supply advantages.

As is currently the case with pharmaceutical companies exploiting the need-based willingness of countries of the Global South to allow large-scale drug testing with comparatively loose restrictions,[8] we can anticipate a certain "colonial" mindset of AI companies when negotiating lower local standards of reliability, explainability, and accuracy in deploying or testing their equipment (in the following we will concentrate on explainability standards as a unique issue to AI-DSS and AI governance more generally). In this chapter, we will show that AI governance is facing a moral dilemma. On the one hand, global AI governance and their ethics are largely influenced by male, rich, and powerful people,[9] which might lead to a regulatory monopoly that needs to be overcome. Otherwise, highly context-dependent concerns like expert scarcity may be worsened. On the other hand, postcolonial power structures and imperialist "residue" have led to "universal" standards which have created long-term epistemic, technological, and economic dependencies for those communities who scramble to fulfil those standards in the first place. They do not only lack the technologies to help themselves, but they now are also expected to have technologies that serve a standard far beyond their current capabilities. Thus, they are reliant on those who have both the technologies and introduced those standards. To find a path to a more just use of medical AI (diagnostic tools, therapeutic devices), we ought to be cognisant of the inherent unequal power distributions, financial interests, societal biases, and other structural injustices that negatively affect a given healthcare system.

The case discussed in this chapter is the one of explainability of AI-DSS. The chapter aims to demonstrate the lack of debate around these challenges from the perspective of philosophy of technology and AI ethics. The calls for considering questions of justice and fairness in AI governance are becoming louder;[10] however, we find the topic to be woefully under-researched. To rectify this, we first introduce the issue at hand and explain how global AI explainability standards for the use of AI-DSS are relevant to questions of justice. We then turn towards refining the subjects of these injustices and argue that they should be understood as collectives rather than populations. This allows for a more precise and intersectional view of those who are affected by structural injustices of different kinds. The main objective of our paper is to demonstrate the need to critically reflect on the current processes of how medical AI is developed, how it is certified and ethically appraised, and how it is distributed. For this, we analyse a slate of concerns regarding these current processes and offer some potential solutions.

2.2 AI-DSS in the Light of Justice

In this section, we outline the discourse on the global governance of AI-DSS and explain why, in the context of healthcare, we find this discourse to be disconnected from justice. In particular, we argue that justice must play an integral part in discussions surrounding the uses and explainability standards of AI (cf. also Heilinger's immanent critique of AI ethics).[11] The relatively high standards for explainability, as well as for accuracy and transparency, in the Global North could hamper the development and distribution of medical AI in less equipped areas. Prescribing such standards seems justified in expert-abundant regions but the justification may fail when considering context-dependent factors such as expert scarcity. However, at the moment, the standards are predominantly elaborated by the Global North and the corporations that engage in the development of medical AI-DSS.[12] Therefore, lowering these standards to supply "anything" implies that the Global North determines the acceptability standards for medical equipment to be used in the Global South. In consequence, not considering the context and demands of regional inequalities may introduce a regulatory monopoly in medical policymaking which violates demands of relational justice.[13] If expert-scarce regions were to offer sound arguments to use certain AI systems, these reasons should not be ignored.

2.2.1 The Advantages and Perils of Global AI Governance

This chapter takes an ideal theory stance. We are aware that our proposal, in practice, may raise issues in policymaking and legislation that must contend with practical challenges and limitations. Future work will need to address these dimensions from non-ideal conditions. Our aim is to provide a more fundamental deliberation-guiding perspective on the problem of AI governance.

The ever more ubiquitous application of AI in everyday life and in medical care specifically has inspired a movement of efforts to regulate and standardise AI. This is usually referred to as "AI governance" and includes a collection of rules, ethical and technical principles, democratically discussed policies, and legal frameworks, all aiming at the regulation of the development and application of AI-based systems.[14] Some of these are local, while most others have global or universal validity claims. Ethical principles to build and use AI are taken to represent universally applicable moral principles[15] or at least taken to be grounded on strong political validity claims.[16] The efforts for a global AI governance are often motivated to create ethically binding principles for worldwide operating institutions and corporations (or at least for worldwide applied AI-based devices). Thus, they are intended to function – if properly observed – as quality-guaranteeing frameworks and baselines for any AI.

We can also observe the efforts for a global AI governance in discussions surrounding medical technologies, and especially medical AI. Many of these principles prescribe that medical AI must respect individual choices and support human users rather than rationalise their influence away and into the purview of an opaque technology. Transparency and some demands of replicability also pose limits to the process of sourcing and handling medical data, limiting excessive or dubious data-gathering schemes. Moreover, explainability requirements are meant to ensure the ability of physicians to responsibly provide patients a diagnosis,[17] who in turn can informedly consent to the treatment following the AI-provided diagnosis.[18]

If global AI governance is pursuing these principles, why would anyone object to or criticise them besides their content? This is because global AI governance is at risk of reproducing especially privileged points of view, and rather than being an inclusive, democratic process of participation of all kinds of stakeholders, it is often the result of either elite scientific deliberations or, if it is participatory, it usually involves the industry, political, and scientific participants that follow certain agendas.[19]

Hagendorff points out that, with some exceptions, many of these proposals are indeed written by largely male, rich, and powerful groups of people.[20] It is, therefore, unavoidable that some of the proposals are based on considerations – including considerations about what is important or valuable and considerations about how the proposals should be implemented – that mirror their standpoint. For that reason, the demand that global AI governance must indeed be global, intersectional, and fair has been growing in relevance.

As stated before, some of the rules currently proposed for governing AI extend to medical AI, while others are explicitly concerned with the digitisation of medical processes and the implementation of medical AI technologies. We claim that the latter may also fall under the limits and problems of global AI governance and thus deserve a closer look. We will provide such a look in the following sections.

2.2.2 Why Justice Matters

Global AI governance is largely motivated by considerations of global justice. Implementing global standards may be an important means of implementing global equality. While there are many theories of justice, for the scope of this chapter, we will briefly contrast distributive justice in the sense of Rawls with relational justice in the sense of Anderson. Put simply, from a stance of distributive justice, a just society is a society in which the principle of *fair equality of opportunity* and the *difference principle* are met. This means, first, that the distributions of goods are independent of non-moral factors and enable each and everyone's self-realisation; and second, the distributions of goods do not discriminate against the worst-off.[21] From a stance of relational justice, however, a just society is a society in which its members are in a mutual relation of equality and recognise one another as moral equals. Therefore, relational justice also demands the distribution of certain goods to a certain degree, namely, to the extent that the basis to *function* as an equal member of society is given to all and no unjustified hierarchies and dependencies evolve.

In the context of AI-DSS in healthcare, justice considerations are mostly concerned with biased and discriminating systems.[22] But the more general discourse on justice in healthcare may entail interesting insights when discussing moral implications of AI-DSS in the healthcare domain. As unequal distributions in healthcare cause otherwise avoidable and significant harm, it is widely recognised that the redistribution of healthcare knowledge and resources has a special priority.[23] Access to healthcare is essential to securing health and to a flourishing life. Thereby, health and healthcare are major concerns for theories of justice. Both distributive and relational justice scholars attribute similar levels of importance to health and, consequently, to the access to healthcare services. While proponents of distributive approaches to justice identify health as a presumptive condition of equality of opportunity,[24] proponents of relational approaches to justice recognise health among the conditions for individuals to function as moral equals.[25] Therefore, it seems like an egalitarian point of view necessitates implementing global standards for healthcare to realise equality of opportunity, the difference principle, and moral equality. Hence, to equalise healthcare and consequently health conditions globally, the demands made in global governance of AI that generally distribute equal rights and demands across the board are justified. However, global AI governance, as pointed out in Section 2.2.1, currently does not integrate everyone equally, thereby clashing with demands of relational equality and calling into question the overall acceptability of the governance framework. Given that AI-DSS offers chances to provide healthcare services for regions suffering from expert scarcity, one should carefully examine context-dependent arguments for explainability standards in healthcare, potentially suggesting context-dependent explainability standards.

2.2.3 Towards Context-Dependent Explainability Standards?

Healthcare is not equally distributed. There are expert-abundant and expert-scarce regions, with very different access means to treat and inform patients. In expert-scarce regions, injustices cannot be overcome by providing access to healthcare, as the existing inequalities are not caused by a mere lack of supply, but by structural disadvantages. Such disadvantages can only be remedied through the redistribution of knowledge from those regions with expert abundance. To ensure sustainable, enduring, and just access to medical services and healthcare, any region should have its own "home-grown" supply of doctors and medical equipment – a certain medical autarky. However, while yielding such an ideal solution and struggling slowly towards its realisation, the redistribution of experts and expert-producing infrastructure is not feasible within a sensible time frame.

AI-DSS now has the capacity to work as a provisional remedy for these structural disadvantages and it is, therefore, worth discussing the potentials and pitfalls of AI-DSS in equalising healthcare standards across regions.[26] AI-DSS could, for instance, diagnose breast cancer, indicate diabetic retinopathy through eye scans,[27] as well as conduct complex analyses of tomography scans[28] without the presence of a human expert. AI-DSS can also provide further treatment recommendations[29] and thereby extend access to healthcare to those previously suffering from lack of access.

Yet still, AI-DSS does have epistemological pitfalls. Implementing AI-DSS in expert-scarce regions would require standards of explainability that differ from the prevalent standards in expert-abundant regions,[30] standards that stem from discussions on the global AI governance level. These global standards can limit the applicability of some AI-DSS to provide medical help, as they are set from a generally wealthy perspective on what we should ideally expect from medical explanations. Lowering normative explainability standards to fit local needs caused by expert scarcity, hence, would yield better access to healthcare services, but it might also open the gates to some critical slippery slopes that we will elaborate on later in more detail.

The issue with explainability standards (as well as others) set by global perspectives, and the dilemma resulting from efforts to undermine these have similarities to pharmaceutical trials. There is abundant evidence[31] that companies from "resource rich" nations have been using clinical trials in resource-poor nations to outsource the risks while keeping the benefits in the richer nations. The chance that equally influential global AI corporations, from equally rich nations, are utilising any changes or exceptions to the global AI governance frameworks is high. Thus, the risk of corporations using expert-scarce areas to improve their devices deemed insufficient, while only bringing the technology back to expert-rich areas to lastingly improve their healthcare, is real. In order to obtain a better grasp on how to spell out these risks, we now analyse the subject of those AI governance decisions.

2.3 From Health-Insecure Populations to Health-Insecure Collectives

To clarify the subjects of our inquiry, i.e., those who are both affected by a set of standards as well as the candidates for setting their own standards, we propose some terminological choices. In debates about structural injustices, "vulnerable" is typically used to identify groups who are at risk of those injustices. If a structurally unjust pattern of treatment is detected, we may call those groups that are at higher risk of being affected by it "vulnerable groups" (in contrast to those groups who may benefit from structurally unjust patterns).

In contrast to this use, in clinical trials, the term refers to those groups who may be impaired to fully consent to participating in a trial.[32] Impairment of the ability to consent is often associated with the mental capacity to fully appreciate the potential consequences of consenting to laid out processes and the explicit agreement to the risks associated with these consequences. However, in clinical trials, this does not only include those who lack the cognitive capacity to properly consent (e.g., children, people with dementia, and unconscious people), but also those who are in economic, social, or otherwise contextual pressure situations that may create a problematic or consent ability-undermining incentive structure (e.g., incarcerated people or those in urgent need).

The subjects of our investigations are, indeed, vulnerable groups. However, as they are both potentially subject to structurally unjust treatments as well as emergency situations, it may impair their ability to consent to treatment with certain AI-DSS, as they are in urgent need and cannot reasonably be expected to reject a treatment. Furthermore, the classification of a group as vulnerable comes with a certain discursive baggage that we aim to avoid. At the same time, such classification is somewhat imprecise for discussions surrounding health due to its dual use. To pronounce both of these dimensions – the precariousness of their situation as well as them being at the receiving end of a structurally unjust healthcare system – we call these groups "health-insecure" (and those who are not subject to these conditions, conversely, "health-secure").

The term "group" is equally unclear, as it can refer to any kind of randomly chosen collection of individuals. To clarify that we consider a group a unity that shares a certain practical bond, and that often understands itself as a subject of this particular bond, we use the term "collectives". Instead of referring to "populations", which is the more popular term in discussions about international dimensions of justice, "collectives" allow for a conceptualisation of a group as equally at risk. "Population" may be a politically more expedient term, as a population is subject to a certain jurisdiction; however, collectives share reasons. And the kind of reasons we are discussing here are, on the one hand, the fact that they are on the receiving end of healthcare inequalities and are affected by the lack of effort to correct these inequalities. And on the other hand, the fact that they demand to be taken seriously regarding their own preference and chosen standards. For example, when Penu, Boateng, and Owusu discuss the standards of explainability in Sub-Saharan Africa, they do not refer to the populations of the countries constituting the region, but rather to the collective that will be subject to their deliberations: the future patients being diagnosed and treated with AI-DSS.[33] Therefore, we ought to discuss AI-DSS, the rules for their explainability, and requirements for their use from the perspective of collectives.

A health-insecure population, e.g., undersupplied people in expert-scarce areas, may consist of, no matter how carefully assessed, a group of consent-apt persons. But this ought not to suggest that this population is to be considered consent-apt at large. That is, the consent to apply lower standards of explainability to address scarcity in medical expertise does not sufficiently rely on an individual's agreement. It may result from/in unjustified authority, itself constituting a concern of relational justice. Populations, in this political understanding, are collections of individuals, while a collective has a certain identity of being a collective. In this sense, any self-governance of a population is merely the summary of all the individuals' opinions, not necessarily regarding the group's overall efforts. In collectives, self-governance is understood as a group effort, irreducible to mere individual opinions. Thus, the subjects of both structural injustice as well as the rule-setting and self-governing entities of our investigation are health-secure and health-insecure collectives (HSCs and HICs). If globally set standards are to be replaced by local standards, as demonstrated by some cases of local explainability,[34] these decisions must be made with collectives that set their own standards in the light of relational equality.

There are many concerns about the ability to have relationally equal exchanges between purveyors of AI-DSS on the one hand, and HICs seeking relief on the other hand. We discuss these from a post-colonial perspective (that incorporates historically grown injustices) in the next section.

2.4 An Emerging Post-Colonial Dilemma

Power imbalances suggest relations of authority. If a person has authority over another, their mutual equality is in question. From a stance of relational justice, the unequal relations between members of a society, not necessarily nation bound,[35] require justification that is sufficient for those who are under the authority.[36] This includes authority as a relation in which the subject to authority follows the directives of the authority. We work from the assumption that authority is only ever justified if the circumstances and exertion of such authority fulfil one of these conditions: either it constitutes a service which one is free to accept if following the directive presumably procures a better result than following one's own reasons[37] or, authority is given by the democratic collective in which everyone can equally co-decide on a directive that is acceptable to all.[38] The former option typically emerges in situations of different levels of expertise, the latter in administering a democratic state. In Section 2.3, we argued that to justify lower standards of explainability, democratic collectives must co-decide on the process. Under these conditions, local relative standards of explainability can be justified within the collectives. However, we did not make a claim on the justification *between* collectives.

In the next subsection, we will examine whether lower standards of explainability for HICs may maintain or even introduce illegitimate power imbalances.

2.4.1 Post-Colonial Medical Aid

Post-colonial literature emphasises the maintenance of oppressive structures and inequalities between former colonisers and former colonised ones under the cloak of aid or development programmes. Not only should one evaluate inequalities in healthcare through the socio-historical perspective of post-colonialism,[39] the same holds for the governance of AI.[40] This renders the issue of AI in healthcare relevant on two fronts: historically inherited inequalities and structural injustices.

Our proposal, to allow for lower standards of explainability in HICs, may in fact result in a dilemma of this post-colonial concern. In order to overcome the regulatory monopoly of the former colonisers and to reduce inequalities in health security, allowing lower standards of explainability in formerly colonised collectives is under discussion. However, a reasonable worry may be that techno-solutionist help might replace actual long-term aid (e.g., through the redistribution of knowledge and resources by education and enhanced distributional equality) and create long-term dependencies of HICs on HSCs. Moreover, as AI-based systems are mostly produced by corporations with global reach in health-secure contexts, these corporations will most probably have little incentive to diligently work on developing more explainable and better-performing systems. As long as the HICs remain dependent on their AI-based systems, their focus will be limited to their system complying with the local relative standards of HICs. Like the global reach of pharmaceutical companies, tech corporations only have the rules of global AI governance and their national translations to limit them. Yet, these rules are questionable and of limited effect.

2.4.2 Replacement of Subsidiary Improvements

The proposal under discussion is that HICs should be enabled to participate in the governance of AI in the sense that they may democratically decide on the use of AI-DSS to improve local healthcare situations. However, such participatory inclusion may co-exist with structural inequalities.[41] The mere use of AI-DSS will certainly neither erase the inequalities between HICs and HSCs regarding the impact of HICs on global AI governance nor will it address the structural problem of unequal distributions of knowledge and resources. But we did argue that it may diminish inequalities in healthcare (Section 2.2). Hence, while the health security of HICs may increase, the regulatory, epistemic, and wealth hierarchies between HICs and HSCs will remain largely unchanged. Hence, another concern may be that the proposal leads to shallow replacements on resolving the more fundamental, structural inequalities, by providing techno-solutionist help. The significance of this concern becomes more prominent when combined with the concerns on dependence of monopolies and big data.

2.4.3 Monopolies and Big Data

Big AI companies are already largely influential. It is safe to assume that illegitimate power imbalances between HICs and the companies in negotiations of medical standards for medical AI will show in the results; it may make the entire process of creating "relationally just" medical AI supplies seem as a form of domination.[42] The entities able to provide the infrastructure needed for AI-DSS are most likely private corporations in the field of big data. However, the commercial field of big data suffers from a significant tendency of monopolisation,[43] as both the amount of already collected data (the starting point) and the computing infrastructure for processing large amounts of data significantly impact the success of the development of data-reliant technologies. AI-DSS is one of such technologies. It is usually based on machine-learning algorithms and relies on huge corpora and computational power.[44] Especially in medicine, due to the sensibility of the data and the reasonable normative requirements for data collection,[45] the problem of data collection may impede smaller companies and research teams from entering the applied development of AI-DSS. Collecting data and conducting clinical trials in many iterations is expensive, paired with the need for labelling and training, cost becomes a critical factor for monopolisation. Furthermore, as AI-DSS are mostly commercial technologies, they tend to rely on proprietary code and data. Proprietary code and data will impede HICs to develop their own technology, and further reduce the transparency on the method of operation of the system. Consequently, commercial AI-DSS, which is assumed to use proprietary code and data, could introduce a dependency of HICs on the providers. Due to the lack of competition and alternatives, providers have little to no reason, other than goodwill, to improve their technology.

The same holds for the provision of the technology itself. But why would that be a problem if the technology still improves the healthcare situations of the collectives? Dependencies introduce power imbalances as the dependent (the HIC) must follow the provider's directives. To stick to our case, the collective cannot easily change the provider if it decides that the offered system is no longer good enough (*monopoly*), neither can it improve the system by itself (*proprietary code and data*) nor easily develop its own system (*replacement of subsidiary improvements*) or even stop using the system (*medical need*). Thus, the HIC will not be able to decide on the directives to act upon freely; it will become dependent on the providers.[46] Therefore, democratic legitimation would not hold. For the dependency to be legitimate, one must assume that the providers offering the supposedly best systems or HICs must be enabled to provide the AI-DSS by themselves by redistributing the knowledge on how to develop AI-DSS and by non-proprietary code and data.

2.4.4 The Problem of Epistemic Dependency

Our argument on the dilemma of global explainability standards emphasises the epistemic dependency of collectives on corporations from HSCs. We argue that this lacks democratic legitimation. However, healthcare has a widely accepted and morally acceptable set of epistemic dependencies when it comes to expert–non-expert relationships. In general, a patient is epistemically dependent on the physician. Following Raz, understanding authority as a service, this may be justified by the fact that the physician presumably knows better than the patient and follows the best reasons to act upon. That is, the patient may assume the physician to give directives in his or her own interest. Does an analogous argument hold for the epistemic dependency of HICs on private corporations? Such corporations' supposed reasons to act upon are motivated by making profit. Thus, the collectives may have better reasons to act upon than the corporations, in improving the quality of the product. But they might lack, due to further unjustified inequalities in the global distribution of knowledge and resources, the capacity to do so. Thereby, we cannot assume such epistemic dependency to be justifiable.

All these deliberations may allow for *ad-hoc* responses and fixes. Some regulatory requirements in some spots, some moral assertions in others could be conceived to be providing the necessary means to keep this system permissible. However, we contend that the dilemma discussed here – the pressure of global standards of AI governance vs. the need for differentiated standards (of, *e.g.*, explainability) – is not morally problematic in and of itself.

These dilemmas persistently emerge as the current system leans towards inequality and requires constant redistribution, violating fundamental principles of equality. Thus, even while being fixed constantly, the source of the dilemma, not its solution, appears to be the more fundamental issue at stake. Ultimately, techno-capitalism, as the identified source of our dilemma, ought to be put into focus for further investigation.

2.5 Concluding Remarks and Prospects

Although good reasons for context-dependent standards of explainability can be identified in the light of justice, the risks of neo-colonial structures in global AI governance have turned out to be a serious concern. The unjustified power that tech companies have over collectives, the companies' entrenchment strategies to maintain said power through monopolies and proprietary code and data, and the almost certain exploitation of changes in internationally binding standards, all exacerbate the risk of keeping HICs insecure. The fact that a collective is being supplied with merely sufficient technology to cover the worst inequalities without ever enabling them to develop their own healthcare infrastructure is not relational equality. For the demands of such an account of justice, collectives must be allowed to make their decisions but without the immediate pressure of having to make decisions in need. Thus, the imperative to help where help is needed is still very much in force, requiring HSCs to provide medical aid without entangled discussions about explainability standards.

Lastly, these demands suggest a pluralist account of AI governance with different regions setting standards according to their own needs.[47] We should endorse this path for AI governance.

To remedy the immediate suffering of HICs, the only way forward is one of a dual strategy that is demanding of HSCs, mostly rich states of the global north, to show actual commitment. Not only in enabling HICs to choose their own standards without having them fall victim to globally acting tech companies' incentive to push these lower standards, but at the same time to create a healthcare infrastructure in those places that is self-sustaining. This way, HICs may become healthcare independent, or at least not further dependent on the whim of HSCs and tech companies, and thus are enabled to set their own standards.

These demands make apparent that injustices in health security are not an isolated field that can be resolved on its own through ethical demands. It comes about through historically rooted global inequality and is perpetuated through power imbalances and, as such, can only be fully overcome if there are structural changes in how we relate to each other.

Funding Statement

The research for this chapters was funded by the project ELSA-AID (grant number 01GP1910A) of the German Federal Ministry of Education and Research (Bundesministerium für Bildung und Forschung (BMBF)).

Notes

1 Anderson ES, 'What Is the Point of Equality?' (1999) 109 Ethics 287.
2 Heilinger JC, *Cosmopolitan Responsibility* (De Gruyter 2020) <https://library. oapen.org/handle/20.500.12657/23628> accessed 28 February 2023; Zhuang X, 'World Citizenship and Global Health' in Bhakuni H and Miotto M (eds.), *Justice in Global Health: New Perspectives and Current Issues* (Routledge 2023).
3 Voigt K, and Wester G, 'Relational Equality and Health' (2015) 31 Social Philosophy and Policy 204, 211.
4 Ibrahim A and others, 'Artificial Intelligence in Digital Breast Pathology: Techniques and Applications' (2020) 49 The Breast 267.
5 Tang A and others, 'Canadian Association of Radiologists White Paper on Artificial Intelligence in Radiology' (2018) 69 Canadian Association of Radiologists Journal 120; Abràmoff MD and others, 'Pivotal Trial of an Autonomous AI-Based Diagnostic System for Detection of Diabetic Retinopathy in Primary Care Offices' (2018) 1 Digital Medicine 1.
6 Abràmoff MD and others (n 5).
7 As a complete introduction falls out of the scope of this chapter, to the interested reader, we recommend further readings to the problem of explainability of AI and its normative standards. For instance, Mittelstadt B, Russell C and Wachter S, 'Explaining Explanations in AI', Proceedings of the conference on fairness, accountability, and transparency (2019) provide a good introduction to the problem of explainability in AI, initiating a flourishing debate on the normative standards on explainability standards for AI as compared to human (cf. e.g. Zerilli J and others, 'Transparency in Algorithmic and Human Decision-Making: Is There a Double Standard?' (2019) 32 Philosophy & Technology 661; Kempt H, Heilinger JC and Nagel SK, 'Relative Explainability and Double Standards in Medical Decision-Making' (2022) 24 Ethics and Information Technology 20). Consequently, we started a debate on normative explainability standards, comparing different areas and levels of expert scarcity/abundance in our previous work (cf. Kempt H, Freyer N and Nagel SK,

'Justice and the Normative Standards of Explainability in Healthcare' (2022) 35 Philosophy & Technology 100).

8 Salhia B, and Olaiya V, 'Historical Perspectives on Ethical and Regulatory Aspects of Human Participants Research: Implications for Oncology Clinical Trials in Africa' (2020) JCO Global Oncology 959.

9 Hagendorff T, 'The Ethics of AI Ethics: An Evaluation of Guidelines' (2020) 30 Minds and Machines 99.

10 Png MT, 'At the Tensions of South and North: Critical Roles of Global South Stakeholders in AI Governance', 2022 ACM Conference on Fairness, Accountability, and Transparency (Association for Computing Machinery 2022) <https://doi.org/10.1145/3531146.3533200> accessed 28 February 2023; Mohamed S, Png MT and Isaac W, 'Decolonial AI: Decolonial Theory as Sociotechnical Foresight in Artificial Intelligence' (2020) 33 Philosophy and Technology 659.

11 Heilinger JC, 'The Ethics of AI Ethics. A Constructive Critique' (2022) 35 Philosophy & Technology 61.

12 Mohamed S, Png MT and Isaac W (n 10); Png (n 10); Taylor L, 'Public Actors Without Public Values: Legitimacy, Domination and the Regulation of the Technology Sector' (2021) 34 Philosophy and Technology 897.

13 Png MT (n 10).

14 For an overview and review of proposed regulatory frameworks, see Lewin Schmitt, 'Mapping Global AI Governance: A Nascent Regime in a Fragmented Landscape' (2022) 2 AI and Ethics 303; For an analysis of ethical frameworks, see Hagendorff (n 9).

15 See for example Tasioulas J, 'First Steps Towards an Ethics of Robots and Artificial Intelligence' (30 June 2019) <https://papers.ssrn.com/abstract= 3413639> accessed 28 February 2023; Floridi L, and Cowls J, 'A Unified Framework of Five Principles for AI in Society', Machine Learning and the City (John Wiley and Sons, Ltd 2022) <https://onlinelibrary.wiley.com/doi/abs/10. 1002/9781119815075.ch45> accessed 28 February 2023.

16 'Ethics Guidelines for Trustworthy AI | Shaping Europe's Digital Future' (8 April 2019) <https://digital-strategy.ec.europa.eu/en/library/ethics-guidelines-trustworthy- ai> accessed 28 February 2023.

17 Grote T, and Berens P, 'On the Ethics of Algorithmic Decision-Making in Healthcare' (2020) 46 Journal of Medical Ethics 205.

18 McDougall RJ, 'Computer Knows Best? The Need for Value-Flexibility in Medical AI' (2019) 45 Journal of Medical Ethics 156.

19 Png MT (n 10); Bender EM and others, 'On the Dangers of Stochastic Parrots: Can Language Models Be Too Big?', Proceedings of the 2021 ACM Conference on Fairness, Accountability, and Transparency (Association for Computing Machinery 2021) <https://doi.org/10.1145/3442188.3445922> accessed 28 February 2023.

20 Hagendorff T (n 9).

21 Rawls J, *A Theory of Justice - Ethics: Contemporary Readings* (Belknap Press/ Harvard University Press 1971).

22 Giovanola B, and Tiribelli S, 'Beyond Bias and Discrimination: Redefining the AI Ethics Principle of Fairness in Healthcare Machine-Learning Algorithms' (2022) AI and Society <https://www.scopus.com/inward/record.uri?eid=2-s2.0-8513 0223028&doi=10.1007%2fs00146-022-01455-6&partnerID=40&md5=cbf9f4 fea4d79be1ea2fff4d7eef6bd5>.

23 Daniels N, *Just Health Care* (Cambridge University Press 1985); Daniels N, *Just Health: Meeting Health Needs Fairly* (Cambridge University Press 2007); Wolff J,

'The Demands of the Human Right to Health' (2012) 86 Aristotelian Society Supplementary Volume 217; 'General Comment No. 14 (2000), The Right to the Highest Attainable Standard of Health (Article 12 of the International Covenant on Economic, Social and Cultural Rights)' <https://digitallibrary.un.org/record/425041> accessed 28 February 2023.

24 Rawls J (n 21); Daniels (n 23).
25 Anderson ES (n 1); Voigt K, and Wester G (n 3).
26 Kempt H, Freyer N and Nagel SK (n 7).
27 Abràmoff MD and others (n 5).
28 De Fauw J and others, 'Clinically Applicable Deep Learning for Diagnosis and Referral in Retinal Disease' (2018) 24 Nature Medicine 1342.
29 Somashekhar SP and others, 'Watson for Oncology and Breast Cancer Treatment Recommendations: Agreement with an Expert Multidisciplinary Tumor Board' (2018) 29 Annals of Oncology 418.
30 Kempt H, Freyer N and Nagel SK (n 7).
31 see Salhia B and Olaiya V, 'Historical Perspectives on Ethical and Regulatory Aspects of Human Participants Research: Implications for Oncology Clinical Trials in Africa' [2020] JCO Global Oncology 959.
32 Shivayogi P, 'Vulnerable Population and Methods for Their Safeguard' (2013) 4 Perspectives in Clinical Research 53.
33 Penu O, Boateng R and Owusu A, 'Towards Explainable AI(XAI): Determining the Factors for Firms' Adoption and Use of XAI in Sub-Saharan Africa' (2021) AMCIS 2021 TREOs <https://aisel.aisnet.org/treos_amcis2021/35>.
34 Kempt H, Freyer N, and Nagel SK (n 7).
35 Heilinger JC, (n 2).
36 Forst R (ed.), *Justice, Democracy and the Right to Justification: Rainer Forst in Dialogue* (1st edn, Bloomsbury Publishing Plc 2014) <https://www.bloomsburycollections.com/book/justice-democracy-and-the-right-to-justification-rainer-forst-in-dialogue> accessed 28 February 2023.
37 Raz J, *The Morality of Freedom* (Clarendon Press 1986).
38 Anderson ES, (n 1) 312ff.
39 Packard RM, *Post-Colonial Medicine – Medicine in the Twentieth Century* (Taylor and Francis 2000).
40 Png MT (n 10).
41 Cleaver F, 'Paradoxes of Participation: Questioning Participatory Approaches to Development' (1999) 11 Journal of International Development 597.
42 Taylor L (n 12).
43 Hindman M, *The Internet Trap: How the Digital Economy Builds Monopolies and Undermines Democracy* (Princeton University Press 2018); Klinge TJ and others, 'Augmenting Digital Monopolies: A Corporate Financialization Perspective on the Rise of Big Tech' (2022) Competition & Change 10245294221105572.
44 Bender EM and others (n 19).
45 Mittelstadt BD, and Floridi L, 'The Ethics of Big Data: Current and Foreseeable Issues in Biomedical Contexts' in Mittelstadt BD and Floridi L (eds), *The Ethics of Biomedical Big Data* (Springer International Publishing 2016) <https://doi.org/10.1007/978-3-319-33525-4_19> accessed 28 February 2023.
46 Taylor L (n 12).
47 See Okolo CT, Dell N and Vashistha A, 'Making AI Explainable in the Global South: A Systematic Review', ACM SIGCAS/SIGCHI Conference on Computing and Sustainable Societies (COMPASS) (Association for Computing Machinery 2022) <https://doi.org/10.1145/3530190.3534802> accessed 28 February 2023 for a review on explainability in the 'global south'.

Bibliography

Abràmoff MD and others, 'Pivotal Trial of an Autonomous AI-Based Diagnostic System for Detection of Diabetic Retinopathy in Primary Care Offices' [2018] 1 npj Digital Medicine 1.

Anderson ES, 'What Is the Point of Equality?' [1999] 109 Ethics 287.

Bender EM and others, 'On the Dangers of Stochastic Parrots: Can Language Models Be Too Big?', Proceedings of the 2021 ACM Conference on Fairness, Accountability, and Transparency (Association for Computing Machinery 2021) 10.1145/34421 88.3445922 accessed 28 February 2023.

Cleaver F, 'Paradoxes of Participation: Questioning Participatory Approaches to Development' (1999) 11 Journal of International Development 597.

Daniels N, *Just Health Care* (Cambridge University Press 1985).

Daniels N, *Just Health: Meeting Health Needs Fairly* (Cambridge University Press 2007).

De Fauw J and others, 'Clinically Applicable Deep Learning for Diagnosis and Referral in Retinal Disease' [2018] 24 Nature Medicine 1342.

'Ethics Guidelines for Trustworthy AI | Shaping Europe's Digital Future' [8 April 2019] <https://digital-strategy.ec.europa.eu/en/library/ethics-guidelines-trustworthy-ai> accessed 28 February 2023.

Floridi L, and Cowls J, 'A Unified Framework of Five Principles for AI in Society', Machine Learning and the City (John Wiley and Sons, Ltd 2022) <https://online library.wiley.com/doi/abs/10.1002/9781119815075.ch45> accessed 28 February 2023.

Forst R (ed), *Justice, Democracy and the Right to Justification: Rainer Forst in Dialogue* (1st edn, Bloomsbury Publishing Plc 2014) <https://www.bloomsburycollections. com/book/justice-democracy-and-the-right-to-justification-rainer-forst-in-dialogue> accessed 28 February 2023.

'General Comment No. 14 (2000), The Right to the Highest Attainable Standard of Health (Article 12 of the International Covenant on Economic, Social and Cultural Rights)' <https://digitallibrary.un.org/record/425041> accessed 28 February 2023.

Giovanola B, and Tiribelli S, 'Beyond Bias and Discrimination: Redefining the AI Ethics Principle of Fairness in Healthcare Machine-Learning Algorithms' [2022] AI and Society <https://www.scopus.com/inward/record.uri?eid=2-s2.0-85130223028&doi=10.1007%2fs00146-022-01455-6&partnerID=40&md5= cbf9f4fea4d79be1ea2fff4d7eef6bd5>

Grote T and Berens P, 'On the Ethics of Algorithmic Decision-Making in Healthcare' [2020] 46 Journal of Medical Ethics 205.

Hagendorff T, 'The Ethics of AI Ethics: An Evaluation of Guidelines' [2020] 30 Minds and Machines 99.

Heilinger JC, *Cosmopolitan Responsibility* (De Gruyter 2020) <https://library.oapen. org/handle/20.500.12657/23628> accessed 28 February 2023.

Heilinger JC, 'The Ethics of AI Ethics. A Constructive Critique' [2022] 35 Philosophy & Technology 61.

Hindman M, *The Internet Trap: How the Digital Economy Builds Monopolies and Undermines Democracy* (Princeton University Press 2018).

Ibrahim A and others, 'Artificial Intelligence in Digital Breast Pathology: Techniques and Applications' (2020) 49 The Breast 267.

Kempt H, Freyer N and Nagel SK, 'Justice and the Normative Standards of Explainability in Healthcare' (2022) 35 Philosophy & Technology 100.

Kempt H, Heilinger JC and Nagel SK, 'Relative Explainability and Double Standards in Medical Decision Making' (2022) 24 Ethics and Information Technology 20.

Klinge TJ and others, 'Augmenting Digital Monopolies: A Corporate Financialization Perspective on the Rise of Big Tech' [2022] Competition & Change 10245294221105572

McDougall RJ, 'Computer Knows Best? The Need for Value-Flexibility in Medical AI' [2019] 45 Journal of Medical Ethics 156.

Mittelstadt B, Russell C and Wachter S, 'Explaining Explanations in AI', Proceedings of the conference on fairness, accountability, and transparency, 2019.

Mittelstadt BD, and Floridi L, 'The Ethics of Big Data: Current and Foreseeable Issues in Biomedical Contexts' in B. D. Mittelstadt and L. Floridi (eds), *The Ethics of Biomedical Big Data* (Springer International Publishing 2016) 10.1007/978-3-319-33525-4_19 accessed 28 February 2023.

Mohamed S, Png MT and Isaac W, 'Decolonial AI: Decolonial Theory as Sociotechnical Foresight in Artificial Intelligence' [2020] 33 Philosophy and Technology 659.

Okolo CT, Dell N and Vashistha A, 'Making AI Explainable in the Global South: A Systematic Review', *ACM SIGCAS/SIGCHI Conference on Computing and Sustainable Societies (COMPASS)* (Association for Computing Machinery 2022) 10.1145/3530190.3534802 accessed 28 February 2023.

Packard RM, *Post-Colonial Medicine – Medicine in the Twentieth Century* (Taylor and Francis 2000).

Penu O, Boateng R and Owusu A, 'Towards Explainable AI(XAI): Determining the Factors for Firms' Adoption and Use of XAI in Sub-Saharan Africa' [2021] AMCIS 2021 TREOs <https://aisel.aisnet.org/treos_amcis2021/35>

Png MT, 'At the Tensions of South and North: Critical Roles of Global South Stakeholders in AI Governance', 2022 ACM Conference on Fairness, Accountability, and Transparency (Association for Computing Machinery 2022) 10.1145/3531146.3533200 accessed 28 February 2023.

Rawls J, *A Theory of Justice – Ethics: Contemporary Readings* (Belknap Press/Harvard University Press 1971).

Raz J, *The Morality of Freedom* (Clarendon Press 1986).

Salhia B and Olaiya V, 'Historical Perspectives on Ethical and Regulatory Aspects of Human Participants Research: Implications for Oncology Clinical Trials in Africa' [2020] JCO Global Oncology 959.

Schmitt L, 'Mapping Global AI Governance: A Nascent Regime in a Fragmented Landscape' [2022] 2 AI and Ethics 303.

Shivayogi P, 'Vulnerable Population and Methods for Their Safeguard' [2013] 4 Perspectives in Clinical Research 53.

Somashekhar SP and others, 'Watson for Oncology and Breast Cancer Treatment Recommendations: Agreement with an Expert Multidisciplinary Tumor Board' [2018] 29 Annals of Oncology 418.

Tang A and others, 'Canadian Association of Radiologists White Paper on Artificial Intelligence in Radiology' [2018] 69 Canadian Association of Radiologists Journal 120.

Tasioulas J, 'First Steps Towards an Ethics of Robots and Artificial Intelligence' <https://papers.ssrn.com/abstract=3413639> accessed 28 February 2023.

Taylor L, 'Public Actors Without Public Values: Legitimacy, Domination and the Regulation of the Technology Sector' [2021] 34 Philosophy and Technology 897.

Voigt K and Wester G, 'Relational Equality and Health' [2015] 31 Social Philosophy and Policy 204.

Wolff J, 'The Demands of the Human Right to Health' [2012] 86 Aristotelian Society Supplementary Volume 217.

Zerilli J and others, 'Transparency in Algorithmic and Human Decision-Making: Is There a Double Standard?' [2019] 32 Philosophy & Technology 661.

Zhuang X, 'World Citizenship and Global Health', in H. Bhakuni and M. Miotto, *Justice in Global Health: New Perspectives and Current Issues* (Routledge 2023).

PART II

Responsibility for Justice: Law, Civil Society, and the Private Sector

3

EVERYTHING IS UNCONSTITUTIONAL

Contesting Structural Violence in Health Systems with Legal Mobilisation

Luciano Bottini Filho

3.1 Introduction

The justiciability of the right to health and the role of Courts in promoting justice in a health system has long been a matter of contention.[1] Examples of misuse of resources or unsatisfactory scope of judicial review have abounded and, in some jurisdictions, litigation is still not a commonly trusted step towards social change particularly where access to high-cost medical technologies is concerned.[2] It is important to be clear on the judicial interventions that can be pursued by using human rights in courts and the power of these judicial actions to create change beyond individual litigants. An intractable problem in some jurisdictions is the predominant use of individual litigation as compared to structural lawsuits, where the latter is regarded as more beneficial to reducing inequalities.[3]

In this chapter, I present a model of structural litigation uncovering entrenched structural violence in health systems and compare it to lawsuits seeking individual remedies or direct satisfaction of health services or goods. Structural violence, in this chapter, is understood as encompassing different forms of systemic constraints (of economic, social, cultural, or political order) brought to bear against individuals (generally in marginalised situations) as limitations to their full potential in society (in this case, in health outcomes).[4]

Structural violence was originally introduced in a general sense by Galtung, in the 1960s, who defined it as any form of hindrance to potential human realisation arising from institutions or a set of circumstances, which cannot be individually ascribed to a single person or agent.[5] Since then, this early formulation was embraced as a heuristic device to contest health

DOI: 10.4324/9781003399933-6

disparities, particularly after the anthropological work of Paul Farmer.[6] It has been employed across different contexts as indirect form of violence through common patterns of discriminatory oppression, power inequalities, marginalisation, and endured suffering in social conflicts.[7] For instance, traditional examples of structural violence as negative circumstances in a health system are racism and discrimination against migrants.

By considering structural violence in a health system, I review a useful model of litigation taking a transformative justice lens to directly address those prevalent and systemic causes of social injustice. As a form of human rights experimentalism, I discuss some recent jurisprudential constructions in Brazil, where there is a growing recognition of the possibility of finding the entirety of healthcare policies unconstitutional, which, I suggest, should be viewed as a viable instrument of transformation in a health system. This unconventional type of declaration, noting a systemic level of failure demanding a complete policy review, is a practical possibility in envisaging mechanisms of transformative justice in health systems. Such an approach would be different in its form and objectives from structural orders for rights enforcement and would prioritise exposing existing forms of structural violence in defining the remedy or forming the claim by litigants. This progressive usage of courts can be posited despite the challenges surrounding the justiciability of the right to health and other social policies, even with very limited declaratory interventions. In this sense, I present the pathway for this model constituted by two contributing factors for strategic litigation: a) a procedural mechanism allowing for structural litigation, and b) active legal consciousness supported by authoritative knowledge demonstrating the effects or incidence of structural violence in a health system. The convergence of these factors engenders "opportunity structures" (the structural conditions for claim formation and positive outcomes) that may enable court decisions centred on structural violence in a health system.[8]

This chapter proceeds in seven steps. The first three sections concern the conceptual relations between structural violence and structural litigation and outline the advantages of legal claims that foreground structural violence. Section 3.2 explores the notion of structural violence in a health system. Section 3.3 traces the relationship between structural violence and transformative justice and Section 3.4 ties together transformative justice with court interventions as an understated association in structural judicial remedies for health systems. The remaining parts review the structural opportunities that have been found in practice with a case study in Brazil on healthcare policies and transgender rights. Section 3.5 describes the limited application of structural violence in judicial practice thus far, while Section 3.6 presents the procedural opportunity to build such claims with the doctrine of unconstitutional state of affairs. Section 3.7 describes how the doctrine has been used to challenge structural violence against transgender rights in the Brazilian health system. Section 3.8 outlines the remaining opportunity structures (legal consciousness and authoritative knowledge as to the manifestation of structural violence) necessary for a similar type of decision advanced by the court in the case study.

3.2 Structural Violence in Health Systems

The notion that widespread harmful forces in society (characterised by inequalities in the organisation of politics, economy, and so on) have an impact on health has been long recognised in public health practice. To a degree, this has been reflected in the much more predominant efforts on social determinants of health, though social structures in this strand of research or policy guidance do not have a strong connotation of political blame or wrongful perpetration of injustice. Social determinants of health stand as a more neutral observation in social epidemiology.[9] In comparison, structural violence has a reproaching undertone of active creation of avoidable injustice by institutions and social arrangements.

This more reproaching framing of the society inflicting structural violence is to a large extent a fruit of Paul Farmer's work. The genealogy of Farmer's application of structural violence in the healthcare sector is well established by Herrick and Bell, tracing it back to an article published in 1996.[10] Ever since, Farmer has been a leading voice against systemic injustice in healthcare, by popularising the term (as a matter of fact but also as theoretical development from Galtung), most notably with the HIV pandemic and health crisis in Haiti.[11] Farmer adopts structural violence in health as a construct in which human harms are inflicted by the social arrangements that determine how a society functions, such as economy and politics.[12] This view of structural violence is a synthesis of social structures and violence, in which "arrangements are structural because they are embedded in the political and economic organization of our social world; they are violent because they cause injury to people".[13]

In becoming more conversant with the idea of structural violence, a rising number of medical practitioners and public health experts have realised that their work demands interventions of a structural nature since treating patients alone would not cure social failings responsible for institutionalised health inequalities and vulnerabilities.[14] Today, on a smaller scale than social determinants of health, structural violence is often cited in critiquing poor health system performance and rampant inequalities or in justifying alternative measures to prevent the social causes of public health emergencies or the discrimination of marginalised groups in healthcare.[15] This has been done, however, not without criticism of its conceptual vagueness and of the fact that structural conditions, such as racism, may have different meanings or experiences in history. The notion of structural violence is also unclear because it is difficult to be reproduced as part of a controlled environment or through experiments and is often employed without a consistent use or standard operationalisation within research.[16]

For the purposes of structural litigation, as discussed in this chapter, the contribution of the notion of structural violence to healthcare litigation is that it is a guiding claim to confront the pervasive contextual causes of poor health outcomes. To shape structural claims, structural violence does not necessitate being fully pre-determined and can be individualised within a particular case brought before courts through local legal mobilisation. As will be discussed later, with possible structural remedies claims can at least assist in uncovering negative circumstances from their invisibility and in de-normalising expressions of structural violence viewed as natural, inevitable, or excessively intangible.[17]

3.3 From Structural Violence to Transformative Justice Measures

Having highlighted the relationship between structural violence and health systems, I begin by considering the recognition of such negative forces as an agenda of transformation of policies and State conduct in what has been described both in the literature and social activism as "transformative justice".[18] This model of contemplating social change will be, in the later sections, associated with structural claims. The thrust to acknowledge structural violence as a strategy for social change in policymaking comes from the need for action on the causes behind ongoing wrongdoings or harms, so it is important for courts to directly address them, especially if they are to develop structural approaches.

As a practical process, the transformative insight has been applied by advocates and civil organisations acting against harmful circumstances in a community, but not merely to obtain relief or immediate redress for individual violations. This ideal outcome has been pursued specifically in relation to a number of policies, such as female incarceration, land redistribution, child abuse prevention, abolitionism campaigns, penal system reform, and gender violence.[19] Such common usages of transformative justice, as I distinguish here, are not underscored by a systematic and uniform theory of justice and the notion does not have a consistent use, save for the association with the term structural violence as being pivotal to change. The action-oriented usages of the term, therefore, are largely part of the actors' own formulations.

And while the awareness of structural violence has led to different transformative justice practices (*e.g.*, criminal justice restorative approaches), the premise of structural violence in healthcare has rarely been discussed under the aegis of a theory of transformative justice. The attempts to define transformative justice became more systematically connected to structural violence with Gready and Robins' recommendation to use "transformative justice" to overcome the shortcomings or failures of traditional platforms of peace and reconciliation in the field of transitional justice.[20] The move to transformation from transition has gained more traction with their attempt to differentiate between the two types of justice.[21] For Gready and Robins, the transformative model had the added value of tackling the root causes of democratic failure or human rights abuses, in particular the lack of concern for economic and social rights.[22] Several effects have been regarded as transformative in this agenda (addressing economic and social inequalities, aiming for long-term deeper change, etc.) but the central feature of the model is to respond to structural violence.[23]

Therefore, both approaches to transformative justice detailed here (the theoretically developed approach in reaction to transitional justice and the more flexible approach found in advocacy or policy initiatives) respond to structural violence and demonstrate the importance of turning to the major structural causes of oppression or inequalities in advocacy and social mobilisation.

There is no well-developed theory of transformative justice for economic and social rights adjudication, but some commentators appear to refer to social transformation or change as a goal of litigation. For instance, in appreciating the political role of courts in social change, the concept of "social transformation" was described by Roberto Gargarella as "the altering of structured inequalities and power relations in society that reduces the weight of morally irrelevant circumstances, such as socio-economic status/class, gender, race, religion or social orientation".[24]

To build a transformative justice ethos into a health system with strategic litigation, we should pay attention to how courts can approach structural violence and become involved with claims at a structural level. In what follows, I will examine the common considerations about the structural dimension of litigation. I will then move to doctrinal developments in Brazil where in a case involving transgender rights the Supreme Court declared the whole health system unconstitutional. The case aims to provide an example of a structural opportunity.

3.4 Transformative Courts in Health: Connecting Structural Orders with Structural Violence

Thus far, I have suggested that there is mounting recognition of the toll of structural violence in heath. I observed that structural violence has been described as a pervasive source of inequalities and has influenced academic and non-academic responses towards the structural causes of social problems. From this perspective, I now examine the potential commonalities between structural court orders and the approach of a transformative agenda centred on structural violence.

In Farmer *et al*'s view, the most appropriate way to tackle structural violence in public health is to undertake structural interventions (which were not explicitly expressed as including court orders).[25] The interventions, to this effect, were conceived as complex programmes going further from conventional clinical care by investing in services at home to account for lingering barriers in access to healthcare such as nutrition, housing, and other basic needs. But courts can also structurally intervene in judicial review pertaining to health matters, just that these interventions have not oriented towards the idea of structural violence *per se*. The scope for structural remedies through Courts is not as specific as a structural health intervention in Farmer's example of first-line clinical work combined with more expansive social care. Sructural interventions in judicial studies refer to complex policy rulings denominated as "structural orders", which are defined by Boyle as "a remedial response to a systemic problem".[26] Structural judicial remedies have been discussed in policies involving resources, administrative powers, and public services, and more commonly under economic and social rights realisation. Individual litigation for economic and social rights has shown negative distributive effects and poor implementation, which has led to calls for structural remedies.[27] This category of rights can be responded to with a number of remedies like damages, declarations of incompatibility or invalidity, interim injunctions, and other creative dialogical forms of judicial supervision of government progress.[28] There is increasing debate on the nature of the enforcement of economic and social rights and whether judges should commit to weak or strong remedies to ensure social change.[29] Weak remedies consist of declarations and non-intrusive interventions that allow the State to find appropriate means without replacing political decisions.[30] Strong remedies interfere with or define a policy by specifying immediate measures.[31] Some have argued that weak remedies are more appropriate but only if they could be enforced with feedback or follow-up from the Courts regarding the progress made by legislators or the government, essentially demonstrating judicial supervision under institutional dialogue.[32]

Regardless of the model of structural remedy employed, the success of structural litigation still depends on the pathways and institutional factors ranging from how claims are formed to their procedures, decision-making, and implementation in a political system.[33] In both modalities, positive impact and capacity to remedy social wrongs are still the object of research and disagreement. Authors depend on the ability of courts, jurisdiction, and method of research to draw their conclusions on the choice of structural remedy.[34] But commentators can be reluctant about the ability of courts to stipulate the right structural remedy or set out major policy reforms to produce positive change.[35] However, as mentioned earlier, courts usually do not turn to the issue of the existence of any structural aspect before determining a remedy under a judicial decision. So how should courts come to terms with structural violence as a desirable standard of adjudication for systematic forms of rights violations in health system contexts?

Existing disagreements related to the usage and impact of structural orders are significant, but the approach to structural violence in court decisions for a health system would not necessarily require complex orders. To be clear, I do not place emphasis on decisions that are highly complex in their execution or nature or have a plethora of remedies combined to address structural violence. Whether courts should adopt weak or strong forms of remedies following recognition of structural violence is not pertinent to the scope of this analysis and may require further local studies that measure impact and implementation. What is important to take into account is the fact that even though scholars have fixated upon the efficacy or suitability of structural orders (weak or strong, or both), they have never inquired about the added value of having a structural approach with regard to both the claim and judicial reasoning. The existence of violations based on structural violence is independent of the complexity of the available remedies (weak or strong) and may only hinge on a court's capacity to make declarations about the incidence of structural violence contributing to rights violations or on a litigant's ability to form claims aimed at structural violence.

In theory, structural violence could be recognised and remedied by declarations or judicial statements of incompatibility (the weak route), especially when these declarations and statements target discriminatory policies that can be rectified by formal orders. The symbolic effect of these remedies is well described in the literature, and structural orders of a declaratory nature can at least portray structural violence, and its silent effects, as a material reality that requires immediate action.[36]

In the following section, I consider how rights-based judgments in healthcare have failed to bring to light structural violence. I also note that chronic resource scarcity or economic deficit often stand in the way of structural interventions. And, for that reason, further variations of structural violence affecting health systems (*e.g.*, those of abstract, cultural, or ideological nature and those connected to gender bias, racism, ableism, anti-indigenous movements, etc.) have a much less prominent role in judicial reasoning. Moreover, a large portion of the healthcare litigation considered by the literature (in particular in Latin American jurisdictions) comprises individual claims aimed at treatment coverage (*e.g.*, access to drugs), instead of structural determinants such as market deregulation or inefficient financing.[37] Therefore, other than the economic barriers to affording therapies, structural violence is unlikely to be deeply engaged by courts.

3.5 Searching for Structural Violence in Healthcare Litigation

The foregoing discussion indicates that the structural turn by courts witnessed to date has not been followed by a careful inquiry into structural violence. At best, the turn merely suggests that courts are at times willing to be involved with systematic problems (multiple or persistent violations) and issue decisions that target different aspects of State non-compliance.[38] It can be argued, then, that structural violence is poorly framed within structural litigation – or at least that there are few cases that give due consideration to structural violence.

Therefore, judges tend to focus primarily on establishing complex remedies by judicial orders directed against a background of massive violations (in a number of victims or cases) than determining a suitable intervention in response to an explicitly identified form of structural violence. In healthcare, few courts have effectively addressed rights violations by passing structural orders towards major health systems reform, let alone having made statements on structural violence.[39] Most commonly, courts issue simple remedies for immediate relief for healthcare needs raised by the petitioner.

An example of this type of legal approach is found with the Angola migrants case that came before the African Human Rights Commission. In *Institute for Human Rights and Development in Africa* v. *The Republic of Angola*, the Commission recommended that the State "take measures to ensure that all persons in detention are provided with proper medical examination and medical treatment and care" after finding rights violations of non-nationals arrested for immigration purposes in Angola.[40] But the analysis of the facts was restricted to the healthcare facilities and services provided in the detention centre, without considering the structural violence perpetrated by the State as a hostile environment to migrants perceived as threats to national interests. It is worth noting that the events related to this case took place within the context of *"Operação Brilhante"*, a governmental operation aimed at curbing the entry of foreigners into diamond mining zones to serve local economic interests. Thus, the hostile environment or negative rhetoric towards migrants in general (and not only in prisons) was a process of structural violence. And yet it was not addressed from the perspective of a health systems reform seeking a non-discriminatory environment.[41]

Another good example comes from cases of sexual and reproductive rights, where structures of inequalities leading to human rights violations are not meaningfully addressed despite litigation having a clear structural character. In Uganda, with the Constitutional Petition n. 16, the Supreme Court did find a violation of the right to health for the government's failure to take sufficient steps to ensure essential medical services for maternal care.[42] In its reasoning, however, the Court centred its analysis on individual episodes of healthcare failure and on addressing the availability of services and the responsibility to timely ensure access to healthcare for maternal health. The Court, therefore, missed the chance to go beyond "technical fixes" of healthcare delivery and acknowledging the existence of structural determinants of gender inequality and addressing such structural determinants by, for example, imposing a duty to re-evaluate and reform the maternal health programmes in a gender-sensitive manner.[43]

Similarly, a narrative of structural problems raising multiple rights violations is found in the decision T-760 by the Supreme Court of Justice of Colombia in 2008.[44] The focus here was on the State's inability to manage the flow of resources necessary to satisfy urgent requests from patients unable to meet treatment costs due to extreme poverty. T-760 is known to be a case in point in policy reform through health systems litigation, as the Court here had both ordered a host of steps for the government to comply with its duty to provide medicines and retained control over the implementation of the decision. The structural problem, however, was only partially addressed, as the remedy (a monitored order to implement policy reforms for access to treatments) was designed to ensure sufficient transfer of funds to healthcare, and not to reform deeper economic policies, the neoliberal mindset, or the imbalance in economic powers that jeopardised the affordability and financialisation of the health system.

It cannot escape one's attention that economic and material questions in the implementation of economic and social rights remain a central obstacle serving as a counter-argument for the justiciability of such rights. As most structural decisions in this domain are recent or extraordinary, there is no robust evidence of the failure or inaptitude of these remedies when complex policies demand substantive resources. The progress in universal health coverage in Colombia following T-760 has so far achieved mixed results. While higher spending on health has been reported, the health budget has not grown in line with the Court's demand and the criticism persists that patients continue to resort to courts for a policy that would be better suited to be run by governments.[45] However, as mentioned before, structural violence is not limited to lack of financing and resources and, if the economic and material gridlocks are difficult to overcome by judicial interventions, there are cultural and socio-political forms of structural violence that may still be addressed by courts.

Forms of structural violence can at the very least be judicially acknowledged, which many courts do not attempt to do. Part of this problem is how the claims are articulated by litigants and decided by courts. There are judicial conditions to be met under constitutional or legal frameworks, including legal standing, legal basis, and the necessary correlation between the damage and the conduct. Given such conditions, the link between the circumstances of structural violence and the right to health is suppressed so that courts can reach a decision within the legal boundaries. The approach taken by judges precludes any assessment of factors regarded as structural violence – it is enough to determine whether access to healthcare has been guaranteed, despite evidence as to the root causes for any claim.

3.6 Declaring a Health System Wholly Unconstitutional – A Structural Pathway for Health Policies

To move away from a more limited rights violation/satisfaction approach, courts need to engage with the structural aspect of healthcare policies. Here I will set out a framework for structural violence claims in health. The first condition is a pre-existent legal route for courts to entertain collective claims or examine matters at a structural level in a jurisdiction (rather than specific local public bodies). Here an example from Brazilian courts and the flourishing "state of unconstitutional affairs" doctrine is illustrative. The state of unconstitutional affairs was first proposed by the Colombian Constitutional Court and later imported by their Brazilian counterparts. The Colombian Court made this declaration for the first time, in 1994, in examining a case about social security funds for teachers who were never appropriately covered.[46] Since then the Court has issued this declaration only 10 times, but in such cases, the rulings have prompted significant attention over the structural causes of ongoing massive violations and helped victims' access to justice.[47]

In Brazil, this jurisprudential construct was raised more than a decade later, in 2009, with ADPF-347. The case was lodged by the Socialism and Liberty Party, soliciting a declaration of unconstitutionality with respect to the prison system in Brazil, on the grounds of the precarious conditions and excessive and indiscriminate placement of criminal defendants in custody.[48] A similar case was simultaneously brought before the same court, requesting collective compensation for the overcrowding in the criminal system. In response to these cases, the Supreme Federal Court for the first time took the view that the Colombia doctrinal approach could be applied to the prison system. The decision set out the requirements for such a declaration within the same parameters of the Colombia doctrine: a) generalised violations of fundamental rights; b) inaction or recurrent and persistent incapacity of State authorities to remove those violations; and c) the need for overcoming those transgressions in a manner that involves multiple authorities and State powers.[49] If compared to typical rights-based (individual) approaches, it can be seen that the declaration is directed towards the entirety of a policy or factual situation, not a law, individual decision, or single petitioner violation.

These procedural conditions allow litigants to approach the structural causes of healthcare inequalities and failures through a pathway more expedient to transformative justice. Rather than individually redressing specific violations (related to denial of healthcare or access to a particular treatment), this doctrine allows courts to tackle systematic problems in a policy without relying on a direct violation approach. By "direct violation approach", I mean that each individual situation is taken as the infringement of obligations of result, rather than indirect violations of intermediary and circumstantial structures related to obligations of conduct (means to achieve substantive results) which include eliminating forms of structural violence that interfere with the realisation of rights.[50]

As it can thus be inferred, this doctrine can be instrumental for the aspirations of transformative justice in a health system, since it paves the way to achieve health transformations without the need of establishing several individual rights violations. That helps to expose the existence of structural violence across various levels of healthcare as a systemic pattern (as opposed to redressing individual, episodical, or isolated forms of healthcare failures by immediate direct relief, such as a specific group of prisoners or a treatment for certain patients).

3.7 A Structural Violence Claim: Trans-persons and Health System Marginalisation in Brazil

After the establishment of the doctrine of the state of unconstitutional affairs as a legal possibility, Brazilian litigants have tested this legal path to respond to massive health violations. I now explore a case contesting structural violence against transgender people in the Brazilian public healthcare system (known as "Sistema Único de Saúde", or "Unified Health System" in English).

Lodged before the Brazilian Supreme Court by the Brazilian Workers' Party, the case was argued on the basis that the cis-normative structure of the whole healthcare services was inherently unconstitutional, calling for a national-level judicial intervention.[51] From this perspective, the main contention was that the national public health services were developed in a manner so as to capture the assumptions of the "ordinary person" based on cis-gender accounts of health provisions, sex, and reproduction divisions between men and women. This model disregarded the characteristics of a spectrum of transgender persons whose gender identity may have been adjusted by self-declaration or in the civil register without a full transitioning medical procedure. Transgender men and women who kept their natal sex or sex assigned at birth, therefore, had been denied access to healthcare by being refused or unable to book services or by not being referred to the appropriate specialist practice, in particular for sexual and reproductive services. One important concern in this model of care was the production of hospital birth certificates not compliant with transgender needs, by limiting parenthood to binary categories of "father" and "mother" without transgender-conforming options with neutral language or self-identified information.

Cisgenderism, as observed in this case, is a form of structural violence characterised by "the cultural and systemic ideology that denies, denigrates, or pathologizes self-identified gender identities that do not align with assigned gender at birth as well as resulting behaviour, expression, and community".[52] In health systems, institutionalised cisgenderism may create barriers or even lead to the denial of care for patients who do not conform to pre-conceived ideologies of the natural or ordinary body. Transgender patients may be unable to approach medical professionals with their own experiences and particular clinical knowledge which may be neglected in favour of most accepted evidence or established care routines.[53]

The case began after the Federal Public Defenders Office had issued, to no avail, a recommendation to the government to remove barriers to healthcare access affecting transgender patients who had not undergone reassignment surgery. The Worker's Party, a popular left-wing political party in Brazil, then lodged a complaint after attempts to request that the Ministry of Health revise its services to appropriately cater to transgender persons' specific experiences.

According to the Party's submission, the overall configuration of public healthcare services was essentially a prevalent violation of the rights to life and to health, and a direct breach of the dignity principle under Brazilian constitutional law. The party maintained that the government was aware of the discriminatory effects on users who used a gender different from their birth assignment and, considering the ongoing mismanagement and omissions across the population, a state of unconstitutional affairs should be declared. Two injunctions were pleaded for by the petitioners: a) immediate elimination of discriminatory divisions or patient triage in healthcare services, allowing for patients without gender reassignment to book or be referred to care consistent with their self-declared gender, and b) that maternity and birth delivery services should produce transgender-sensitive birth certificates which use the parent designation concordant with each transgender parent self-reporting or post-reassignment designation.[54]

Those arguments were supported by the petitions of *amicus curiae* as part of advocacy groups and public defenders mobilisation, who framed the violation as a complex and interlinked form of State violation of the right to health. Such a narrative fits neatly with the concept of structural violence by virtue of generalised transphobia, bias, and discrimination cutting across the entire health system. The issue with transgender access to healthcare in Brazil is placed within a background of multiple factors of violence and stigmatisation beyond healthcare. Healthcare marginalisation is compounded by structural determinants such as domestic abuse, psychological oppression, job market exclusion, and risk of murder.

In agreeing with the petitioners' submission, in July 2021, justice Gilmar Mendes made two interim orders granting the complaint requests: a) Healthcare services must reprogramme their records, booking systems, and patient protocols to allow for transgender people to receive adequate healthcare independent of their self-declared or registered gender identity, and b) birth certificates for transgender parents should refer to birth givers/parturient to avoid binominal classification of father and mother.[55] Until January 2023, the case is *sub judice* and there is no available data on the implementation of the decision. Just as in the Colombian experience, judicial progress may take years.

3.8 Other Opportunity Structures in Brazil: Evidence Attribution and Legal Consciousness

Having presented the transgender constitutional case in Brazil, I will analyse circumstances that facilitate the procedural structural route open to litigants, namely, established evidence of structural violence and active legal consciousness about systemic causes of injustice. These two factors are interdependent and shall be examined successively.

First, the prospect of employing strategic litigation to challenge healthcare structural violence by reviewing the constitutionality of an entire health system largely depends on how courts will be able to find the existence of social harm stemming from those omnipresent adverse circumstances. In other words, to respond to structural violence, litigants would have to provide compelling evidence of harm from intangible and generalised structures such as gender bias, racism, xenophobia, ableism, classism, etc.

The Brazilian Supreme Court has incidentally and tacitly agreed with the applicant's evidence in the motion contending that there is a vicious structure in the health system determined by cisgenderism. Similarly, for this strand of litigation on account of structural violence to stand a chance in other courts, litigants should be able to demonstrate, according to the relevant standards of proof, that those social forces do exist and, simultaneously, establish their connection with health outcomes or poor health system administration amounting to a rights violation. This is conceivably an innovative frontier in developing strategic litigation for transformative justice in health systems, by collecting evidence of structural violence as a central argument for judicial intervention. However, this is not much different from what has been undertaken, for instance, in climate litigation evidence making.

To draw a parallel with climate change litigation, structural violence may entail a similar evidential burden to determine the relationship between broader human activities and government policy culminating in a specific reduction in health outcomes for certain affected groups. With climate change, litigants were supported by studies under the field of "attribution science", which identify the correlation or causation between state policies, pollution levels, and the cumulative effect of nature's degradation caused by progressive global warming and changes in the ecosystem.[56] This body of knowledge permitted judges to acknowledge the predicted environmental harm and engage with complex economic and political measures, imposing preventive and reparative orders for environmental damages. These predicted harms are relatively invisible and not attributable to a single agent or source, just as structural violence in a health system.

The consequences of structural violence in a health system are not far from what has been conceived in the climate change literature by disclosing forms of social harm. This was illustrated by the expert consensus argued at the Brazilian Supreme Court by the Federal Public Defender Office and sexual diversity advocacy groups.[57] Petitions from the *amicus curiae* called attention to academic research and literature to demonstrate the predicament of transgender individuals through qualitative assessment of Brazilian health services.[58] Preconceptions against transgender people by healthcare professionals were classified as "trans broken arm syndrome", an unconscious inclination to believe that any health condition follows from the patient's transgender identity.[59] This body of knowledge was employed as a means to make concrete such invisible structures.

Alongside academic evidence, the second main enabling condition was the already active legal consciousness around transgender rights in Brazil. Legal consciousness is attributed to the capacity of the rights holders to understand and make sense of their experiences through legal concepts and mechanisms.[60] There was an already established set of constitutional precedents in favour of transgender rights, such as the case in which the crime of racism (to practice, induce, or incite discrimination or bias for some protected categories) was read to protect transgender people even though the statute had no express reference to this group.[61] Thus, Brazilian courts had already established a positive environment for legal challenges; litigants and courts were in constant legal mobilisation. The exact role of legal consciousness via constitutional precedents in this case is a matter of further research.

3.9 Conclusion

Why would a court declare an entire health system unconstitutional? I have suggested in this chapter that there are good reasons for at least having a declaratory decision revealing the invisible power of structural violence and laying bare those patterns of injustice as incompatible with the rule of law and constitutional order. The symbolic effects of such limited intervention can be further investigated, but the position and status of patients in a health system can theoretically undergo a dramatic alteration. If, for instance, a court issues an order declaring the entire health system biased or discriminatory towards black people, several scenarios can follow. Would doctors police their own behaviour given the flaws in the system, and would they do so independently of government efforts or recommendations? Would the media take interest in covering the dysfunctional health system? Would black patients be more cognisant of their oppression and exercise leverage in accessing healthcare?

There are several limitations in pursuing structural claims anchored in structural violence. For one, the concept of structural violence in a health system is clouded by uncertainties (though litigants can detect their own sources of structural violence on a case-by-case basis by delimiting and giving proof of them). Additionally, in the judicial review arena, the range of structural orders made available by courts is the product of institutional variables that litigation alone cannot control, in particular the procedural standing and other rules that enable access to justice at a structural level. These limitations are considered closely by judicial review scholars, but there has been little interest in considering claims under structural violence. The example of the ruling in Brazil is the result of a combination of circumstances beyond constitutional doctrine. In that case, the litigants were prepared to challenge the state of affairs through law and had credible knowledge of the health system's structural problem. Other health systems and jurisdictions can test similar approaches, but of utmost importance would be the capacity of local litigants to identify and articulate claims of structural violence. They must gather evidence and knowledge to inform courts of the contested problem and encourage adjudicators to intervene structurally.

With the foregoing discussion, I attempted to illustrate the potential of structural claims grounded in or directed towards structural violence. Despite the persistent problems of litigation as a tool for social transformation, it is possible to devise elements of transformative justice (broadly conceived) when pursuing strategic litigation around structural violence perpetrated by or within a health system. If a form of transformative justice practice by courts is to be established for a health system, it is essential to understand how this can be integrated into litigants' mobilisation and judicial discourse. By deploying population data and specific academic analysis, structural violence can be presented before courts as a preventable or actionable cause of human rights violation. In the same way that science has allowed the flourishing of climate change lawsuits, research can unearth the impact of structural violence in specific health outcomes across different minoritised groups. For instance, there is a growing association between structural violence and inequalities in health outcomes for migrants, ethnic minorities, and women owing to a discriminatory setting induced by deliberate political choices.[62] At a minimum, courts can follow a model of transformative justice (understood as a theory of change against structural violence) and experiment with more frontal judicial declarations of systematic incompatibility of an entire health system with fundamental principles of a state.

Compared to individual claims on the right to health, structural lawsuits covering state-wide healthcare policies are still in their early days and must be closely investigated for prospective social impact. An advantage of this form of lawsuit is the prospect of concentrating efforts against the entire health system at once. This is particularly advantageous where deficient policies and shared governance operate at different regional and local levels of jurisdiction in a large territory. Further research advancing the body of knowledge of systemic issues in a health system for litigants, in partnership with public health experts and anthropologists, may translate research into claimable evidence for structural violence in constitutional complaints against national health policies. Research on structural violence will assist litigants in designing their petitions to claim structural remedies and will guide courts to appropriate judicial orders. Judicial decisions in such cases can, at the very least, make visible the surreptitious materialisation of structural violence and open the door for testing further structural remedies.

Notes

1 See *e.g.*, Andia TS and Lamprea E, 'Is the Judicialization of Health Care Bad for Equity? A Scoping Review' (2019) 18 International journal for equity in health 1; Biehl and others, 'Judicialization 2.0: Understanding Right-to-Health Litigation in Real Time' [2018] Global Public Health 1; Yamin AE and Gloppen S (eds), *Litigating Health Rights: Can Courts Bring More Justice to Health?* (Harvard University Press 2011); Flood CM and Gross A, 'Litigating the Right to Health: What Can We Learn from a Comparative Law and Health Care Systems Approach' (2014) 16 Health and Human Rights 62.
2 In Latin America, see cases from Costa Rica, Brazil, Uruguay, and Colombia: Norheim OF and Wilson BM, 'Health Rights Litigation and Access to Medicines: Priority Classification of Successful Cases from Costa Rica's Constitutional Chamber of the Supreme Court' (2014) 16 Health and Human Rights 47; Hawkins B and Rosete AA, 'Judicialization and Health Policy in Colombia: The Implications for Evidence-Informed Policymaking: Judicialization and Health Policy in Colombia' (2019) 47 Policy Studies Journal 953; Virgilio Afonso Da Silva and Fernanda Vargas Terrazas, 'Claiming the Right to Health in Brazilian Courts: The Exclusion of the Already Excluded?' (2011) 36 Law & Social Inquiry 825.
3 See Everaldo Lamprea-Montealegre, 'Stopping a Litigation Epidemic: Lessons from Colombia and Brazils Highest Courts', *Local Maladies, Global Remedies* (Edward Elgar Publishing 2022).
4 See Bandy X. Lee, 'Structural Violence', *Violence: An Interdisciplinary Approach to Causes, Consequences, and Cures* (Wiley 2019) 123.
5 Galtung J, 'Violence, Peace, and Peace Research' (1969) 6 Journal of Peace Research 167.

6 See *e.g.*, Farmer PE, 'Pathologies of Power', *Pathologies of Power* (University of California Press 2004); Paul Farmer, 'An Anthropology of Structural Violence' (2004) 45 Current anthropology 305; Farmer PE and others, 'Structural Violence and Clinical Medicine' (2006) 3 PLoS medicine e449.

7 For common elements of structural violence usages, see Jackson B and Sadler LS, 'Structural Violence: An Evolutionary Concept Analysis' (2022) 78 Journal of Advanced Nursing 3495, 3503.

8 These enabling factors may be also called "legal opportunity structures" or "actor's opportunity structures". See Lehoucq E and Taylor WK, 'Conceptualizing Legal Mobilization: How Should We Understand the Deployment of Legal Strategies?' (2020) 45 Law & Social Inquiry 166, 183; Gloppen S, 'Studying Courts in Context: The Role of Non-Judicial Institutional and Socio-Political Realities' [2015] Closing the Rights Gap from Human Rights to Social Transformation 297–301.

9 On the distinction between these terms, see Herrick C and Bell K, 'Concepts, Disciplines and Politics: On 'Structural Violence'and the "Social Determinants of Health"' (2020) 32 Critical Public Health 295, 303–304; Fernando De Maio and David Ansell, '"As Natural as the Air Around Us": On the Origin and Development of the Concept of Structural Violence in Health Research' (2018) 48 International Journal of Health Services 749, 750.

10 Herrick and Bell (n 9) 297; Farmer PE, 'On Suffering and Structural Violence: A View from Below' (1996) 125 Daedalus 261.

11 Farmer, 'An Anthropology of Structural Violence' (n 6).

12 Farmer PE and others (n 6) 1686.

13 ibid.

14 Zakrison TL, Valdés DM and Muntaner C, 'Social Violence, Structural Violence, Hate, and the Trauma Surgeon' (2019) 49 International Journal of Health Services 665.

15 See e..g: Sirleaf M, 'Ebola Does Not Fall from the Sky: Structural Violence & International Responsibility' (2018) 51 Vand. J. Transnat'l L. 477, 483–88; Hamed S and others, 'Racism in European Health Care: Structural Violence and Beyond' (2020) 30 Qualitative Health Research 1662, 1663–64.

16 De Maio and Ansell (n 9) 754.

17 Winter Y, 'Violence and Visibility' (2012) 34 New Political Science 195, 196; Rylko-Bauer B, 'Structural Violence, Poverty, and Social Suffering' in Brady D and Burton LM (eds), *The Oxford Handbook of the Social Science of Poverty* (Oxford University Press 2016) 55–56.

18 For practioners' usages see *e.g.*, Kim ME, 'From Carceral Feminism to Trans-formative Justice: Women-of-Color Feminism and Alternatives to Incarceration' (2018) 27 Journal of Ethnic & Cultural Diversity in Social Work 219; Kershnar S and others, 'Toward Transformative Justice' (generation FIVE 2007) 5 <http://%3A%2F%2Fwww.generationfive.org%2Fwp-content%2Fuploads%2F2013%2F07%2FG5_Toward_Transformative_Justice-Document.pdf&usg=AOvVaw1tXeSxfnbDhFJL3nFF5yqI> accessed 1 November 2022. On academic theoretical frameworks, see *e.g.*, Gready P and Robins S, 'From Transitional to Transformative Justice: A New Agenda for Practice' (2014) 8 International Journal of Transitional Justice 339.

19 Kim (n 18); Kershnar and others (n 18).

20 Gready and Robins (n 18).

21 ibid.

22 ibid.

23 Evans M, 'Structural Violence, Socioeconomic Rights, and Transformative Justice' (2016) 15 Journal of Human Rights 1, 7–8; Dáire McGill, 'Tackling Structural Violence through the Transformative Justice Framework', *Transitional and Transformative Justice* (Routledge 2019).

24 Domingo P, 'Introduction' in Gargarella R, Domingo P and Roux T (eds), *Courts and Social Transformation in New Democracies* (Routledge 2017) 2.

25 Farmer and others (n 6) 1689.

26 Boyle K, 'Academic Advisory Panel Briefing Paper Access to Remedy–Systemic Issues and Structural Orders 30 November 2020'.

27 See Ferraz OLM, 'Harming the Poor through Social Rights Litigation: Lessons from Brazil' (2010) 89 Texas Law Review 1643, 1664; Brinks DM and Gauri V, 'The Law's Majestic Equality? The Distributive Impact of Judicializing Social and Economic Rights' (2014) 12 Perspectives on Politics 375, 375.

28 Roach K, *Remedies for Human Rights Violations: A Two-Track Approach to Supra-National and National Law* (Cambridge University Press 2021) 408–53. Roach K, 'Remedies and Accountability for Economic and Social Rights' in Langford M and Young K(eds), *The Oxford Handbook of Economic and Social Rights* (Oxford University Press).

29 Ibid. See also: Landau D, 'Choosing between Simple and Complex Remedies in Socio-Economic Rights Cases' (2019) 69 University of Toronto Law Journal 105; Dixon R, 'Creating Dialogue about Socioeconomic Rights: Strong-Form versus Weak-Form Judicial Review Revisited' (2007) 5 International Journal of Constitutional Law 391.

30 Tushnet M, 'Social Welfare Rights and the Forms of Judicial Review' (2003) 82 Texas Law Review 1895, 1909.

31 ibid 1911–12.

32 Roach K, 'Dialogic Remedies' (2019) 17 International Journal of Constitutional Law 860.

33 Gloppen (n 8) 292–97.

34 Sano H, 'Evidence in Demand: An Overview of Evidence and Methods in Assessing Impact of Economic and Social Rights' (2014) 32 Nordic Journal of Human Rights 387, 391–92; Gloppen S, 'Legal Enforcement of Social Rights: Enabling Conditions and Impact Assessment' (2009) 2 Erasmus L. Rev. 465, 474–79; Langford M, 'The Impact of Public Interest Litigation: The Case of Socio-Economic Rights' (2021) 27 Australian Journal of Human Rights 505; Brinks and Gauri (n 27).

35 On the weak and strong debate, see Landau (n 29). On the pitfalls of structural adjudication, see Weaver RL, 'The Rise and Decline of Structural Remedies' (2004) 41 San Diego Law Review 1617, 1628–31; Boyle K, *Economic and Social Rights Law: Incorporation, Justiciability and Principles of Adjudication* (Routledge 2020) 16–25.

36 On the symbolic effect and positive aspects of litigation by improving relational position of litigants, see Vitale D, 'The Relational Impact of Social Rights Judgments: A Trust-Based Analysis' (2022) 42 Legal Studies 408.

37 See note 2.

38 See *e.g.*, Huneeus A, 'Reforming the State from Afar: Structural Reform Litigation at the Human Rights Courts' (2015) 40 Yale Journal of International Law 1, 13–17.

39 Colombian case T-760, discussed in this chapter, is reputed to be one of the closest forms of structural claim in health. See Hawkins and Rosete (n 2); Lamprea E, Forman L and Chapman AR, 'Structural Reform Litigation, Regulation and the Right to Health in Colombia', *Comparative Law and Regulation* (Edward Elgar Publishing 2016); Alicia Ely Yamin and Oscar Parra-Vera, 'How Do Courts Set Health Policy? The Case of the Colombian Constitutional Court' (2009) 6 PLoS Medicine e1000032.

40 *Institute for Human Rights and Development in Africa (on behalf of Esmaila Connateh & 13 others) v. Angola*, 292/04, African Commission on Human and Peoples' Rights, May 2008.

41 On the negative rhetoric and poor health access of migrants in Angola, see e.g: Human Rights Council, Report of the Special Rapporteur on the human rights of migrants on his mission to Angola, (A/HRC/35/25/Add.1) 25 April 2017, paras 66–67.

42 Constitutional Petition N. 16 (Maternal Health Care), Center for Health, Human Rights and Development (CEHURD), Prof. Ben Twinomugisha, Rhoda Kukiriza, Inziku Valente v. Attorney General – Constitutional, 2020.

43 Grown C, RG Geeta and Pande R, 'Taking Action to Improve Women's Health through Gender Equality and Women's Empowerment' (2005) 365 The Lancet 541; Alicia Ely Yamin, 'From Ideals to Tools: Applying Human Rights to Maternal Health' (2013) 10 PLoS Medicine e1001546, 1–2.

44 Corte Constitucional de Colombia (2008) Sala Segunda de Revisión, Sentencia T-760. July 31, 2008. Magistrado Ponente: Manuel José Ceped

45 Restrepo-Zea JH, Casas-Bustamante LP and Espinal-Piedrahita JJ, 'Cobertura Universal y Acceso Efectivo a Los Servicios de Salud:¿ Qué Ha Pasado En Colombia Después de Diez Años de La Sentencia T-760?' (2020) 20 Revista de Salud Pública 670, 673–76.

46 C.C., Oct. 20, 1998 Sentencia T-590/98, https://www.corteconstitucional.gov.co/relatoria/1998/t-590-98.htm (Colom.); C.C., May 26, 1998 Sentencia SU-250/98, https://www.corteconstitucional.gov.co/relatoria/1998/SU250-98.htm (Colom.); C.C., Apr. 28, 1998, Sentencia T-153/98, https://www.corteconstitucional.gov.co/relatoria/1998/t-153-98.htm (Colom.).

47 Espinosa MJG and Lozano GO, 'The Unconstitutional State of Affairs Doctrine' in Jackson VC and Dawood Y (eds), *Constitutionalism and a Right to Effective Government?* (Cambridge University Press 2022).

48 ibid.

49 Lopes Filho JM and Augusto Maia IC, 'The Use of Foreign Precedents and the State of Unconstitutional Things Declaration by the Federal Supreme Court' (2018) 117 Revista Brasileira de Estudos Politicos 219; Machado C and Oliveira LPS, 'Unconstitutional State of Affairs and the Protection of Minimum Rights in Brazil' (2018) 4 Revista Juridica 166.

50 I draw this distinction from the literature on international human rights obligations. See Chapman AR, 'A Violations Approach for Monitoring the International Covenant on Economic, Social and Cultural Rights' (1996) 18 Human Rights Quarterly 23; Wolfrum R, 'Obligations of Result Versus Obligations of Conduct' in Arsanjani MH and Reisman WM (eds), *Looking to the future: essays on international law in honor of W. Michael Reisman* (Martinus Nijhoff Publishers 2011).

51 Supremo Tribunal Federal (ADPF 787), 28 June 2021.

52 Lennon E and Mistler BJ, 'Cisgenderism' (2014) 1 Transgender Studies Quarterly 63, 63.

53 Ansara YG, 'Cisgenderism in Medical Settings: Challenging Structural Violence Through Collaborative Partnerships' in Ian Rivers and Richard Ward (eds), *Out of the ordinary: Representations of LGBT lives* (Cambridge Scholars Publishing 2012).

54 ADPF 787 (note 50), p. 3.

55 ADPF 787 (note 50), pp. 36–37.

56 See *e.g.*, Lloyd EA and Shepherd TG, 'Climate Change Attribution and Legal Contexts: Evidence and the Role of Storylines' (2021) 167 Climatic Change 1.

57 See ADPF/787, Pedido de ingresso como amicus curiae (21089/2022) and Pedido de ingresso como amicus curiae (60218/2021).

58 See *e.g.*, de Carvalho Pereira LB and Chazan ACS, 'O Acesso Das Pessoas Transexuais e Travestis à Atenção Primária à Saúde: Uma Revisão Integrativa' (2019) 14 Revista Brasileira de Medicina de Família e Comunidade 1795.

59 Research reference alluded to in one of the amicus curiae petitions. See ADPF/787 (21089/2022, note 55, pp. 7-8) and ibid 11.
60 See. Chua LJ and Engel DM, 'Legal Consciousness Reconsidered' (2019) 15 Annual Review of Law and Social Science 335, 336.
61 Lei n° 7.716, de 5 de janeiro de 1989, art. 20; Supremo Tribunal Federal (ADO 26), 13 June 2020.
62 See *e.g.*, Rabin J and others, 'Anti-immigration Policies of the Trump Administration: A Review of Latinx Mental Health and Resilience in the Face of Structural Violence' (2022) 22 Analyses of Social Issues and Public Policy 763.

Bibliography

Andia TS and Lamprea E, 'Is the Judicialization of Health Care Bad for Equity? A Scoping Review' (2019) 18 *International Journal for Equity in Health* 1.

Ansara YG, 'Cisgenderism in Medical Settings: Challenging Structural Violence Through Collaborative Partnerships' in I. Rivers and R. Ward (eds.), *Out of the Ordinary: Representations of LGBT Lives* (Cambridge Scholars Publishing 2012).

Biehl J and others, 'Judicialization 2.0: Understanding Right-to-Health Litigation in Real Time' [2018] *Global Public Health* 1.

Boyle K, *Economic and Social Rights Law: Incorporation, Justiciability and Principles of Adjudication* (Routledge 2020).

Boyle K, (2021). Academic Advisory Panel Briefing Paper Access to Remedy – Systemic Issues and Structural Orders (National Task Force on Human Rights Leadership, The Scottish Government) 30 November 2020, available at https://storre.stir.ac.uk/retrieve/83ce5341-cc71-43dd-98ad-72be806d9a10/BOYLE%20Systemic%20Issues%20and%20Structural%20Orders%20Briefing%20Paper.pdf

Brinks DM and Gauri V, 'The Law's Majestic Equality? The Distributive Impact of Judicializing Social and Economic Rights' (2014) 12 *Perspectives on Politics* 375.

Chapman AR, 'A Violations Approach for Monitoring the International Covenant on Economic, Social and Cultural Rights' (1996) 18 *Human Rights Quarterly* 23.

Chua LJ and Engel DM, 'Legal Consciousness Reconsidered' (2019) 15 *Annual Review of Law and Social Science* 335.

Da Silva VA and Terrazas FV, 'Claiming the Right to Health in Brazilian Courts: The Exclusion of the Already Excluded?' (2011) 36 *Law & Social Inquiry* 825.

de Carvalho Pereira LB and Chazan ACS, 'O Acesso Das Pessoas Transexuais e Travestis à Atenção Primária à Saúde: Uma Revisão Integrativa' (2019) 14 *Revista Brasileira de Medicina de Família e Comunidade* 1795.

De Maio F and Ansell D, '"As Natural as the Air Around Us": On the Origin and Development of the Concept of Structural Violence in Health Research' (2018) 48 *International Journal of Health Services* 749.

Dixon R, 'Creating Dialogue about Socioeconomic Rights: Strong-Form versus Weak-Form Judicial Review Revisited' (2007) 5 *International Journal of Constitutional Law* 391.

Domingo P, 'Introduction' in R. Gargarella, P. Domingo and T. Roux (eds.), *Courts and Social Transformation in New Democracies* (Routledge 2017).

Espinosa MJC and Lozano GO, 'The Unconstitutional State of Affairs Doctrine' in Vicki C Jackson and Y. Dawood (eds.), *Constitutionalism and a Right to Effective Government?* (Cambridge University Press 2022).

Evans M, 'Structural Violence, Socioeconomic Rights, and Transformative Justice' (2016) 15 *Journal of Human Rights* 1.

Farmer PE, 'On Suffering and Structural Violence: A View from Below' (1996) 125 *Daedalus* 261.

Farmer PE, 'An Anthropology of Structural Violence' (2004) 45 *Current anthropology* 305.

Farmer PE, 'Pathologies of Power', *Pathologies of Power* (University of California Press 2004).

Farmer PE and others, 'Structural Violence and Clinical Medicine' (2006) 3 *PLoS Medicine* e449.

Ferraz OLM, 'Harming the Poor through Social Rights Litigation: Lessons from Brazil' (2010) 89 *Texas Law Review* 1643.

Flood CM and Gross A, 'Litigating the Right to Health: What Can We Learn from a Comparative Law and Health Care Systems Approach' (2014) 16 *Health and Human Rights* 62.

Galtung J, 'Violence, Peace, and Peace Research' (1969) 6 *Journal of Peace Research* 167.

Gloppen S, 'Legal Enforcement of Social Rights: Enabling Conditions and Impact Assessment' (2009) 2 *Erasmus Law Review* 465.

Gloppen S, 'Studying Courts in Context: The Role of Non-Judicial Institutional and Socio-Political Realities' [2015] *Closing the Rights Gap from Human Rights to Social Transformation*.

Gready P and Robins S, 'From Transitional to Transformative Justice: A New Agenda for Practice' (2014) 8 *International Journal of Transitional Justice* 339.

Grown C, Gupta GR and Pande R, 'Taking Action to Improve Women's Health through Gender Equality and Women's Empowerment' (2005) 365 *The Lancet* 541.

Hamed S and others, 'Racism in European Health Care: Structural Violence and Beyond' (2020) 30 *Qualitative Health Research* 1662.

Hawkins B and Alvarez Rosete A, 'Judicialization and Health Policy in Colombia: The Implications for Evidence-Informed Policymaking' (2019) 47 *Policy Studies Journal* 953.

Herrick C and Bell K, 'Concepts, Disciplines and Politics: On 'Structural Violence' and the "Social Determinants of Health"' (2020) 32 *Critical Public Health* 295.

Huneeus A, 'Reforming the State from Afar: Structural Reform Litigation at the Human Rights Courts' (2015) 40 *Yale Journal of International Law* 1.

Jackson B and Sadler LS, 'Structural Violence: An Evolutionary Concept Analysis' (2022) 78 *Journal of Advanced Nursing* 3495.

Kershnar S and others, 'Toward Transformative Justice' (generation FIVE 2007) http://%3A%2F%2Fwww.generationfive.org%2Fwp-content%2Fuploads%2F2013%2F07%2FG5_Toward_Transformative_Justice-Document.pdf&usg=AOvVaw1tXeSxfnbDhFJL3nFF5yqI accessed 1 November 2022.

Kim ME, 'From Carceral Feminism to Transformative Justice: Women-of-Color Feminism and Alternatives to Incarceration' (2018) 27 *Journal of Ethnic & Cultural Diversity in Social Work* 219.

Lamprea E, Forman L and Chapman AR, 'Structural Reform Litigation, Regulation and the Right to Health in Colombia', *Comparative Law and Regulation* (Edward Elgar Publishing 2016).

Lamprea-Montealegre E, 'Stopping a Litigation Epidemic: Lessons from Colombia and Brazils Highest Courts', *Local Maladies, Global Remedies* (Edward Elgar Publishing 2022).

Landau D, 'Choosing between Simple and Complex Remedies in Socio-Economic Rights Cases' (2019) 69 *University of Toronto Law Journal* 105.

Langford M, 'The Impact of Public Interest Litigation: The Case of Socio-Economic Rights' (2021) 27 *Australian Journal of Human Rights* 505.

Lehoucq E and Taylor WK, 'Conceptualizing Legal Mobilization: How Should We Understand the Deployment of Legal Strategies?' (2020) 45 *Law & Social Inquiry* 166.

Lennon E and Mistler BJ, 'Cisgenderism' (2014) 1 *Transgender Studies Quarterly* 63.

Lloyd EA and Shepherd TG, 'Climate Change Attribution and Legal Contexts: Evidence and the Role of Storylines' (2021) 167 *Climatic Change* 1.

Lopes Filho JM and Augusto Maia IC, 'The Use of Foreign Precedents and the State of Unconstitutional Things Declaration by the Federal Supreme Court' (2018) 117 *Revista Brasileira de Estudos Politicos* 219.

Machado C and Oliveira LPS, 'Unconstitutional State of Affairs and the Protection of Minimum Rights in Brazil' (2018) 4 *Revista Juridica* 166.

McGill D, 'Tackling Structural Violence through the Transformative Justice Framework', *Transitional and Transformative Justice* (Routledge 2019).

Norheim OF and Wilson BM, 'Health Rights Litigation and Access to Medicines: Priority Classification of Successful Cases from Costa Rica's Constitutional Chamber of the Supreme Court' (2014) 16 *Health and Human Rights* 47.

Rabin J and others, 'Anti-immigration Policies of the Trump Administration: A Review of Latinx Mental Health and Resilience in the Face of Structural Violence' (2022) 22 *Analyses of Social Issues and Public Policy* 763.

Restrepo-Zea JH, Casas-Bustamante LP and Espinal-Piedrahita JJ, 'Cobertura Universal y Acceso Efectivo a Los Servicios de Salud:¿ Qué Ha Pasado En Colombia Después de Diez Años de La Sentencia T-760?' (2020) 20 *Revista de Salud Pública* 670.

Roach K, 'Dialogic Remedies' (2019) 17 *International Journal of Constitutional Law* 860.

Roach K, *Remedies for Human Rights Violations: A Two-Track Approach to Supra-National and National Law* (Cambridge University Press 2021).

Roach K, 'Remedies and Accountability for Economic and Social Rights' in M. Langford and K. Young (eds.), *The Oxford Handbook of Economic and Social Rights* (Oxford University Press).

Rylko-Bauer B., 'Structural Violence, Poverty, and Social Suffering' in D. Brady and L. M. Burton (eds.), *The Oxford Handbook of the Social Science of Poverty* (Oxford University Press 2016).

Sano H-O, 'Evidence in Demand: An Overview of Evidence and Methods in Assessing Impact of Economic and Social Rights' (2014) 32 *Nordic Journal of Human Rights* 387.

Sirleaf M, 'Ebola Does Not Fall from the Sky: Structural Violence & International Responsibility' (2018) 51 *Vand. J. Transnat'l L.* 477.

Tushnet M, 'Social Welfare Rights and the Forms of Judicial Review' (2003) 82 *Texas Law Review* 1895.

Vitale D, 'The Relational Impact of Social Rights Judgments: A Trust-Based Analysis' (2022) 42 *Legal Studies* 408.

Weaver RL, 'The Rise and Decline of Structural Remedies' (2004) 41 *San Diego Law Review* 1617.

Winter Y, 'Violence and Visibility' (2012) 34 *New Political Science* 195.

Wolfrum R., 'Obligations of Result Versus Obligations of Conduct' in M. H. Arsanjani and W. Michael Reisman (eds.), *Looking to the Future: Essays on International Law in Honor of W. Michael Reisman* (Martinus Nijhoff Publishers 2011).

X. Lee B, 'Structural Violence', *Violence: An Interdisciplinary Approach to Causes, Consequences, and Cures* (Wiley 2019).

Yamin AE, 'From Ideals to Tools: Applying Human Rights to Maternal Health' (2013) 10 *PLoS Medicine* e1001546.

Yamin AE and Gloppen S (eds.), *Litigating Health Rights: Can Courts Bring More Justice to Health?* (Harvard University Press 2011).

Yamin AE and Parra-Vera O, 'How Do Courts Set Health Policy? The Case of the Colombian Constitutional Court' (2009) 6 *PLoS Medicine* e1000032.

Zakrison TL, Milian Valdés D and Muntaner C, 'Social Violence, Structural Violence, Hate, and the Trauma Surgeon' (2019) 49 *International Journal of Health Services* 665.

4

FRAMING NOMA

Human Rights and Neglected Tropical Diseases as Paths for Advocacy

Alice Trotter and Ioana Cismas

4.1 Introduction

Search the internet for 'noma' and information about the world's best restaurant located in Copenhagen, Denmark will likely be returned first. Also sharing this name is a little-known disease that affects people living in conditions of extreme poverty across Africa, Asia, and Latin America.[1] Noma, the disease, is a devastating gangrenous condition that starts inside the mouth and is estimated to affect around 140,000 individuals every year.[2] It is both preventable and, when diagnosed early in young children, highly treatable.[3] When noma develops undetected, however, the disease spreads very quickly to the structures surrounding the mouth. This may lead to the destruction of the skin, muscle, and bone of the person's face.[4] The untreated mortality rate for noma, last reported by the World Health Organization (WHO) in 1998 and still used today, estimates that up to 90% of children do not survive the full onset of this disease.[5]

Surviving children carry the experience of noma on their faces for a lifetime. People affected by the disease are known to encounter social isolation, stigmatisation, and discrimination, as well as difficulties with speaking, eating, and seeing.[6] It is thought that there may be as many as 770,000 people living with these long-lasting sequelae.[7] Given noma's strong association with malnutrition and extreme poverty, as well as the isolation many survivors may experience, it is likely that current epidemiological understandings of the disease underestimate the reality of noma today.[8]

We are not the first authors to contrast the accessibility of information about a restaurant with the (in)accessibility of information on a

DOI: 10.4324/9781003399933-7

malnutrition-related disease.[9] Indeed, a noma survivor and advocate recently started his presentation on the disease by referencing the famous Danish restaurant.[10] Making this connection is one way of communicating – or 'framing' – the depths of noma's neglect to specific audiences. The contrast also serves as an illustration of the focus of this chapter itself: the examination of noma's framing in health, humanitarian, and human rights circles.

The aim of this chapter is to evaluate two of the most recent framings of noma – as a human rights issue and as a neglected tropical disease (NTD) – and to consider how these frames have, and could be, leveraged to enhance advocacy and generate policy change at international level and on the ground to tackle noma and support survivors. We posit that developing awareness of the purpose and perception of these frames – whilst also continuing existing inquiries into noma's epidemiology, prevention, and treatment – is essential in lifting the veil of neglect that has long encircled noma globally and in many national contexts.

This chapter reports the findings of a research project that combined desk-based and empirical research to examine noma's framing as a human rights issue and as an NTD.[11] A narrative review of the literature on social and political theories of framing served to structure a series of key informant interviews. Twenty medical, humanitarian, and human rights practitioners from inter- and non-governmental organisations were purposively sampled for their expertise on noma to participate in 'elite' interviews. With the consent of our participants, these interviews were recorded, transcribed, and thematically analysed. In reporting the contributions of our participants, we honour the requests of both those who requested full anonymity as well as those individuals who preferred to be identified in the research outputs.

Structurally, the chapter is divided into four parts. Following this introduction, the second part draws on an interdisciplinary literature to define framing and identify its possible purposes as a means of communication. Using the findings of this review, we then configure our examination of existing research, expertise, and outputs on noma. The third part examines 'frames' of noma that have been variously prominent over the last four decades: the medicalised and humanitarian frames, as well as the human rights and NTD frames. Our focus is on the 'who' (the framers), the 'why' (the purpose of the framing), and the 'what' (the outcome sought and/or accomplished) in respect to the identified frames. The penultimate section of the article draws together the findings of the narrative literature review with those of the key informant interviews to reflect on the significance of the intermingling of the discussed frames for enhancing future advocacy efforts on noma. The conclusion reflects on the NTD and human rights frames' compatibility and complementarity.

4.2 What is (in) a Frame?

Framing theory departs from the premise that an issue or topic may be "viewed from a variety of perspectives".[12] Frames animate this process, as rhetorical devices created and advanced by actors with the intention to communicate specific understandings of an issue and to target the generation of specific responses. Media outlets, national governments, social movements, and transnational advocacy networks have all been framers – *the who*' in our three-part analysis – that sought to utilise framing processes for a variety of reasons – '*the why*'.[13] Some actors design and deploy frames to "mobilise adherents and constituents" for a particular cause or to "demobilise antagonists".[14] Other framers, such as activist groups, seek to construct "shared understandings of the world ... that [then] legitimate and motivate collective action".[15] As will be discussed in the following sections, when this perspective is applied to the noma agenda, it is possible to discern the influence of the professional identity of the frame-*r* on the purpose and outcome of the frame-*ing*.

Scholars underscore the versatility of framing as an advocacy tool. For Jorgensen and Steier, a frame is a means of advancing "one possible view" on an issue, while Merry notes the utility of frames as tools for "packaging and presenting ideas".[16] When read together, these definitions highlight that a frame is not comprised of an issue in and of itself, but refers to different features of a given substantive issue. As such, the practice of framing involves a "selection" of particular features of the issue at hand and the highlighting of their "salience" with the aim of prompting specific reactions from target audiences.[17]

That the same issue can be communicated in different ways to different audiences and for different reasons is a cornerstone of both the theory and practice of framing. Keck and Sikkink provide one illustration of this in their analysis of land-use rights in the Amazon rainforest. The authors observe that the rights in question, "took on an entirely different character and gained quite different allies when viewed in a deforestation frame than in either social justice or regional development frames".[18] It is clear that multiple framings of the same issue can co-exist, either simultaneously or over an extended period of time. There may be tensions between these frames, or stakeholders may leverage differences in the focus of the frames to stimulate and influence action. This process is, however, predicated upon framers being able to formulate an issue in such a way that speaks to the interests of the intended audience. As Snow and Benford summarise, "the potency of a frame depends on its relevance to the targeted population".[19] Thus, the greater degree of relevancy, the more likely a frame will affect discursive and material changes – 'the what' or outcome in this chapter's analysis. As the following section discusses, in the context of the noma agenda there is some evidence of the former – with narrative changes emerging – and, with the progression of the NTD campaign, we consider it likely that material changes will come to greater fruition over the course of the next decade.

4.3 Frames of Noma in Operation

Attention now turns to consider the frames of noma that continue to operate both locally, in affected states, and internationally, across health, humanitarian, and human rights fora. In doing so, the analytical focus is on the framers (who), their aim (why), and the outcomes of the framing process (what). Because of the limited literature on noma, this section of the article is supported by reflections on both our own and our research participants' experiences. At this stage, it is necessary to disclose the authors' positionality – Cismas has been involved in noma's framing as a human rights concern since 2009 and in all subsequent efforts to support noma's inclusion on the WHO list of NTDs,[20] while Trotter has been a principal researcher on one of the most recent major interdisciplinary research projects on noma.[21] In undertaking our examination of noma's framing in this article, we will therefore engage with our own work reflexively, and thus necessarily critically.

4.3.1 The 'Traditional' Frames: Medicalised and Humanitarian Frames

Noma's framing as both a medicalised and humanitarian issue has since the early 1990s directed how various stakeholders identified and acted on the disease. Practice has closely intertwined these frames, which have been drawn together by the specific medical, social, and economic circumstances that are thought to give rise to noma.[22] This is reflected in the assemblage of approaches required to prevent and treat the disease. As one interview participant observed, noma sits a bit in-between emergency-medical and humanitarian-development interventions.[23]

The medicalised and humanitarian frames were brought into being – not coincidentally – by charities, medical, and humanitarian actors. Two evolutive characteristics relating to both the purpose and outcome of these frames are of relevance to our discussion: the locality and scope of interventions.

Non-governmental organisations with a charitable and/or medical character, such as Sentinelles, the Dutch Noma Foundation, Facing Africa, Hilfsaktion Noma e.V., and Winds of Hope engaged in humanitarian- and medicalised-based framings of noma with the specific purpose of raising funds in the Global North to resource surgical 'missions' to Sub-Saharan Africa. These organisations primarily delivered surgical interventions in areas where noma was known to occur, and some temporary relocated individuals to European hospitals for treatment.[24] The importance of this work should not be underestimated: treatment was offered to people at all five stages of noma. Another important strand of work focused on noma's aetiology, which despite efforts remains to this day unknown.[25]

In time, the locality and scope of interventions took a different, and we would argue more sustainable meaning. The focus of the movement – which by the mid-2000s also included Health Frontier Laos, Médecins Sans Frontières (MSF), and other members of the NoNoma Federation – shifted to incorporate capacity building of local actors and the prevention of noma as central features. Efforts to build local medical (including surgical) knowledge and structures have led, for example, to the establishment of noma health centres in Burkina Faso and Niger[26] and to the creation of the first specialist hospital for noma patients in Sokoto, Nigeria.[27] Medical professionals spoke about the social determinants and consequences of noma – in particular, poverty, and malnutrition.[28] Awareness-raising campaigns were developed targeting healthcare professionals and traditional healers working in communities across a dozen countries in Africa.[29] For example, brochures were developed and circulated by WHO's Regional Office for Africa (WHO AFRO) to depict and explain the stages of noma.

It is not surprising that in the 30 years since the emergence of these frames an evolution has occurred in their purpose and outcomes. The medicalised-humanitarian frame has not remained temporally or spatially rigid. This fluidity is characteristic of framing in practice.[30] Benford and Snow observe that once in circulation, frames are in a continuous process of being, "constituted, contested, reproduced, transformed and/or replaced".[31]

In the case of noma, one example of this is evident in the changing practices around the provision of specialist reconstructive surgery for children who had developed, and survived, the latter stages of the disease. Where previously people were brought to Europe to undergo reconstructive treatment, normative practice has moved towards a more localised model, with specialist medical care facilities established in several Sub-Saharan African states. This has enabled individuals to undergo reconstructive treatment in-county, often accompanied by their families as they move through surgical and rehabilitation pathways at clinics staffed by both local and Global North surgeons. The benefits of doing so are clear: aftercare takes place in relatively familiar, accessible environments, more local staff receive specialised training and participate in care provision, and the scope of the care provided is expanded and benefits many more people at risk or affected by noma.[32] A related example is the recognition of the agency of local actors. In Nigeria, the Noma Children's Hospital – set up by the Nigerian Ministry of Health in Sokoto and supported by MSF since 2014 – regards community-based services as a central pillar of its model of care. In addition to local health workers, leaders and members of community are seen as vital for noma's prevention and treatment in a more sustainable manner.[33] Similarly, an evaluation report of the WHO Africa Regional Programme on Noma Control notes that "with the support of Hilfsaktion ... the programme trained 5000 health workers (doctors, nurses, midwives, community health workers and medical assistants) in 10 countries to be able to carry out preventive and management actions".[34]

Put differently, a shift in focus has evidently begun, engendering, or accepting, local ownership of the processes aimed to prevent and treat noma. Finally, then, and without seeking to take away from the importance of charity-led work – indeed, in the past, often surgical missions sponsored by charities and staffed by Global North doctors were the only avenue to medical intervention for many who experienced noma in the Global South – it is important to observe that the discourse had, on occasion, signalled a 'white saviour' trope. This approach is problematic both morally, as well as from the point of view of sustainability of interventions.[35]

4.3.2 Noma's More Recent Framings: Human Rights and NTDs

The human rights and NTD framings of noma have emerged in the last 15 years. These frames are, therefore, comparatively recent occurrences and the process of their development is ongoing. As there is very little research that directly examines these frames of noma, the following discussions are both pro- and retrospective, recognising the trajectory of current advocacy whilst also reflecting on our own and our research participants' experiences with these framing processes.

The analysis of the human rights and NTD frames of noma must begin with one of their earliest iterations: the 2012 Human Rights Council Advisory Committee (HRCAC) *Study on severe malnutrition and childhood diseases with children affected by noma as an example* (hereafter, HRCAC Study).[36] The HRCAC is formed of independent experts who are mandated to provide research-based advice to the United Nations (UN) Human Rights Council, the main intergovernmental UN body tasked with the protection of human rights. In the HRCAC Study, noma was for the first time presented as a cause and effect of human rights violations, with the Committee *also* going on to request that the WHO recognise noma as an NTD.[37]

The Committee was not, however, the first mechanism of the UN to underscore the links between the human rights and NTD frames more generally. In 2007, Paul Hunt, the then Special Rapporteur for the right to health stated that "neglected diseases are both a cause and consequence of human rights violations".[38] This association is often mutually reinforcing, for as Hunt goes on to observe, "failure to respect certain rights increases the vulnerability of individuals ... to neglected diseases [and] people affected by neglected diseases are vulnerable to violations of their human rights".[39] Whilst we recognise both this intermingling of the two frames, and that undertaken by the HRCAC, for the cogency of the analysis, this section will first consider noma's communication as a human rights concern, and then as a NTD.

4.3.2.1 Which Human Rights Frame, with What Purpose, and What Outcomes?

In formulating the human rights frame of noma, the HRCAC Study described the disease as, "the most brutal face of poverty and malnutrition in children ... thus giv[ing] rise to some of the worst violations of the rights of child".[40] As is characteristic of a violations-based approach to human rights framing, the Study goes on to recognise governments of both affected and donor states as the principal duty bearers for acting against the prevalence of noma and addressing discrimination experienced by survivors.[41] The identification of these actors as bearers of legal obligations, as well as the evocative language used to emphasise accountability, aligns the Study with 'naming and shaming' practices often employed in human rights campaigns.[42] These practices are typically carried out by non-governmental organisations seeking to identify and denounce perpetrators of violations with the aim of establishing accountability, ensuring redress for victims and survivors, and preventing further abuse.[43]

Why then did the HRCAC pursue this *specific* approach? Among our research participants, the rationale underpinning the HRCAC's decision to adopt a rights-based – and specifically a violations-based – framing of noma was undisputed. Indeed, this framing was perceived to be intuitive – not just because of the professional identity of the framer, a body working on human rights, but because of the nature and circumstances of the disease itself. As one interviewee noted, the majority of noma cases seen today are "children who are born into these basic human rights violations".[44] The individuals developing noma are those whose rights to adequate food, sanitation, and health are not realised, and who, in their large majority, will have their right to life itself violated.[45] Another interview participant specifically urged due consideration of the right to life of people affected by noma:

> ... it's important we don't forget that everyone has a right to live. [Noma] is not only a disease, not only malnutrition, but it's a matter of life itself ... somehow you see not only the life of a child [but] you also see their death. You see what you never see in someone. You see the skull, you see the bones, and you see the potential death of the person.[46]

As this interview excerpt so vividly demonstrates, a significant moral impetus continues to animate the noma agenda, cutting across the medicalised, humanitarian, and human rights frames. Indeed, according to the author of the HRCAC Study, who is also one of the co-authors of this article, the Committee sought to use a human rights violations-based framing of noma to leverage the moral authority embodied by the wider human rights agenda. Yet, the HRCAC's overarching goal was, as Cismas notes:

> To speak to the consciousness of governments and, importantly, that of the WHO. We [the HRCAC] wanted to see them taking action on the ground, *not because it was the charitable thing to do but because they have human rights obligations under international treaty and customary law to do so.* We wanted to see accountability.[47]

If the PANEL (Participation, Accountability, Non-Discrimination and Equality, Empowerment, and Legality) principles are taken to embody the human rights approach, the HRCAC concentrated on legality – anchoring action and policies on noma in legal rights – and accountability – monitoring of states' activity on noma and providing remedy when that activity falls short. Specifically, the HRCAC was preoccupied with how both legality and accountability were being frustrated by the restricted locality and limited thematic scope of noma-related activities.

In the early 2000s, following a decision of the Regional Consultative Committee, the noma programme was transferred from WHO headquarters in Geneva to WHO AFRO – specifically to the oral health department.[48] Stakeholders expressed concerns, reported in the HRCAC Study, that this relocation would likely serve to institutionally invisibilise people at risk or affected by noma who lived *outside* the African continent.[49] Recent scholarship continues to emphasise that noma's prevalence remains under-explored in Latin America, Asia, and specifically the Indian subcontinent.[50]

A human rights frame, then, connects the absence of monitoring and institutional attention paid to noma in these regions with the human rights violations that individuals living in these areas and affected by the disease are *likely* to experience.[51] The likelihood is not theoretical, if we argue by analogy with the lived experiences of those in Sub-Saharan Africa affected by noma,[52] and based on the limited evidence from existing studies focusing on Asia.[53] As such, a whole range of human rights are at stake, certainly the right to health, but also the rights to food, water and sanitation, housing, education, life, freedom of expression, the right of children with disabilities to a full and decent life, and the overarching right to equality and non-discrimination.[54] Human rights framing also points to the fact that states, as primary duty bearers under international human rights law, are failing these individuals.

As such, the HRCAC aim was to widen the geographical scope of inter-ventions beyond sub-Saharan Africa and the thematic focus beyond medi-calised interventions to include considerations of the lived experiences of rights holders – whether at risk or survivors of noma – and of the obligations that states have towards these individuals. Adopting such an expansive approach would, therefore, enable stakeholders to address noma through the lens of structural power imbalances that manifest themselves in poverty and discriminatory patters, and thus connect the disease with broader agendas that seek to tackle these – the human rights movement evidently, but also, at the time, the Millennium Development Goals.[55]

The examination of whether noma's framing as a human rights concern has materialised into concrete outcomes must recognise that its two objectives – acknowledgement by states of their human rights obligations in respect to individuals at risk of noma and survivors as *rights holders*, and the global institutionalisation of noma's prevention and treatment – were undoubtedly ambitious. They require significant, almost paradigmatic shifts in the way that stakeholders think and act on noma. As we look back over the decade since the HRCAC study was published, it is perhaps unsurprising that the objectives of the human rights frame cannot be said to have been fully achieved in either state practice or institutionalisation processes. Yet, there are three significant advances that should be noted.

The HRCAC's focus on legality has been echoed by some scholarly works – interestingly published in medical journals[56] – research projects[57] and WHO publications.[58] These portray individuals affected by noma as rights holders, often emphasising their victimhood as people whose rights have been violated. The WHO AFRO's Step-by-Step Guide to Develop National Action Plans for Noma Prevention and Control in Priority Countries presents a more complex understanding of noma survivors than was seen before. The guide includes the objective of "reintegration of noma survivors and their families into society", centring lived experiences, as well as seeking to ensure reintegration in educational institutions and workplaces, and to facilitate small business opportunities and partnerships with community groups and development initiatives.[59] Finally and crucially, authorities are encouraged to seek noma survivors' input in noma prevention and control activities, including by enlisting them as community health workers.[60] This indeed reflects a fuller understanding of the human rights approach, one that engenders the empowerment and participation of those whose rights are affected by noma in policy processes that directly concerns them.

In terms of accountability efforts, the Human Rights Council acknowledged in a 2012 resolution the work conducted by the HRCAC on noma, and explicitly encouraged states to implement the *Human Rights Principles and Guidelines to improve the protection of children at risk or affected by malnutrition, specifically at risk of or affected by noma*.[61] This instrument had been developed by the Committee and annexed to its 2012 Study as an embodiment of a human rights approach to tackling noma and addressing discrimination against survivors. Subsequently, UN treaty bodies had taken up noma in their periodic country reviews.[62] The Committee on

Economic, Social and Cultural Rights (CESCR) and the Committee on the Rights of the Child (CRC) – the treaty bodies tasked with monitoring state parties' compliance with the International Covenant on Economic, Social and Cultural Rights (ICESCR) and the Convention on the Rights of the Child (CRC) respectively – have asked Burkina Faso, Ethiopia, and Eritrea to report on the prevalence of noma in their populations.[63]

Have states embraced noma's human rights framing? In response to the above-mentioned UN treaty bodies' review, a marked contrast is evident, with Eritrea on the one hand, and Burkina Faso and Ethiopia on the other. Eritria denied the very existence of noma within its borders.[64] Ethiopia and Burkina Faso, however, engaged constructively with the CRC and the CECSR, respectively.[65] The latter explained how it partnered with non-governmental organisations and the WHO in the "fight against noma", what progress it has made, and interestingly that it "advocated the inclusion of noma in the list of neglected tropical diseases".[66]

Whilst no general conclusion can be drawn from these few examples of state practice as to whether states assume their human rights obligations in respect to individuals experiencing noma, one observation is in order. States that have engaged with humanitarian organisations or charities – as did both Burkina Faso and Ethiopia – and had worked with the WHO to develop noma programmes – the case of the former – are more likely to not deny the existence of the disease, and thus not seek to further invisbilise survivors. In turn, this may place them in a better position to see the utility of and assume a human rights approach to noma.

Nigeria's practice provides further evidence for the above observation: steps taken to address noma could be interpreted and presented as an indicator of a state's progress toward the realisation of international human rights obligations. Various Nigerian state actors in collaboration with intergovernmental and non-governmental partners have taken active roles in shaping multi- and cross-scalar action on noma. Nigeria is one of several African states to have established national action plans in collaboration with the WHO, and the disease has been incorporated into the curriculum of medical schools.[67] It has also sought to develop public awareness of the disease through an annual 'National Noma Day'.[68] During the third commemoration of the day in 2019, the federal government declared its commitment to eliminating the disease in Nigeria by 2030.[69] This in-country action has been undertaken alongside interventions in the international health agenda: with the support of MSF, the Nigerian Ministry of Health has taken the lead on preparing the dossier of evidence for submission to the WHO Strategic Advisory Group calling for noma to be recognised as an NTD. Full circle then, at a side-event presentation during the COP26 summit held in autumn 2021 when a representative of the Nigerian delegation noted that the human rights to food, health, and education are vulnerabilised when a person develops noma.[70] These actions of Nigeria, which have occurred at different scales and in different fora serve to demonstrate that when states take steps to address noma, they are less likely to be adverse to applying a human rights approach to noma – a discussion to which we shall return in the next section of this chapter.

Finally, then, the above-mentioned dossier of evidence, which has been submitted to the WHO in January 2023, cites human rights obligations as one of the justificatory grounds for the inclusion of noma in the WHO list of NTDs.[71]

4.3.2.2 NTD as Noma's Self-Evident Frame and Framers, yet with What Outcome?

As several interview participants observed, the rationale of communicating noma as an NTD is evident: noma meets each of the four criteria of a NTD. The disease:

1 predominantly affects people living in conditions of poverty, and causes important morbidity and mortality in these populations, therefore justifying a global response;
2 affects people living in tropical and subtropical areas;
3 is immediately amenable to broad control; and
4 and has been neglected in the field of research.[72]

Noma's inclusion on the formal WHO list of NTDs would, therefore, be a recognition of fact. It would also be the logical and purposeful step to pursue, with the derivation of a range of benefits immediately clear. Drawing in part on the trajectories of other neglected diseases formally recognised by the WHO, interview participants noted that the visibility, awareness, and funding of noma in the international health agenda would likely increase.[73] NTDs have, as one interviewee noted, become "an established brand" which attaches certain commitments from inter-, national, and corporate actors in the global health community.[74] Gaining the WHO's recognition of noma as an NTD would, then, "carry a lot of weight", according to another participant.[75] This would be a highly positive development, likely amplifying awareness within the global health community, expanding attention and political commitment in national health policy, and increasing funding for in-field programming.

Despite noma's framing as an NTD being self-evident, as noted above, at the time of writing, its inclusion on the WHO NTD list remains an objective to be formally reached. Indeed, as two experts in the field describe it, noma remains a "neglected-neglected tropical disease".[76]

What can explain this? There may have been a number of possible factors at work. First, the HRCAC Study – which, recall, recommended noma's inclusion on the WHO NTD list – did not have its intended *immediate* impact. While some states had shown an interest, the buy-in had not been cultivated due to lack of human and financial resources. The hope was that a multi-stakeholder, cross-regional coalition would emerge that championed noma's formal listing as a WHO NTD. Whilst this did not materialise immediately in the years after the HRCAC's report publication, MSF had taken up work on noma in Sokoto, Nigeria. This led to more systematic attention being paid to noma within the organisation: a large, influential humanitarian actor had thus entered the noma advocacy stage.

Second, there was a resistance to declaring noma an NTD from some WHO member states (important voluntary contributors to the organisation's budget) and from within the WHO itself. We understand this to have occurred in a context of insufficient resources and capacity that the WHO Department of Control of Neglected Tropical Diseases was facing (and indeed continues to face to this day).[77] Jean Ziegler, former member of the HRCAC, wrote of a high-level meeting with a Swiss public health official:

[they] refused to present any resolution on noma to the World Health Assembly, [arguing that] 'there are already far too many diseases on the checklist'. WHO's representatives in the field are already overwhelmed. They hardly know what to do next. Adding another disease to the list – don't even think about it.[78]

Thus, the NTD framing of noma had to contend with a counter-framing: the competition between diseases for human and foremost financial resources. It is unlikely that the institutional challenges that were described by Ziegler nearly a decade ago have been resolved. However, the inclusion of snakebite envenoming on the NTD list in 2017 continues to give reason for optimism.[79]

Third, noma fell prey to the vicious circle of imperfect data. Data on noma's incidence and prevalence dates to the 1990s and is objectively imperfect. As to the circle: when advocates had previously raised noma's inclusion in the WHO NTDs list, advocations were rebutted as 'premature' given lack of data systematically evidencing the disease's impact on populations. More data and more recent data, it was argued, were needed to prove the necessity of noma being listed as an NTD. As to the viciousness of the circle: NTDs by their very definition *will* have imperfect data because they are neglected by research. To gain better data, noma will have to not be neglected by researchers. This very point was brought home in the dossier of evidence in support of noma's addition to the WHO NTD list.[80]

Who then are noma's NTD framers? The NTD frame blends humanitarian and medical approaches to diseases which, in the case of noma, are the fields where the majority of actors are working to provide immediate and long-term interventions. Whilst the process of *framing* noma as an NTD may have been initiated by the HRCAC in 2012, the intervening years have seen medical experts and humanitarian practitioners take up the agenda, ground it in empirical evidence, and launch strategic advocacy efforts. In 2017, an interdisciplinary, multi-actor advocacy task force was established, and a few meetings were held at MSF's headquarters in Geneva with, among others, representatives of Sentinelles, GESNOMA, and MSF – some of the individuals present had been involved in the successful snakebite dossier.

Some four years later, MSF launched an official campaign for noma's recognition as an NTD, appointed a researcher to draft the dossier of evidence, and a journalist and award-winning documentary filmmaker as campaign manager. Notably, whilst run by MSF, the campaign has become paradigmatic in its inclusion of a range of stakeholders: from medical experts, humanitarians, charities who had long worked on noma, human rights practitioners, and to, most importantly, noma survivors themselves.[81]

The progression of the campaign over the last three years offers the most concrete indication yet that noma's position in the international health agenda may be about to change. One key moment was the World Health Assembly's approval of a landmark oral health resolution in May 2021 that proposed exploring noma's inclusion in the next cycle of the NTD roadmap.[82] Another crucial event is marked by the submission of the dossier of evidence by Nigeria and 30 cross-regional co-sponsoring states. 2023 is likely to be a year to watch for noma.

It would not be amiss to ask: what changed in the past decade? The epidemiological data on noma has seen little progress[83] – yet, advocates seem, and rightly so, to have broken the vicious circle of imperfect data we discussed earlier. Noma remains as deadly *and* can be cured as inexpensively if treated in the early stages – again, advocates appear to have had greater success in persuading states and WHO structures of this fact. This may have assuaged some concerns in particular of those who resisted noma's inclusion on the WHO list due to (legitimate) concerns relating to limited human and financial resources. The conclusion appears inescapable: what changed and enabled the progress in noma advocacy that we currently witness has less to do with the disease itself and more to do with its framers. Nigeria, the largest country in Africa by population size and GDP, is leading the campaign for noma's listing. MSF, one of the most important and influential humanitarian organisations, has provided support, expertise, and resources to develop the dossier of evidence and the advocacy campaign – in doing so, it has built bridges between decades of work of noma medical experts, of charities and organisations, and human rights professionals and sought to centre the voices of noma survivors.

4.4 Two Inter-Related Reflections for Future Advocacy

Whilst it is not yet possible to identify a definitive outcome, the above discussions combine to suggest that the NTD frame is currently seen as the most effective way to further noma's position in the international health agenda. The inclusion of noma in the WHO NTD list, however, will not be a silver bullet for the eradication of noma and the realisation of the human rights of people who experience and survive the disease. Funding, research, integration in existing mechanisms, new policies, continued political will, and changing of mindsets will all be needed. Drawing on the above analysis, a thematic literature review, and the responses of our interview participants, we offer two reflections for future advocacy practice on noma.

4.4.1 Prioritising the NTD Frame, While Retaining Elements of Other Frames

We posit that when the status of NTD is formally conferred upon noma by the WHO, core elements of the medicalised, humanitarian, and human rights frames must be retained and incorporated within the roadmap process. Over the last 40 years of their operation, the actors engaged in these frames have developed unparalleled knowledge of noma: of its causes and its risk factors, of the treatment of people who have developed noma and their follow-up, of the surveillance of cases and the planning of effective medical as well as socio-economic interventions. They have also funded such work (almost) at the exclusion of state and corporate funding. Further utilising and scaling up these evidence bases will be crucial to develop the global institutionalisation of preventative action and treatment of noma.

The rights-based nature of our own work leads us to advocate in particular for incorporation of the human rights perspective going forward. Doing so will be vital in ensuring that people affected by noma take up positions at the forefront of the agenda and that their lived experiences inform planning and programming at every level – in other words that the empowerment and participation principles become reality. Working to incorporate these principles into practice may, in time, come to guard against over-medicalisation, understood here as application of exclusively or predominately medical knowledge to social problems.[84] Over-medicalisation is likely to have a tunnel-vision effect: looking at noma through medical lenses *only* will focus on its prevention and treatment through medical means *only*, ignoring the structural power imbalances that give rise to noma in the first place and fuel patterns of discrimination.

Edificatory are the comments in reference to leprosy made by Alice Cruz, the UN Special Rapporteur on the elimination of discrimination against persons affected by leprosy and their family members. Leprosy, an NTD formally recognised by the WHO, and noma share similar social consequences for the people they affect.[85] Cruz notes, "we cannot separate the discrimination attached [to this disease] from social and economic justice and inequality".[86] This means that, when programming, actors must look beyond health-related stigma, which is far too often understood by non- and intergovernmental organisations as stigma and discrimination that is restricted to person-to-person interactions.[87] Instead the wider structures of power that condition the social realities of people with NTDs must be acknowledged and addressed. The alternative is to "somehow justif[y] [stigmatisation] as being sort of a natural consequence" of NTDs.[88] On this account then, it is the health conditions that are thought to catalyse the 'social disqualification' of individual people or populations.[89]

This has, to a certain extent, been documented by research into the lived realities of people who have developed noma. A doctoral thesis surveyed 200 people living with sequelae of noma in Niger. Nearly half of those interviewed had encountered instances of discrimination, and over 30% had experienced some form of social exclusion.[90] Another, more recent example sees Kagoné et al. discuss a series of interviews carried out with noma survivors, healthcare professionals, and opinion leaders in Burkina Faso. One individual, who had received medical treatment for noma, spoke of their experiences: "when you are the only one in the village with this disease, you become the village pariah. The stigma drives you crazy and you suffer an unbearable ordeal".[91] As this interview excerpt directly, and crucially, exemplifies, a person's development of noma is not *just* a medical issue. It is, therefore, necessary to recognise and account for the "wider power relations that shape the micro dynamics" of stigma that are experienced by people in their day-to-day lives.[92] We move to follow Cruz in submitting that the human rights agenda may be uniquely placed to expand work on the disease:

> [t]hat is why it is important to have these diseases recognized in the human rights arena ... [because] you can call for other types of intervention ... that attach a cross-sectoral governance mentality.[93]

Widening the scope and focus of interventions on noma through the human rights frame would, we posit, place people, and their rights, at the centre of policy and programming. We recognise, however, that doing so may require a significant reorientation in the practice of non- and intergovernmental organisations both in the field of NTDs and in that of human rights.

4.4.2 Retaining a Human Rights Frame, but Reflexively Refocusing it and Educating Stakeholders

Earlier in this chapter, we discussed the broad-based agreement amongst our interviewees that noma was a human rights issue. This consensus was, however, complicated when we asked our interview participants to consider the effect of the human rights frame in states where noma is known or thought to occur. When responding to this question, the majority of participants leant on a violations-based framing to then express concerns over the perceived repercussions of this. A participant commented that, "it's not pleasant [for governments] ... to hear that there are violations of human rights in their country",[94] while a second suggested that, "it would be like shaming and blaming people who are [decision-makers] in affected countries".[95] There may, therefore, be political connotations of engaging with the human rights frame – or at least in its violation-based form – as one participant hypothesised. If a humanitarian organisation were to adopt this framing, this may mean that: [the organisation] would have to denounce [noma] as a violation of the right to food, and by extension [the organisation] would have to denounce the activities of the state.[96] Doing so in states where the human rights agenda is contentious may result in outcomes that range from the restriction of access for non-governmental organisations to constraining institutional surveillance of cases.[97]

There are three relevant aspects that we wish to highlight in relation to these concerns. First, the tension between a (violation based) human rights approach and (especially emergency) humanitarian action is not a novel phenomenon, and it certainly does not only concern noma. For example, humanitarian bodies such as the UN High Commissioner for Refugees have, historically, resisted calls to embrace a human rights approach for fear of being perceived as politicised and thus compromising its ability to gain humanitarian access to refugees, internally displaced people and other persons of concern to its mandate.[98] This position, of course, has been replaced by a recognition of the complementarity of the human rights and refugee law frameworks, their respective missions, and the importance of context sensitivity. Returning to noma, perhaps no better evidence exists as to the compatibility between the human rights and humanitarian frames than the example provided by state practice. Indeed, as noted earlier, states that are open to working on noma with humanitarian organisations are less likely to shy away from human rights discourses.

The lesson to be learnt by human rights practitioners is that they will have to engage more constructively with humanitarians explaining the synergies between the human rights approach and the medicalised and humanitarian framings of noma.

Second, whilst analysing the answers provided by our interviewees, we observed that often it is not a human rights approach to noma that raises concern, but a particular discourse that associates noma with poverty, and poverty with shame. For example, one participant noted: "noma is a shameful disease in one sense ... a synonym of poverty in many ways ... It would be difficult to admit that your population is suffering from noma".[99]

The 2012 HRCAC Study had indeed explained the correlation between poverty and noma. Whilst adopting discourse often employed by medical doctors and charities working on noma, the Study was insufficiently reflexive and sensitive to the connotations it evoked for affected states, and foremost for individuals experiencing noma. Its intention had been to break the stigma attached to poverty by moving states towards preventing and treating the disease, addressing discrimination experienced by those affected by noma, and power imbalances that give rise to poverty; yet, it may have reinforced the perception of stigma by using such expression as "noma, the face of poverty". It is hoped that a participatory approach, which centres the voices of noma survivors, not only in programming and implementation of noma policies, but also in research and fundraising activities, will avoid such errors. To cite Fidel Strub and Mulikat Okanlawon, who set up the Elysium Noma Survivors Association: "Noma is often referred as the 'Face of Poverty'. We think it more like the face of neglect instead".[100]

Third, it is important to emphasise that 'naming and shaming' approaches are not the only human rights framings. Entman notes that framers may expect to impart common responses across audiences, yet, in reality, the frames they construct are "not likely to have a universal effect on all".[101] Thus, a more positive, progress-based human rights framing may be the more appropriate focus for certain states, such as those already addressing noma or those that are willing to engage in such activities. We believe that such a framing is already evident and yields results, as illustrated by the UN treaty bodies' review processes of Burkina Faso and Ethiopia.

This is not to say that the violations-based frame should be set aside. Rather, both forms of rights-based framing retain utility. As our earlier discussion of the UN treaty body system sought to evince, adopting a violations approach has been beneficial in ensuring that human rights mechanisms *themselves* are attentive to noma. There are signs that this frame has begun to also be embedded institutionally within the WHO – guidance and training material recently published by WHO AFRO have incorporated human rights language when discussing the experiences of people who have developed noma and the need to address discrimination.[102] In contrast, framing action on noma as progress on human rights obligations may function more prospectively, perhaps furthering state buy-in to case surveillance, as well as education and awareness-raising initiatives. It is, then, more a question of deployment of these different iterations of the human rights frame.

Several of our participants suggested that connecting noma with the Sustainable Development Goals (SDGs) may, perhaps, bring the disease under the remit of a different international framework of indicators.[103] Whilst not without their own challenges,[104] the broad scope of the SDGs and the constructive, collaborative dialogues that underpin them may serve to reorientate the current human rights framing of state action on noma toward the notion of progress. As one interview participant noted, doing so will rhetorically present the governments of affected states, "as leaders in the fight against noma and, therefore, in achieving [some of] the SDGs".[105]

4.5 Conclusion: Advocating for Frame Compatibility Due to Their Complementarity

At the conclusion of this article, we posit that developing the relationship between the human rights and NTD framings of noma is the way forward for advocacy and action. Noma, after all, exists at the intersections of health and nourishment, of individualised medical interventions and wider, deeply political systems. Recognising this interconnectedness in practice requires, as one interview participant remarked, stakeholders to remain attentive to the fact that, for noma, the "underlying problem is not medical".[106] This is of course relatively straightforward to write: the reality of doing so is, we recognise, incredibly complex, and the first steps may have to be medical ones. Put differently, the human rights and NTD frames of noma need to find ways to become increasingly compatible because their individual success lies in their complementarity. Not only is it possible for these two overarching framings of noma to co-exist, but we move to suggest that translation of this coexistence into policy and action will be necessary for the long-term advancement of the agenda. Doing so will go some way towards recognising that, as Cruz incisively observed in interview, it is no longer possible to, "separate what is medical from the social, the economic, the cultural, and the political".[107]

Notes

1 See, Srour ML, Marck K, and Baratti-Mayer D, 'Noma: Overview of a Neglected Disease and a Human Rights Violation' (2017) 96 American Journal of Tropical Medicine and Hygiene 2; Baratti-Mayer D, Pittet B, Montandon D et al., 'Noma: an 'infectious' disease of unknown aetiology' (2003) 3 Lancet Infectious Diseases 7; Farley E, Mehta U, Srour ML et al., 'Noma (cancrum oris): A scoping literature review of a neglected disease (1843 to 2021)' (2021) 15 PLOS Neglected Tropical Diseases 12.
2 World Health Organization, 'The World Health Report, Life in the 21st century: A vision for all' (Geneva: World Health Organization 1998) 45; ibid.,

Baratti-Mayer D et al. (2003); Farley E, Ariti C, Amirtharajah M et al., 'Noma, a neglected disease: A viewpoint article' (2021) 15 PLOS Neglected tropical Diseases 6.

3 World Health Organization Regional Office for Africa, 'Information brochure for early detection and management of noma' (Brazzaville: World Health Organization, 2016).

4 Baratti-Mayer D, 'GESNOMA (Geneva Study Group on Noma): an aetiological research on noma disease' (2007) 104 Stomatologie 1.

5 World Health Organization (1998) *supra* note 2, 45; Baratti-Mayer D et al. (2003), *supra* note 1.

6 See for example: Baratti-Mayer D et al. (2003), *supra* note 1; Srour ML et al. (2017), *supra* note 1; Srour ML, Watt B, Phengdy B et al., 'Noma in Laos: stigma of severe poverty in rural Asia' (2008) 96 The American Journal of Tropical Medicine and Hygiene 2.

7 Bourgeois DM, and Leclercq ML, 'The World Health Organization initiative on noma' (1999) 5 Oral Diseases 2; Baratti-Mayer D et al. (2003), *supra* note 1.

8 Galli A, Brugger C, Fürst T et al., 'Prevalence, incidence, and reported global distribution of noma: a systematic literature review' (2022) 22 Lancet Infectious Disease 8.

9 See, Johnson S, 'Noma: the hidden disease known as the 'face of poverty'' *The Guardian* (Online, 2 November 2021). <https://www.theguardian.com/global-development/2021/nov/04/noma-the-hidden-childhood-disease-known-as-the-face-of-poverty> accessed 20 November 2022; Burki T, 'Taking a look at noma' (2020) 20 Lancet Infectious Disease 6.

10 See, Strub's presentation at the conference 'Noma, through the eyes of survivors and scientific evidence – Lifting the neglect from a neglected tropical disease', co-organised by the University of York and Médecins Sans Frontières, House of Commons, London, 11 January 2023.

11 This chapter is one output of a wider research project, 'Noma - The Neglected Disease: An Interdisciplinary Exploration of Its Realities, Burden, and Framing' (The Noma Project) <https://thenomaproject.org/>. The project, which ran from 2019 to 2022, received generous support through research grants and donations provided by public and private institutions. We gratefully acknowledge the Swiss Network for International Studies, Hilfsaktion Noma e.V., the Service de la Solidarité Internationale (SSI) of the Republic and Canton of Geneva, Noma-Hilfe-Schweiz and the Winds of Hope Foundation. The fieldwork re-ported in this paper received full ethical approval, from the University of York's Economics, Law, Management, Politics and Sociology Ethics Committee in November 2019.

12 Chong,D and Druckman JN, 'Framing Theory' (2007) 10 Annual Review of Political Science, 104.

13 Lecheler S, Bos L, and Vliegenthart R, 'The Mediating Role of Emotions: News Framing Effects on Opinions About Immigration' (2005) 92 Journal of Mass Communication Quarterly 4; Pang N, and Goh D, 'Social Media and Social Movements: Weak Publics, the Online Space, Spatial Relations, and Collective Action in Singapore' in Bruns A, Enli G, Skogerbø E et al. (eds), *The Routledge Companion to Social Media and Politics* (1st edn, Routledge 2015), 110.

14 Snow DA, and Benford RD, 'Ideology, frame resonance, and participant mobilization' (1988) 1 International Social Movement Research, 198.

15 McAdam D, McCarthy J, Zald M, et al. (1996), 6, as cited in Keck M, and Sikkink K, 'Transnational advocacy networks in international and regional politics' (1999) 51 International Social Science Journal 159, 90.

16 Jorgenson J, and Steier F, 'Frames, Framing, and Designed Conversational Processes: Lessons From the World Café' (2013) 49 Journal of Applied Behavioral Science 3, 389; Merry SE, *Gender violence, a cultural perspective* (1st edn, Wiley-Blackwell 009), 41.

17 Entman R, 'Framing: Towards Clarification of a Fractured Paradigm' (1993) 43 Journal of Communication 4, 52.

18 Keck M, and Sikkink K, 'Transnational advocacy networks in international and regional politics' (1999) 51 International Social Science Journal 159, 95.

19 Snow DA, and Benford RD (1992) as cited by Boyle EH, *Female genital cutting: cultural conflict in the global community* (1st edn, John Hopkins University Press 2002), 145.

20 On Cismas' work with the UN Human Rights Council Advisory Committee, see < https://www.righttofood.org/work-of-jean-ziegler-at-the-un/noma/>; for more recent work see, *supra* note 11 and <https://pure.york.ac.uk/portal/en/projects/ esrc-iaanoma-neglected-tropical-diseases-and-human-rights-enhanci> accessed 20 November 2022.

21 See, *supra* note 11.

22 See for example: Farley E et al. (2021), *supra* note 1; Marck KW, 'A history of noma, the 'Face of Survivors' (2003) 111 Plastic and Reconstructive Surgery; Farley E, Lenglet A, and Ariti C, 'Risk factors for diagnosed noma in northwest Nigeria: A case-control study, 2017' (2018) 12 PLoS Neglected Tropical Diseases.

23 Cismas I, and Trotter A, 'Research Interview with Claire Jeantet, Noma Campaign Manager, MSF and Inediz Production Company' (2021).

24 See, Shaye DA, Rabbels J, and Adetunji AS, 'Evaluation of the Noma Disease Burden Within the Noma Belt' 20 (2018) JAMA Facial Plastic Surgery 4.

25 See, Baratti-Mayer et al. (2003), *supra* note 1; Baratti-Mayer D, Pittet-Cuenod BM, and Montandon D, 'GESNOMA (Geneva Study Group on Noma): une recherche médicale de point à but humanitaire' (2004) 49 Annales de chirurgie plastique et esthétique 3. Recently, and encouragingly, we see other researchers leading such endeavours: Uzochukwu J, 'Host-Microbiome Interactions, Microbiological etiology, and Nutritional Risk Factors in Noma Disease in Nigeria: A Case Study of the Sokoto Noma Hospital' (PhD thesis, King's College University ongoing).

26 See for example: Kagoné M, Mpinga EK, Dupuis M et al., 'Noma; Experiences of Survivors, Opinion Leaders and Healthcare Professionals in Burkina Faso' (2022) 7 Tropical Medicine and Infectious Disease 7; World Health Organization, 'NGO focus: Sentinelles in Niger' (1997) Noma Contact: Cancrum Oris Network Action 7–8.

27 Isah S, Amirtharajah M, Farley E et al., 'Model of care, Noma Children's Hospital, northwest Nigeria' (2021) 26 Tropical Medicine and International Health 9.

28 See, Enwonwu CO, 'Noma: a neglected scourge of children in sub-Saharan Africa' (1995) 73 Bulletin of the World Health Organization 4, 541–5; Marck KW, *Noma: the face of poverty* (1st edn, MIT-Verlag GmbH 2003); Srour ML et al. (2008), *supra* note 6 539.

29 Farley E, Bala HM, and Lenglet A, "I treat it but I don't know what this disease is': a qualitative study on noma (cancrum oris) and traditional healing northwest Nigeria' (2020) 12 International Health 1; M Kagoné et al. (2022), *supra* note 26.

30 Hoddy ET, and Ensor JE, 'Brazil's landless movement and rights 'from below" (2018) 63 Journal of Rural Studies.

31 Benford RD, and Snow DA, 'Framing Processes and Social Movements: An Overview and Assessment' (2000) 26 Annual Review of Sociology, 628.

32 *supra* note 27.

33 *supra* note 27.

34 World Health Organization Regional Office for Africa, 'Evaluation of the WHO Africa Regional Programme on Noma Control (2013–2017)' (19 January 2019), xiv.

35 See, Irfan F, 'Neo-colonial philanthropy in the UK' (2021) e1726 Journal of Philanthropy and Marketing; Ashdown BK, Dixe A, and Talmage CA, 'The potentially damaging effects of developmental aid and voluntourism on cultural capital and well-being' (2021) 4 International Journal of Community Well-Being.

36 Human Rights Council Advisory Committee, 'Study of the Human Rights Council Advisory Committee on severe malnutrition and childhood diseases with children affected by noma as an example' (24 February 2012) UN Doc. A/HRC/19/73.

37 ibid., para 58 and 66.

38 Hunt P, Stewart R, Mesquita J et al., 'Neglected diseases: a human rights analysis' (2007) WHO, Special Topics in Social, Economic Research Report Series No. 6, 3.

39 ibid.

40 *supra* note 36, para 30.

41 *supra* note 36.

42 See, Hafner-Burton EM, 'Sticks and Stones: Naming and Shaming the Human Rights Enforcement Problem' (2008) 62 International Organization.

43 Ausderan J, 'How naming and shaming affects human rights perceptions in the shamed country' (2014) 51 Journal of Peace Research 1; Meernik J, Aloisi R, Sowell M et al., 'The Impact of Human Rights Organizations on Naming and Shaming Campaigns' (2012) 56 Journal of Conflict Resolution 2.

44 Cismas I, and Trotter A, 'Research Interview with Leila Srour, Pediatrician and Noma expert, Health Frontiers Laos' (2021).

45 *Supra* note 36, para 48; Trotter A, and Cismas I, 'Noma and Human Rights Law – A Doctrinal Legal Analysis with Focus on Burkina Faso, Niger and Laos, Background Study' (2020). <https://static1.squarespace.com/static/5e624ea1b 53d653768470cb6/t/6089546457c5ef56f07fc311/1619612778742/Noma+%26 +Human+Rights+Law_background+study.pdf/> accessed 20 November 2022.

46 Cismas I, and Trotter A, 'Research Interview with Marie-Solène Adamou Moussa-Pham' Scientific Collaborator, Institute of Global Health, University of Geneva, former Programme Manager and Noma Consultant, Fondation Sentinelles' (2021).

47 Trotter A, 'Research Interview with Ioana Cismas, Academic, Human Rights and Noma Expert, Centre for Applied Human Rights, University of York' (2021).

48 World Health Organization Regional Office for Africa, 'Consultative Meeting on Management of the Noma Programme in the African region: Final Report' (Harare, 19–21 April 2001); Bos K, and Marck KW, 'The surgical treatment of noma' (2006) Alphen aan den Rijn, Belvedere/Medidac.

49 *supra* note 36, para 50.

50 See for example: Galli A et al. (2022), *supra* note 8; Srour ML, Farley E, and Mpinga EK, 'Lao Noma Survivors: A Case Series, 2002–2020' (2022) 106 American Journal of Tropical Medicine and Hygiene 4.

51 *supra* note 36, para 50.

52 See, for example: Kagoné M et al. (2022), *supra* note 26; Grema MSM, 'Expériences des individus à risque et survivants du Noma au Niger' (2021) Rapport d'activité.

53 See, Srour ML et al. (2008), *supra* note 6.

54 Trotter A, and Cismas I (2020), *supra* note 45.

55 *supra* note 47.

56 See for example: Srour ML, Marck KW, and Baratti-Mayer D, 'Noma: Neglected, forgotten and a human rights issue' (2015) 7 International Health 3; Srour ML et al. (2017), *supra* note 1.

57 See, for example: Kagoné M et al. (2022), *supra* note 26; Grema MSM (2021), *supra* note 52. These were outputs of the Noma Project, *supra* note 11.

58 The human rights approach is mentioned as one of the evaluation criteria in the 'Evaluation of the WHO Africa Regional Programme on Noma Control (2013–2017)', commissioned by WHO AFRO (19 January 2019), v and xiii. It is not entirely clear though exactly what the human rights approach of WHO AFRO entailed as the report only mentions that 'the Noma program aims to promote human rights, mainly the right to health and life of poor children'.

59 World Health Organization Regional Office for Africa, 'Step by Step Guide to Develop National Action Plans for Noma Prevention and Control in Priority Countries' (Brazzaville: World Health Organization, 2020), 18.

60 ibid.

61 Human Rights Council, 'Resolution 19/3' (19 March 2012), UN Doc. A/HRC/19/L.21, para 50.

62 A practice which had been encouraged by the HRCAC in its 2012 study, see *supra* note 36, guideline 14.

63 See for example: Committee on Economic, Social and Cultural Rights, List of issues in relation to the initial report of Burkina Faso, (30 October 2015) UN Doc. E/C.12/BFA/Q/1, para 22; Committee on Economic, Social and Cultural Rights, Concluding observations on the initial report of Burkina Faso, (12 July 2016) UN Doc. E/C.12/BFA/CO/1, para 32; Committee on the Rights of the Child, List of issues in relation to the fourth periodic report of the State of Eritrea, (10 March 2015) UN Doc. CRC/C/ERI/Q/4, para 4 and 17; Committee on the Rights of the Child, List of issues in relation to the combined fourth and fifth periodic reports of Ethiopia, (22 October 2014) UN Doc. CRC/C/ETH/Q/4-5, para 4 and 12.

64 'With reference to the Committee's request on measures to tackle Noma (part I, para. 17) the case is not known in Eritrea and therefore, the State party had no reason to ask partners such as the World Health Organization (WHO) and the United Nations Children's Fund (UNICEF) for help and support to combat the disease'. Committee on the Rights of the Child, List of issues in relation to the fourth periodic report of the State of Eritrea Addendum - Replies of the State of Eritrea to the list of issues, (7 May 2015) UN Doc. CRC/C/ERI/Q/4/Add.1, para 70.

65 Committee on the Rights of the Child, List of issues in relation to the combined fourth to fifth periodic reports of Ethiopia, Addendum - Replies of Ethiopia to the list of issues, (4 May 2015) UN Doc. CRC/C/ETH/Q/4-5/Add.1, para 48.

66 Committee on Economic, Social and Cultural Rights, List of issues in relation to the initial report of Burkina Faso, Addendum - Replies of Burkina Faso to the list of issues, (21 April 2016) E/C.12/BFA/Q/1/Add.1, paras 81–87. Note also that the Ambassador of Burkina Faso in Geneva had been one of the main panellists at a conference launching the HRCAC 2012 Study.

67 'Nigeria seeks to eliminate severe and often lethal mouth disease' *WHO AFRO News* (Online, 28 July 2022). <https://www.afro.who.int/countries/nigeria/news/nigeria-seeks-eliminate-severe-and-often-lethal-mouth-disease> accessed 20 January 2023.

68 'Nigeria commemorates National Noma Day 2019' *Federal Ministry of Information and Culture, Nigeria* (Online, 19 November 2019). <https://fmic. gov.ng/nigeria-commemorates-national-noma-day-2019/> accessed 20 January 2023.

69 'Nigeria commemorates third noma day – resolves to eliminate disease by 2030' *WHO AFRO News* (Online, 20 November 2019). <https://www.afro.who.int/ news/nigeria-commemorates-third-noma-day-resolves-eliminate-disease-2030> accessed 20 January 2023.

70 Uzoigwe G, 'Making the case for action on Noma' (Presentation, Climate Change, Oral Health and Sustainability: COP 26 Satellite Conference, University of Glasgow, 2 November 2021).

71 Dossier of evidence in support of the addition of noma to the World Health Organization Neglected Tropical Diseases list. Lead Sponsor: Nigeria (January 2023) 18 and 20.

72 These are the formal criteria for recognition as an NTD, as set forward by the World Health Organization, 'Ninth report of the Strategic and Technical Advisory Group for Neglected Tropical Diseases' (Geneva, 12–13 April 2016). For a systematic analysis of how noma meets each of the criteria, see *supra* note 70.

73 See for example: Cismas I, and Trotter A, 'Research Interview with Elise Farley, Epidemiologist, Noma Expert and Researcher for the dossier of evidence, MSF' (2021); Cismas I, and Trotter A, 'Research Interview with Marie-Solène Adamou Moussa-Pham', *supra* note 46; Cismas I, and Trotter A, 'Research Interview with Peter Steinmann, Public Health Specialist and Epidemiologist, Swiss Tropical and Public Health Institute' (2021).

74 Cismas I, and Trotter A, 'Research Interview with Peter Steinmann', ibid.

75 Cismas I, and Trotter A, 'Research Interview with Epidemiologist' (2021).

76 Srour ML, and Baratti-Mayer D, 'Why is noma a neglected-neglected tropical disease?' (2020) PLoS Neglected Tropical Diseases.

77 See, World Health Organization Regional Office for Africa, 'The Expanded Special Project for Elimination of Neglected Tropical Diseases' (Brazzaville: World Health Organization 2021).

78 Ziegler J, *Betting on Famine: Why the World Still Goes Hungry* (1st edn, New Press 2013) 177.

79 'Snake-bite envenoming: a priority neglected tropical disease' (2017) 390 Editorial, The Lancet 10089.

80 *supra* note 71, 23–35.

81 See for example the campaign website of Médecins Sans Frontières, 'What is Noma?' (Médecins Sans Frontières 2020). <https://noma.msf.org/> accessed 11 February 2023.

82 'World Health Assembly Resolution paves the way for better oral health care' *WHO News* (Online 27 May 2021). <https://www.who.int/news/item/27-05-2021-world-health-assembly-resolution-paves-the-way-for-better-oral-health-care> accessed 20 January 2023.

83 Yet, see an important study on noma's epidemiology that seeks to address some of the gaps, Galli A et al. (2022), *supra* note 8.

84 See, Williams S, and Gabe J, 'Peter Conrad: The Medicalisation of Society' in F Collyer (ed), *The Palgrave Handbook of Social Theory in Health, Illness and Medicine* (1st edn, Palgrave Macmillan 2015), 615–627.

85 Report of the Special Rapporteur on the Elimination of Discrimination against Persons Affect by Leprosy and their Family Members (25 May 2018), UN Doc. A/HRC/38/42.

86 Cismas I, and Trotter A, 'Research Interview with Alice Cruz, United Nations Special Rapporteur on discrimination against persons with leprosy' (2021).

87 ibid.

88 *supra* note 86.

89 Weiss MG, Ramakrishna J, and Somma D, 'Health-related stigma: rethinking concepts and interventions' (2006) 11 Psychology, Health and Medicine 3, 277.

90 Hassane IA, 'Impact psycho-sociologique, devenir et réinsertion sociale des patients victimes du Noma' (PhD thesis, Université Abdou Moumouni 2018).

91 Kagoné M et al. (2022), *supra* note 26, 8.

92 *supra* note 86.

93 *supra* note 86.

94 Cismas I, and Trotter A, 'Research Interview with Denise Baratti-Mayer, Noma Expert and Scientific Collaborator, University of Geneva' (2021).

95 *supra* note 23.

96 Cismas I, and Trotter A, 'Research Interview with Christophe Golay, Senior Research Fellow, Geneva Academy of International Law and Human Rights, and Former Advisor of the UN Special Rapporteur on the right to food' (2021).

97 ibid.; Cismas I, and Trotter A, 'Research Interview with Elise Farley', *supra* note 73.

98 See, Mason E, 'UNHCR, Human Rights and Refugees Collection and Dissemination of Sources' (1997) 25 International Journal of Legal Information 35, 39–40.

99 Cismas I, and Trotter A, 'Research Interview with Tropical Medicine Expert' (2021).

100 See, 'Elysium Noma Survivors Association' (2022). <https://www.elysium-nsa.org> accessed 11 February 2023.

101 *supra* note 17, 54.

102 supra note 59; OpenWHO, 'Noma: training of health workers at national and district levels on skin-NTDs' (Training Course, 2022).

103 *supra* note 23; Cismas I, and Trotter A, 'Research Interview with Elise Farley', *supra* note 73; Cismas I, and Trotter A, 'Research Interview with Public Health Expert' (2021).

104 See for example Bowen K, Cradock-Henry NA, Koch F et al., 'Implementing the 'Sustainable Development Goals': towards addressing three key governance challenges – collective action, trade-offs and accountability' (2017) 26–7 Current Opinion in Environmental Sustainability.

105 *supra* note 23.

106 Cismas I, and Trotter A, 'Research Interview with Klaas Marck, Plastic Surgeon and Former Chairman of the Dutch Noma Foundation' (2021).

107 *supra* note 86.

Bibliography

Primary Sources

Committee on Economic, Social and Cultural Rights, Concluding observations on the initial report of Burkina Faso (12 July 2016) UN Doc. E/C.12/BFA/CO/1.

Committee on Economic, Social and Cultural Rights, List of issues in relation to the initial report of Burkina Faso (30 October 2015) UN Doc. E/C.12/BFA/Q/1.

Committee on Economic, Social and Cultural Rights, List of issues in relation to the initial report of Burkina Faso, Addendum - Replies of Burkina Faso to the list of issues, (21 April 2016) E/C.12/BFA/Q/1/Add.1.

Committee on the Rights of the Child, List of issues in relation to the fourth periodic report of the State of Eritrea (10 March 2015) UN Doc. CRC/C/ERI/Q/4.

Committee on the Rights of the Child, List of issues in relation to the combined fourth and fifth periodic reports of Ethiopia (22 October 2014) UN Doc. CRC/C/ETH/Q/4-5.

Committee on the Rights of the Child, List of issues in relation to the fourth periodic report of the State of Eritrea Addendum – Replies of the State of Eritrea to the list of issues (7 May 2015) UN Doc. CRC/C/ERI/Q/4/Add.1.

Committee on the Rights of the Child, List of issues in relation to the combined fourth to fifth periodic reports of Ethiopia, Addendum – Replies of Ethiopia to the list of issues (4 May 2015) UN Doc. CRC/C/ETH/Q/4-5/Add.1.

Dossier of evidence in support of the addition of noma to the World Health Organization Neglected Tropical Diseases list. Lead Sponsor: Nigeria (January 2023).

Human Rights Council, 'Resolution 19/3' (19 March 2012), UN Doc. A/HRC/19/L.21.

Secondary Sources

Monographs

Heger Boyle E, *Female genital cutting: cultural conflict in the global community* (1st edn, John Hopkins University Press 2002).

Marck KW, *Noma: the face of poverty* (1st edn, MIT-Verlag GmbH 2003).

Merry SE, *Gender violence, a cultural perspective* (1st edn, Wiley-Blackwell 2009).

Ziegler J, *Betting on Famine: Why the World Still Goes Hungry* (1st edn, New Press 2013).

Journal Articles and Contributions to Edited Books

'Snake-bite envenoming: a priority neglected tropical disease' (2017) 390 Editorial, The Lancet 10089.

Ashdown BK, Dixe A and Talmage CA, 'The potentially damaging effects of developmental aid and voluntourism on cultural capital and well-being' [2021] 4 International Journal of Community Well-Being.

Ausderan J, 'How naming and shaming affects human rights perceptions in the shamed country' [2014] 51 Journal of Peace Research 1.

Baratti-Mayer D, Pittet, Montandon D, Bolivar I, Bornand JE, Hugonnet S, Jaquinet A, Schrenzel J and Pittet D, 'Noma: an 'infectious' disease of unknown aetiology' [2003] 3 Lancet Infectious Diseases 7.

Baratti-Mayer D, Pittet-Cuenod BM and Montandon D, 'GESNOMA (Geneva Study Group on Noma): une recherche médicale de point à but humanitaire' [2004] 49 Annales de chirurgie plastique et esthétique 3.

Baratti-Mayer D, 'GESNOMA (Geneva Study Group on Noma): an aetiological research on noma disease' [2007] 104 Stomatologie 1.

Benford RD and Snow DA, 'Framing Processes and Social Movements: An Overview and Assessment' [2000] 26 Annual Review of Sociology.

Bos K and Marck KW, 'The surgical treatment of noma' [2006] Alphen aan den Rijn, Belvedere/Medidac.

Bourgeois DM and Leclercq ML, 'The World Health Organization initiative on noma' [1999] 5 Oral Diseases 2.

Bowen K, Cradock-Henry NA, Koch F and Patterson J, 'Implementing the 'Sustainable Development Goals': towards addressing three key governance challenges – collective action, trade-offs and accountability' [2017] 26–7 Current Opinion in Environmental Sustainability.

Bruns A, Enli G, Skogerbø E, Olof Larsson A and Christensen C (eds), *The Routledge Companion to Social Media and Politics* (1st edn, Routledge 2015).

Burki T, 'Taking a look at noma' [2020] 20 Lancet Infectious Disease 6.

Chong D and Druckman JN, 'Framing Theory' [2007] 10 Annual Review of Political Science.

Collyer F (ed.), *The Palgrave Handbook of Social Theory in Health, Illness and Medicine* (1st edn, Palgrave Macmillan 2015).

Entman R, 'Framing: Towards Clarification of a Fractured Paradigm' [1993] 43 Journal of Communication 4.

Enwonwu CO, 'Noma: a neglected scourge of children in sub-Saharan Africa' [1995] 73 Bulletin of the World Health Organization 4.

Farley E, Lenglet A and Ariti C, 'Risk factors for diagnosed noma in northwest Nigeria: a case-control study, 2017' [2018] 12 PLoS Neglected Tropical Diseases.

Farley E, Bala HM and Lenglet A, '"I treat it but I don't know what this disease is": a qualitative study on noma (cancrum oris) and traditional healing northwest Nigeria' [2020] 12 International Health 1.

Farley E, Ariti C, Amirtharajah M, Kamu C, Oluyide B, Shoaib M, Isah S, Adetunji AS, Saleh F, Ihekweazu C, Pereboom M and Sherlock M, 'Noma, a neglected disease: A viewpoint article' [2021] 15 PLOS Neglected Tropical Diseases 6.

Farley E, Mehta U, Srour ML and Lenglet A, 'Noma (cancrum oris): A scoping literature review of a neglected disease (1843 to 2021)' [2021] 15 PLOS Neglected Tropical Diseases 12.

Galli A, Brugger C, Fürst T, Monnier N, Winkler MS and Steinmann P, 'Prevalence, incidence, and reported global distribution of noma: a systematic literature review' [2022] 22 Lancet Infectious Disease 8.

Hafner-Burton EM, 'Sticks and Stones: Naming and Shaming the Human Rights Enforcement Problem' [2008] 62 International Organization.

Hoddy ET and Ensor JE, 'Brazil's landless movement and rights 'from below'' [2018] 63 Journal of Rural Studies.

Hunt P, Stewart R, Mesquita J and Oldring L, 'Neglected diseases: a human rights analysis' [2007] WHO, Special Topics in Social, Economic Research Report Series No. 6.

Irfan F, 'Neo-colonial philanthropy in the UK' [2021] e1726 Journal of Philanthropy and Marketing.

Isah S, Amirtharajah M, Farley E, Adetunji AS, Samuel J, Oluyide B, Bill K, Shoaib M, Abubakar N, de Jong A, Pereboom M, Lenglet A and Sherlock M, 'Model of care, Noma Children's Hospital, northwest Nigeria' [2021] 26 Tropical Medicine and International Health 9.

Jorgenson J and Steier F, 'Frames, Framing, and Designed Conversational Processes: Lessons From the World Café' [2013] 49 Journal of Applied Behavioural Science 3.

Kagoné M, Mpinga EK, Dupuis M, Adamou Moussa-Pham MS, Srour ML, Malam Grema MS, Zacharie NB and Baratti-Mayer D, 'Noma; Experiences of Survivors, Opinion Leaders and Healthcare Professionals in Burkina Faso' [2022] 7 Tropical Medicine and Infectious Disease 7.

Keck M and Sikkink K, 'Transnational advocacy networks in international and regional politics' [1999] 51 International Social Science Journal 159.

Lecheler S, Bos L and Vliegenthart R, 'The mediating role of emotions: news framing effects on opinions about immigration' [2005] 92 Journal of Mass Communication Quarterly 4.

Marck KW, 'A history of noma, the 'Face of Survivors' [2003] 111 Plastic and Reconstructive Surgery.

Mason E, 'UNHCR, Human Rights and Refugees Collection and Dissemination of Sources' [1997] 25 International Journal of Legal Information 35.

Meernik J, Aloisi R, Sowell M and Nichols A, 'The Impact of Human Rights Organizations on Naming and Shaming Campaigns' [2012] 56 Journal of Conflict Resolution 2.

Shaye DA, Rabbels J and Adetunji AS, 'Evaluation of the noma disease burden within the noma belt' [2018] 20 JAMA Facial Plastic Surgery 4.

Snow DA and Benford RD, 'Ideology, frame resonance, and participant mobilization' [1988] 1 International Social Movement Research.

Srour ML, Watt B, Phengdy B, Khansoulivong K, Harris J, Bennett C, Strobel M, Dupuis C and Newton P, 'Noma in Laos: stigma of severe poverty in rural Asia' [2008] 96 The American Journal of Tropical Medicine and Hygiene 2.

Srour ML, Marck KW and Baratti-Mayer D, 'Noma: neglected, forgotten and a human rights issue' [2015] 7 International Health 3.

Srour ML, Marck KW and Baratti-Mayer D, 'Noma: overview of a neglected disease and a human rights violation' [2017] 96 American Journal of Tropical Medicine and Hygiene 2.

Srour ML and Baratti-Mayer D, 'Why is noma a neglected-neglected tropical disease?' [2020] PLoS Neglected Tropical Diseases.

Srour ML, Farley E and Mpinga EK, 'Lao noma survivors: a case series, 2002–2020' [2022] 106 American Journal of Tropical Medicine and Hygiene 4.

Weiss MG, Ramakrishna J and Somma D, 'Health-related stigma: rethinking concepts and interventions' [2006] 11 Psychology, Health and Medicine 3.

United Nations Publications, Reports, Theses, Presentations, and Policy Briefs

Abdou Hassane I, 'Impact psycho-sociologique, devenir et réinsertion sociale des patients victimes du Noma' (PhD thesis, Université Abdou Moumouni 2018).

Human Rights Council Advisory Committee, 'Study of the Human Rights Council Advisory Committee on severe malnutrition and childhood diseases with children affected by noma as an example' (24 February 2012) UN Doc. A/HRC/19/73.

Malam Grema MS, 'Expériences des individus à risque et survivants du Noma au Niger' [2021] Rapport d'activité.

OpenWHO, 'Noma: training of health workers at national and district levels on skin-NTDs' (Training Course, 2022).

Report of the Special Rapporteur on the Elimination of Discrimination against Persons Affect by Leprosy and their Family Members (25 May 2018), UN Doc. A/HRC/38/42.

Trotter A and Cismas I, 'Noma and Human Rights Law – A Doctrinal Legal Analysis with Focus on Burkina Faso, Niger and Laos, Background Study' [2020]. <https://static1.squarespace.com/static/5e624ea1b53d653768470cb6/t/6089546457c5ef56f07fc311/1619612778742/Noma+%26+Human+Rights+Law_background+study.pdf/> accessed 20 November 2022.

Uzochukwu J, 'Host-Microbiome Interactions, Microbiological etiology, and Nutritional Risk Factors in Noma Disease in Nigeria: A Case Study of the Sokoto Noma Hospital' (PhD thesis, King's College University ongoing).

Uzoigwe G, 'Making the case for action on Noma' (Presentation, Climate Change, Oral Health and Sustainability: COP 26 Satellite Conference, University of Glasgow, 2 November 2021).

World Health Organization, 'NGO focus: Sentinelles in Niger' [1997] Noma Contact: Cancrum Oris Network Action.

World Health Organization, 'The World Health Report, Life in the 21st century: A vision for all' (Geneva: World Health Organization 1998).

World Health Organization, 'Ninth report of the Strategic and Technical Advisory Group for Neglected Tropical Diseases' (Geneva, 12–13 April 2016).

World Health Organization Regional Office for Africa, 'Consultative Meeting on Management of the Noma Programme in the African region: Final Report' (Harare, 19–21 April 2001).

World Health Organization Regional Office for Africa, 'Information brochure for early detection and management of noma' (Brazzaville: World Health Organization 2016).

World Health Organization Regional Office for Africa, 'Evaluation of the WHO Africa Regional Programme on Noma Control (2013–2017)' (19 January 2019).

World Health Organization Regional Office for Africa, 'Step by Step Guide to Develop National Action Plans for Noma Prevention and Control in Priority Countries' (Brazzaville: World Health Organization 2020).

World Health Organization Regional Office for Africa, 'The Expanded Special Project for Elimination of Neglected Tropical Diseases' (Brazzaville: World Health Organization 2021).

Newspaper Articles, Websites, and Blogs

'Elysium Noma Survivors Association' (2022). <https://www.elysium-nsa.org> accessed 11 February 2023.

'Nigeria commemorates National Noma Day 2019' Federal Ministry of Information and Culture, Nigeria (Online, 19 November 2019). <https://fmic.gov.ng/nigeria-commemorates-national-noma-day-2019/> accessed 20 January 2023.

'Nigeria commemorates third noma day – resolves to eliminate disease by 2030' WHO AFRO News (Online, 20 November 2019). <https://www.afro.who.int/

news/nigeria-commemorates-third-noma-day-resolves-eliminate-disease-2030>
accessed 20 January 2023.
'Nigeria seeks to eliminate severe and often lethal mouth disease' *WHO AFRO News*
(Online, 28 July 2022). <https://www.afro.who.int/countries/nigeria/news/nigeria-
seeks-eliminate-severe-and-often-lethal-mouth-disease> accessed 20 January 2023.
'World Health Assembly Resolution paves the way for better oral health care' *WHO
News* (Online 27 May 2021). <https://www.who.int/news/item/27-05-2021-
world-health-assembly-resolution-paves-the-way-for-better-oral-health-care> ac-
cessed 20 January 2023.
Johnson S, 'Noma: the hidden disease known as the 'face of poverty'' *The Guardian*
(Online, 2 November 2021). <https://www.theguardian.com/global-development/
2021/nov/04/noma-the-hidden-childhood-disease-known-as-the-face-of-poverty>
accessed 20 November 2022.
Médecins Sans Frontières, 'What is Noma?' (Médecins Sans Frontières 2020).
<https://noma.msf.org/> accessed 11 February 2023.

5

TRADE MARKS AND THE RIGHT TO HEALTH

A Growing Tension

Alvaro Fernandez-Mora

5.1 Introduction

Intellectual property (IP) rights have taken a centre stage in the information economy. As the means of production in the contemporary global marketplace have become increasingly reliant on intangibles, the laws devoted to their production, propertisation, and exploitation have moved closer to the core of cultural, political, and economic debates. The regulation of IP rights is, thus, gradually becoming an arena for ideological contestation in twenty-first-century policy-making that cuts across a wide range of disciplines and interests.

This growing tension is perhaps most salient in relation to public health. The interface between IP and health often makes global news headlines as societies seek to strike the right balance between incentivising innovation by means of strong IP protection, on the one hand, and maximising access to intellectual goods, on the other. Much of this debate revolves around the restrictions placed by patent law on access to life-saving drugs by those who cannot afford them at the premium prices charged by patent holders.[1] In the last few decades, however, another debate at the intersection between IP and health has attracted a substantial amount of interest from a wide range of stakeholders. I am referring to the restrictions imposed on the use of trade marks by measures of public law aimed at reducing the consumption of goods that pose a risk to health, notably advertising bans, health warnings and, more recently, plain packaging.[2]

Tobacco products constitute the paradigmatic example of an industry that has been increasingly targeted by health-furthering trade mark-restrictive measures since the 1960s in an attempt to curb smoking rates in a wide range

DOI: 10.4324/9781003399933-8

of jurisdictions across the globe. These restrictions have proved to be exceedingly litigious, giving rise to a plethora of legal challenges before domestic and regional courts on grounds that they are incompatible with IP rights and the constitutional safeguards put in place to guarantee their protection, notably the fundamental rights to (intellectual) property and/or to freedom of expression.[3]

There is growing evidence that these restrictions are quickly expanding into other industries, notably alcohol and foods high in fat, sugar, and salt (HFSS). The measures adopted to date in these industries are, for the most part and in their current configuration, rather limited when compared to those already in place for tobacco products. But this might be only a matter of time. Evidence would seem to suggest that, in relation to alcohol and HFSS foods, these measures will continue to expand both geographically and in terms of the encroachment that they effect on trade mark rights.[4] This will likely give rise to a fresh wave of litigation across jurisdictions as trade mark owners operating in the alcohol and HFSS foods industries seek to challenge these measures on the grounds of fundamental rights.

Against this backdrop, the aim of this chapter is threefold. First, to explore the range of trade mark-restrictive measures that legislatures worldwide are adopting to curb the consumption rates of unhealthy products, more precisely, advertising bans, health warnings, and plain packaging. These measures will be analysed in a systematic manner with a view to understanding: (a) the rationales for their adoption; (b) how they impinge on trade mark rights; and (c) their ongoing expansion across industries and jurisdictions in an ambitious global mapping effort. Second, this chapter will engage in a comprehensive comparative review of the case law addressing the interaction between trade marks and the right to health in the context of tobacco products since the 1990s by looking at decisions from Canada, the United States, the European Union (EU), Australia, and the United Kingdom. Delving into the existing case law will allow mapping of the core legal arguments that are likely to drive any potential challenges to the validity of future restrictions on trade mark use beyond tobacco products. Third, this chapter will briefly discuss the normative implications of the continued expansion of trade mark-restrictive measures to promote public health.

Proper engagement with these questions requires that we begin by exploring what a trade mark is, including the functions it performs in the marketplace, in Section 5.2. This will be followed by an in-depth analysis, in Section 5.3, of the types of trade mark-restrictive measures that states have adopted since the 1960s to curb the consumption rates of unhealthy products. To this end, Section 5.3.1 will explore advertising bans, Section 5.3.2 will look at health warnings and, finally, Section 5.3.3 will analyse plain packaging. Concluding remarks will follow.

5.2 Trade Marks: Concept and Functions

As a form of IP, trade marks are legal constructs devised to grant ownership over a particular type of intangible, *i.e.*, a distinctive sign allowing a trader to distinguish its goods or services from those of its competitors in the market. Take, for instance, the sign "Coca-Cola", which is used by The Coca-Cola Company to distinguish its signature soft drink from the like products of other soft drink manufacturers, notably PepsiCo Inc., which uses the sign "Pepsi" to identify its cola products. When distinctive signs are used in this manner (*i.e.*, in connection with a particular product so as to distinguish it from competing products), they become trade marks.

Trade marks are afforded protection under IP laws to ensure that they may perform their fundamental function in the marketplace: to distinguish goods and services. Although essential, source identification is by no means the sole function that marks perform in the contemporary marketplace. Firms increasingly demand that marks perform a variety of functions, notably: (a) a quality function, when the mark signals information about quality or reputation; (b) an advertising function, when the mark is used to inform consumers of the characteristics of the branded goods, or to persuade them into buying such goods; and (c) an expressive function, when the mark is able to convey complex meanings of the sort that can be relied upon by individuals for expressive purposes.[5]

Going back to our example, the "Coca-Cola" marks are infused with an image of shared hedonism – when affixed to The Coca-Cola Company's signature drink, they inform consumers of its thirst-quenching, happiness-inducing features, especially when shared with family and friends. The "Coca-Cola" marks perform an advertising function when they are used on advertisements featuring families and friends sharing and drinking "Coca-Cola"-branded drinks at parties and other social gatherings. And they perform an expressive function when a consumer hosting a party uses the "Coca-Cola" marks (through purchasing, drinking, and offering his guests "Coca-Cola"-branded drinks) to express his adherence to the hedonistic and family/friendship values that these marks convey.

5.3 Promoting Public Health through Trade Mark Regulation: Advertising Bans, Health Warnings, and Plain Packaging

As we saw in the Introduction, legislation encroaching on trade mark rights with the aim of furthering public health has been implemented in relation to goods that pose a risk to health since the 1960s. Until recently, these measures consisted for the most part of advertising bans and health warnings targeting the tobacco industry. But this is gradually changing, in two ways. First, the industries targeted are increasingly wider, with advertising bans and health warnings having been adopted or being proposed in relation to a wider range of unhealthy goods, notably alcoholic drinks and HFSS foods. Second, new and more intrusive forms of encroaching on trade mark rights are being adopted to deter consumption of these goods, notably ever-larger health warnings and plain packaging. The following subsections will explore these measures and their ongoing expansion in more detail.

5.3.1 Advertising Bans

Advertising bans prohibit any, and in some cases all, forms of advertising – for instance, advertising on billboards, newspapers, television, internet, point of sale, or even sponsorships. While most advertising bans do not target trade mark use specifically, they arguably have an impact on manufacturers' capacity to realise certain trade mark functions to their full potential, notably the advertising and expressive functions. The Coca-Cola Company would struggle to convey an image of hedonism through its "Coca-Cola" marks if it were not allowed to advertise its products, even though the advertising ban does not, strictly speaking, affect trade mark use. Advertising constitutes the principal communication vehicle between undertakings and consumers in the contemporary marketplace and, thus, plays a crucial role in allowing a mark to develop brand image. This also explains why an advertising ban would have an impact on the expressive function of the "Coca-Cola" marks too, for it would preclude it from developing more complex meanings of the sort required to engage in expressive use of the mark (i.e., hedonism and family/friendship-oriented values).

One form of advertising ban does, however, impinge on trade mark use directly: brand stretching. As a form of indirect advertising, brand stretching prohibits owners of marks of a given product (e.g., tobacco) from using them on other products (e.g., apparel), and vice versa. Proponents of this restriction argue that by using a mark that is commonly associated with an unhealthy good on another product, the mark will both identify the product and indirectly advertise the unhealthy good.

Advertising bans were first introduced in relation to tobacco products in the 1960s. For example, in 1965, the United Kingdom banned cigarette advertisements on television.[6] A similar ban was adopted shortly after, in 1969, in the United States, which also encompassed radio ads.[7] Stricter advertising bans have gradually been adopted in a growing number of jurisdictions, broadening both the channels and strategies proscribed. This has been to a large extent the result of the concerted efforts in the global fight against smoking prevalence spearheaded by the World Health Organisation (WHO), notably by means of the Framework Convention on Tobacco Control (FCTC) in the early 2000s.[8] As of 2021, 57 countries (out of the 195 surveyed by WHO) banned all forms of advertising of tobacco products, whether direct or indirect.[9] Only 40 countries had not adopted any, or only minimal, forms of advertising bans of tobacco products,[10] with the remaining 98 having in place some form of advertising ban (many of which are rather comprehensive).[11]

Beyond tobacco products, advertising bans have been particularly successful in relation to alcoholic drinks (especially when compared with HFSS foods). This is a remarkable achievement given that, in contrast with tobacco products, there is no legally binding regulatory framework in international law for alcohol. The WHO has attempted to institute a series of policy recommendations and objectives by means of its 2010 Global Strategy to Reduce the Harmful Use of Alcohol,[12] as well as its Global Action for the Prevention and Control of Noncommunicable Diseases 2013–2020.[13] However, these instruments are not legally binding. Of the 123 countries surveyed by WHO in 2018, only 35 had no advertising bans in place (located for the most part in the African and Americas regions).[14] Of the remaining 88 countries that had adopted some form of advertising ban for alcoholic drinks, 51 imposed total bans across all channels.[15]

By contrast, advertising bans for HFSS have been adopted only in a handful of jurisdictions. This is in spite of concerted efforts by the WHO, since at least 2010, to ensure that "children [are] free from all forms of marketing of foods high in saturated fats, trans-fatty acids, free sugars, or salt."[16] In 1980, the Canadian province of Quebec became the first jurisdiction to ban the advertising of HFSS foods to children when it adopted a comprehensive prohibition on all "commercial advertising directed at persons under thirteen years of age."[17] Sweden and Norway adopted similar bans in the 1990s.[18] Other jurisdictions that have adopted some form of advertising ban for HFSS foods include Iran,[19] the United Kingdom,[20] Ireland,[21] Chile,[22] Portugal,[23] Taiwan,[24] South Korea,[25] Mexico,[26] Turkey,[27] and Singapore.[28] More limited bans in educational establishments are in place in Hungary, Spain, Costa Rica, Ecuador, Poland, and Uruguay.[29]

Advertising bans of tobacco products have proved exceedingly litigious. In 1995, the Canadian Supreme Court found the comprehensive advertising restrictions imposed by the 1988 Tobacco Products Control Act unconstitutional on grounds that they interfered with tobacco manufacturers' right to freedom of expression, as protected under Section 2(b) of the Canadian Charter of Rights and Freedoms.[30] The challenged Act banned most forms of advertising and promotion of tobacco products, including those that rely heavily on trade mark use, such as brand stretching. According to the Court, the challenged measures encroached on manufacturers' speech rights in a manner that the government had failed to prove was "reasonable and demonstrably justified", as mandated under Section 5.1 of the Charter.[31] In looking for a "causal link between [brand-stretching] and decrease in tobacco consumption", the Court held that "no causal connection existed [...], whether based on direct evidence or logic or reason".[32] As regards the other forms of advertising, the Court was satisfied that a causal link could be established with the objective of reducing tobacco consumption. However, the government had failed to prove that there were no less restrictive means of achieving this objective.

The Canadian Supreme Court would revisit these questions a decade later in response to tobacco manufacturers' challenge to the revised Tobacco Act,[33] finding it compatible with manufacturers' freedom of expression.[34] According to the Court, because the Act as reformulated restricted the scope of the advertising ban in several ways (notably to advertising targeted at young people, as well as lifestyle advertising (*i.e.*, that which seeks to associate a brand with a set of values or a way of life)), it encroached on plaintiffs' speech rights in a justified manner.

In 1998, the EU adopted the Tobacco Products Advertising Directive, which provided that "all forms of advertising and sponsorship [of tobacco products] shall be banned in the [EU]."[35] The validity of the Directive was challenged by tobacco manufacturers on grounds, *inter alia*, that it was incompatible with the protection afforded to freedom of expression under Article 10 of the European Convention of Human Rights (ECHR).[36] Unfortunately, the Court of Justice of the European Union (CJEU) failed to engage with this claim when it annulled the Directive on grounds of improper legal basis under the EC Treaty. Guidance can, however, be found in the opinion of Advocate General (AG) Fennelly. Because the EU had managed to furnish evidence of "a correlation [...] between the banning of advertising and reductions in average per capita tobacco consumption", the AG found most advertising restrictions to legitimately encroach on manufacturers' freedom of commercial expression.[37] The same was not the case, however, for brand stretching. According to the AG, these restrictions on trade mark use amounted to an encroachment on freedom of expression that the EU had failed to properly justify on grounds of public health protection.[38]

In 2001, US tobacco manufacturers would successfully rely on their speech rights to strike down several advertising restrictions imposed on tobacco products from a Massachusetts regulation.[39] Among other prohibitions, the challenged measure: (a) banned all advertising within a 1,000-foot radius of schools or playgrounds; and (b) imposed restrictions on indoor, point-of-sale advertising.[40] Since the type of speech interfered with in this case was of a commercial nature, the Supreme Court applied intermediate scrutiny, under which the regulatory authority must furnish proof that the challenged measure "directly advances" the substantial governmental interest asserted, and is not "more extensive than is necessary to serve that interest."[41] In this case, the defendant was unable to meet this burden and, thus, to justify the constitutionality of either advertising ban.[42]

5.3.2 Health Warnings

Health warnings require trade mark owners to give up a (increasingly higher) percentage of their package space to allow for messages warning consumers of the health risks associated with smoking tobacco products. Consequently, they take up part of the space that would otherwise be available for trade marks. This can lead, in instances where health warnings occupy most of the package space, to marks not fitting, or only in very reduced form. Health warnings are, therefore, particularly problematic when coupled with advertising bans, for product packaging becomes the last remaining billboard for manufacturers to advertise their products on.

Given their larger size, fanciful logos consisting of stylised words or images often bear the heaviest burden. These marks tend to be the most easily recognisable amongst consumers, thus doing most of the heavy lifting not only in terms of distinguishing the goods of one manufacturer from those of its competitors (*i.e.*, origin function), but also of attracting consumers and retaining their custom (*i.e.*, advertising function). As a result, enlarged health warnings can leave right holders with no other choice but to remove some of their logos altogether from the packaging, or to shrink them to such an extent that they lose their ability to properly fulfil these functions. In turn, this can severely impair trade marks' ability to develop brand image, further curtailing its advertising potential and affecting its ability to develop the sort of complex meanings that are required to perform an expressive function. Furthermore, by forcing manufacturers to showcase their marks alongside the unappealing – even gruesome at times – content of health warnings, their marks become associated with a negative image.

Many countries have enacted legislation requiring health warnings for tobacco products since the 1960s. In their early stages, health warnings consisted only of text covering a very limited surface of the packaging of tobacco products. For instance, in 1965, the US mandated that cigarette packets bear the warning "Caution: Cigarette Smoking May Be Hazardous to Your Health" on a side panel.[43] Health warnings have evolved over time, not only in terms of taking up increasing amounts of packaging space, but also in regards to their content, with many jurisdictions nowadays imposing combined health warnings, *i.e.*, graphic warnings alongside text. Once again, the FCTC has played a major role in accelerating the spread of ever-larger health warnings around the globe – under Article 11.1.(b), tobacco products must bear health warnings covering 50% or more of the package space, and no less than 30%, which "may be in the form of or include pictures."[44] Before the adoption of the FCTC in 2003, only two countries (Canada and Brazil) had adopted combined health warnings covering a substantial amount of the package surface.[45] As of 2021, 101 countries required tobacco products to bear large combined health warnings.[46] Of these, at least 70 jurisdictions require health warnings to cover at least 65% of the front and back surfaces (on average), with 17 countries requiring 80% or over.[47] Interestingly, and as countries look for new and innovative ways of reducing smoking rates further, Canada finds itself at the forefront of the fight against tobacco yet again with its recently proposed textual health warning on each individual cigarette.[48]

Although health warnings are being increasingly adopted in industries beyond tobacco products, their prevalence and intensity rarely compare to that of tobacco. This is perhaps most surprising in relation to alcoholic drinks, where health warnings were first introduced in the 1980s (notably by Mexico in 1984,[49] Colombia in 1986,[50] and the United States in 1988).[51] Since then, however, the number of jurisdictions that have adopted health warnings has been relatively small. This is despite the recommendation by the WHO that Member States adopt "labelling [measures for] alcoholic beverages to indicate [...] the harm related to alcohol."[52] Of the 164 countries surveyed by the WHO in 2018, only 65 had adopted some form of health warning for alcoholic beverages (of which only 23 had a legal requirement regarding the size of the warning label).[53] Of these, 56 mandated warning labels on advertisements, and fewer still, 47 imposed health warnings on labels of bottles or containers.[54] The vast majority of warnings consist exclusively of text, with some exceptions where text is accompanied by a small graphic element consisting, in most cases, of a pictogram in the form of a crossed circle over the silhouette of a pregnant woman, a car, or the minimum legal drinking age. Examples in this regard include France, Turkey, Mexico, Argentina, and Lithuania.[55] Importantly, no country has yet adopted enlarged graphic warnings of the type that are so prevalent in relation to tobacco products. Thailand proposed legislation in 2010 to this effect, but it is yet to be implemented.[56]

Health warnings for HFSS foods are even rarer, with only a handful of jurisdictions having adopted them to date. There appears to be increasing momentum in this regard, ever since the UN Special Rapporteur on the right to health emphatically recommended the adoption of front-of-package health warnings for HFSS foods to combat the obesity epidemic.[57] These measures, which consist predominantly of text warning consumers of high levels of calories, sodium, trans fats, saturated fats, sugars, caffeine, and sweeteners, have been adopted in Mexico,[58] Argentina,[59] Uruguay,[60] Chile,[61] Peru,[62] Israel (where health warnings feature both text and a drawing of the relevant excess nutrient type),[63] Colombia,[64] Brazil,[65] Singapore (only in relation to sugary drinks),[66] and Canada (although manufacturers have until 2026 to adapt their packaging to these requirements).[67]

Health warnings of tobacco products have also proved exceedingly litigious. In 1995, the Canadian Supreme Court not only struck down the provisions from the 1988 Tobacco Products Control Act that banned most forms of advertising (as discussed above), but also the requirement that the packaging of tobacco products bear health warnings.[68] It did so, once again, on free speech grounds. The Court was easily satisfied that a causal link could be established between health warnings and the reduction of tobacco consumption, going as far as claiming that "[t]he government is clearly justified in requiring the [manufacturers] to place warnings on tobacco packaging."[69] However, the Court took issue with the requirement that the warnings be unattributed, which it deemed disproportionate.[70] Against this backdrop, it did not come as a surprise when, a decade later, the Court upheld the health warnings mandated by the revised Tobacco Act (despite their considerable enlargement to cover 50% of the principal display surfaces).[71]

Tobacco manufacturers would be more successful in the United States when they challenged, in 2012, the validity of a proposed federal regulation promulgating a set of pictorial health warnings that would be affixed to cigarette packages covering 50% of their front and back surfaces.[72] In *R.J. Reynolds Tobacco Company* v. *FDA*, the Court of Appeals for the District of Columbia Circuit was easily satisfied that the challenged regulation compelled tobacco manufacturers to express the government's views towards the health risks posed by tobacco products and, thus, interfered with their First Amendment rights.[73] As is most often the case with encroachments on commercial speech, the Court applied intermediate scrutiny. Because the government failed to "provide[...] a shred of evidence – much less 'substantial evidence' [...] – showing that the graphic warnings will 'directly advance its interest' in reducing the number of Americans who smoke", the challenged regulation was held to be unconstitutional.[74]

In a more recent decision, the federal government's enlarged health warnings for cigars were found to be constitutional on grounds that they effected a justified encroachment on manufacturers' First Amendment rights.[75] Compared to *Reynolds*, the proposed health warnings for cigars were considerably less intrusive on manufacturers' speech rights because they consisted of text rather than images, and only covered 30% of the front and back surfaces of packages.[76] It was precisely on this basis that the Court decided, after acknowledging that the proposed health warnings interfered with manufacturers' speech, to assess the constitutionality of the required warnings under lower-level scrutiny (*i.e.*, that which applies to purely factual and uncontroversial information). Under this rather deferential standard, the regulatory authority must simply show that the proposed measure is "reasonably related" to the pursued aim and is not "unjustified or unduly burdensome."[77] According to the Court, where the graphic health warnings in *Reynolds* had been "controversial" and "inflammatory", the textual warnings required for cigars were "unambiguous and unlikely to be misinterpreted by consumers."[78]

Enlarged health warnings (covering 65% of the front and back surfaces of tobacco packages) were also challenged by tobacco manufacturers before the CJEU in 2016 on grounds that they contravened the principle of proportionality – interestingly, they were not challenged on the basis of the right to (intellectual) property nor to freedom of expression.[79] In dismissing the plaintiffs' claim, the CJEU concluded that the health warnings: (a) were not arbitrary in light of the international standards and recommendations set out under the FCTC; and (b) given their contribution to public health, they did not have a "disproportionate impact on the ability of manufacturers to communicate information about the product concerned to consumers", for there was still sufficient space available for manufacturers to affix their marks.[80] Further guidance can be found in AG Kokott's opinion in this case.[81] Importantly, the AG analysed whether the restrictions imposed by enlarged health warnings were compatible with manufacturers' fundamental right to freedom of expression as protected under Article 10 ECHR.[82] In her view, the challenged warnings effected a proportionate interference with speech for two reasons: (a) they promote public health, "which has been recognised as having a particularly high importance"; and (b) they impact commercial expression, which is deserving of limited protection under the ECHR.[83]

5.3.3 Plain Packaging

Since 2011, several countries have gone even further in their efforts to reduce the consumption of goods that pose a threat to health through the adoption of plain packaging measures. By prohibiting the use of marks consisting of logos and shapes, and severely restricting the manner in which word marks can be used, plain packaging constitutes the ultimate form of trade mark-restrictive, health-furthering legislation. But plain packaging imposes additional requirements, notably: (a) the external appearance of the package cannot be embellished; and (b) all packages must conform to certain requirements of size and shape, have a matt finish and feature a drab dark brown colour (which is deemed to be an unpleasing colour for humans). Furthermore, plain packaging is usually coupled with legislation requiring that packages bear enlarged health warnings covering from 75% to 90% of its surface (a percentage that varies depending on the jurisdiction).

Adoption of such a sweeping measure is justified on the need to preclude trade marks from performing their advertising function altogether in relation to unhealthy products. As we saw in the context of health warnings, fanciful marks are better suited to attracting and retaining consumers, hence the total ban imposed by plain packaging on the use of logos and other figurative marks, as well as shape marks. Absent use of these marks, however, advertising is far from the only function that is affected.[84]

Because only word marks can now be used, and they must appear on a prescribed area of the packet and in a standardised size and font, right holders can hardly develop any form of brand image in plain packaging scenarios, hence preventing these marks from performing their expressive function too. Proponents of plain packaging argue that this is consistent with the aim pursued by this measure, which seeks to preserve the core, source-identifying function of marks to the exclusion of all other functions. The objection that is often raised to this line of reasoning is that plain packaging goes too far in its goal of targeting solely the ancillary functions of trade marks. Because plain packaging is so restrictive of trade mark use, its encroachment on the advertising and expressive functions of marks overlaps with the origin function to the extent that they are all hollowed out.[85]

Plain packaging has thus far only been adopted in relation to tobacco products. Although the text of the FCTC does not contain any reference to plain packaging, the Guidelines for Implementation of Article 11 FCTC recommend its adoption by Member States.[86] In 2011, Australia became the first country to enact plain packaging for tobacco products.[87] The rate at which plain packaging is expanding to other jurisdictions, especially since the Dispute Settlement Body of the World Trade Organisation found this measure to be compliant with international trade rules in 2018, is unprecedented.[88] If by 2018 only 9 countries had adopted plain packaging legislation (Australia, France, the United Kingdom, Norway, Ireland, New Zealand, Hungary, Uruguay, and Slovenia),[89] by 2021 this figure had gone up to 21 (Saudi Arabia, Turkey, Thailand, Canada, Belgium, Israel, Singapore, Netherlands, Denmark, Guernsey, Jersey, and Myanmar).[90] An additional three countries have plain packaging in practice, due to importing tobacco products from a jurisdiction that requires plain packaging (Monaco, Cook Islands, and Niue).[91] And at least 13 jurisdictions are formally considering it (Armenia, Chile, Costa Rica, Finland, Georgia, Iran, Malaysia, Mauritius, Mexico, Nepal, South Africa, South Korea, Spain, and Sri Lanka).[92]

There is no evidence of plain packaging having extended to other industries to date, as many had feared. The most noteworthy attempt to date to introduce plain packaging beyond tobacco products was undertaken by Indonesia in 2014 in relation to alcohol (only for drinks with an alcohol volume over 20%), although it failed to materialise.[93] Admittedly, comments by policymakers, expert recommendations, and demands from public health advocates have made news headlines in recent years.[94] Despite the attention-grabbing headlines, no country has taken steps to date to formally introduce plain packaging in relation to goods other than tobacco. And it appears unlikely that it will expand into other industries, at least for the foreseeable future.

A decade ago, some authors framed the prohibition imposed by South Africa on the use of humanised figures on the packaging of baby milk formula under the rubric of plain packaging.[95] This raises the question of whether Mexico's recent prohibition on the use of cartoons or children's characters on the packaging of HFSS foods ought to be characterised as plain packaging.[96] This seems far-fetched, however, judging by the less severe restrictions that these measures impose on trade mark use when compared to plain packaging. Admittedly, these measures can have a substantial impact on the use of marks registered for these classes of goods when they consist of, or contain, some of the forbidden graphic elements described in the respective regulations – some of which may be extremely valuable.[97] However, this measure is not even close to prohibiting the use of any and all non-word marks for HFSS foods, let alone imposing standardised requirements of the sort that can severely threaten the distinctive function of marks.

Plain packaging legislation has been challenged in several jurisdictions to date, but unsuccessfully. The first such challenge was brought by tobacco manufacturers before the High Court of Australia on grounds that the restrictions imposed by the domestic Plain Packaging Act on their trade marks amounted to an acquisition of property under the takings clause of the Constitution.[98] The Court began by acknowledging that: (a) plaintiffs' marks ought to be deemed property under Australian law; and (b) the impugned measures constituted a taking of their property. However, to merit constitutional protection, property must not only be taken from the plaintiffs, but the benefit accruing to the government as a result of the acquisition must be proprietary in character.[99] In denying that this had been the case, the Court held that the "imposition of controls on the packaging and presentation of tobacco products does not involve the accrual of a benefit of a proprietary character to the [government] which would constitute an acquisition."[100]

In 2016, the High Court of England and Wales also dismissed tobacco manufacturers' challenges to the validity of the domestic plain packaging regulations on all counts, including that it did not infringe plaintiffs' fundamental right to (intellectual) property.[101] The Court began by acknowledging that the impugned measure interfered with claimants' right to property. After careful consideration, it held that plain packaging does not effect an expropriation of plaintiffs' rights, but rather amounts to a form of control of use (where, in light of the case law of the European Court of Human Rights, the proportionality principle and the duty to compensate apply less strictly).[102] The next step in the inquiry involved applying a fair balance test to determine whether plaintiffs were entitled to compensation as a result of having their property subjected to a control of use. The Court was easily persuaded that the balancing exercise weighed against tobacco manufacturers, for two reasons. First, plaintiffs' proprietary interests ought to give way to the right to health of UK citizens, which is deserving of a high level of protection. Second, claimants' proprietary interests sought "to promote a product that is internationally recognised as pernicious and which leads to a health 'epidemic'."[103] Tobacco manufacturers' appeal to this decision would also be unsuccessful several months later.[104]

5.4 Conclusion

Health-furthering, trade mark-restrictive measures have been adopted in a growing range of jurisdictions and in relation to a growing number of unhealthy goods – notably alcohol and FHSS foods – since they were first introduced for tobacco products in the 1960s. Advertising bans, health warnings, and plain packaging are, thus, becoming an increasingly popular choice in public authorities' regulatory toolkit for the promotion of public health. One fundamental reason for their growing popularity is their effectiveness in disincentivising the consumption of unhealthy goods. Despite the protracted and controversial debates surrounding the evidentiary burden that governments must meet for these measures to be justified under constitutional and human rights instruments, the overwhelming majority of experts agree that advertising bans, health warnings, and plain packaging have contributed to a reduction in smoking prevalence.[105]

The promotion of public health brought about by trade mark-restrictive measures comes at a cost, however. Not so much for the public authorities that impose them (another key factor that explains their growing popularity across jurisdictions, although one that is rarely discussed), but rather for rightsholders. Courts have been instrumental in ensuring that health-promoting policies targeting trade mark use remain economical for public authorities by systematically rejecting affected trade mark owners' compensatory claims – especially those grounded on expropriation arguments under the right to (intellectual) property, which could prove extremely onerous.

And yet courts across a wide range of jurisdictions have consistently agreed with manufacturers of tobacco products that the restrictions placed on trade mark use by these measures have a bearing on both their proprietary and expressive interests. To date, however, most such interferences with trade mark owners' fundamental rights have been found to be compatible with constitutional and human rights instruments. It is difficult to disagree with most of these findings, especially as they relate to the advertising function of marks. As we have seen, there are compelling reasons to ensure that the right to health takes precedence over trade marks' ability to attract and persuade consumers into buying goods that pose a risk to their health.

Things become less clear-cut where the origin and expressive functions of trade marks are interfered with. Advertising bans and moderate health warnings (*i.e.*, covering up to 65% of the package surface) will rarely encroach on the origin function of marks, and any encroachment on their expressive function will likely be justified in light of the countervailing health objective sought by these measures. However, the restrictions on trade mark use imposed by large health warnings (*i.e.*, covering over 65% of the package surface) and plain packaging will easily have a spillover effect beyond the advertising function of marks and into their origin and expressive functions. Because such restrictive measures strike closer to the core of the fundamental rights to (intellectual) property and to freedom of expression, the burden of proof imposed on public authorities to justify their compatibility with constitutional and human rights instruments ought to be higher.

Given the addictiveness of tobacco products and their severe impact on health (including on non-smokers through second-hand smoke), there is room to argue that both large health warnings and plain packaging can, when narrowly tailored to their intended aim, constitute proportionate restrictions on the rights to property and to freedom of expression of trade mark owners. This is especially true of jurisdictions where the margin of discretion afforded to the legislature under freedom of expression is broader, such as in Europe. This balancing exercise should, however, prove more onerous for public authorities facing challenges to the validity of any such measures in relation to alcoholic drinks and FHSS foods.

When compared with tobacco products, alcohol and FHSS foods share certain characteristics that can weigh against a finding of proportionality. First, most alcohol users and consumers of FHSS foods do so safely, that is, in moderate amounts and showing no patterns of addiction. This is not true of tobacco products, the extreme addictiveness of which prevents most smokers from doing so only occasionally.[106] Second, except in cases of pregnancy, the negative impact that alcohol and FHSS food intake can have on human health does not extend beyond the consumer. At least not directly (*i.e.*, as a by-product of the unhealthy good that bystanders are forced to ingest), as is the case with second-hand smoking.[107] Third, consuming alcohol and FHSS foods can have some benefits on human health (*i.e.*, moderate alcohol intake has been found to reduce the risk of cardiovascular disease, and FHSS foods can constitute a – albeit limited – source of nutrient intake).[108] Fourth, as we saw earlier, the legal obligations imposed by international instruments on the promotional and labelling requirements of alcoholic drinks and FHSS foods do not yet compare to those imposed for tobacco products under the FCTC. Fifth, the historical, cultural, and social significance of alcohol and FHSS foods intake in no way compares to widespread perceptions on smoking and tobacco products, where the latter is increasingly vilified and perceived as an anti-social activity.

Notes

1 See, amongst others: Harris D, 'TRIPS after Fifteen Years: Success or Failure, as Measured by Compulsory Licensing' (2011) 18 Journal of Intellectual Property Law 367; Hestermeyer H, *Human Rights and the WTO: The Case of Patents and Access to Medicines* (OUP 2008).

2 Elsmore M, 'Trademarks, Tobacco, Health: Brokerage by Fundamental Rights?' in A Alemanno and E Bonadio (eds), *The New Intellectual Property of Health Beyond Plain Packaging* (Edward Elgar 2016); Farley CH and DeVaney K, 'Considering Trademark and Speech Rights through the Lens of Regulating Tobacco' (2015) 43 AIPLA Quarterly Journal 289; Davison M and Emerton P, 'Rights, Privileges, Legitimate Interests, and Justifiability: Article 20 of TRIPS and Plain Packaging of Tobacco' (2014) 29 American University International Law Review 505.

3 For an in-depth exploration of how trade mark rights interact with speech, see Fernandez-Mora A, 'A Counterintuitive Approach to the Interaction Between Trademarks and Freedom of Expression in the US and Europe: A Two-Way Relationship' (2021) 39 Berkeley Journal of International Law 293.

4 The rate at which trade mark-restrictive measures have expanded beyond tobacco products in the last decade, both in terms of jurisdictional reach and the encroachment that they effect on trade mark use, reveals a clear upward trend that is bound to continue. These measures and their evolution will be explored in more detail in Section 5.3.

5 Much has been written on the functions theory in EU trade mark law, for instance: Fernandez-Mora A, 'Trade Mark Functions in Business Practice: Mapping the Law Through the Search for Economic Content' (2021) 52 IIC 1370; Kur A, 'Trade Marks Function, Don't They? CJEU Jurisprudence and Unfair Competition Practices' (2014) 45 IIC 434; Senftleben M, 'Function Theory and International Exhaustion: Why It Is Wise to Confine the Double Identity Rule in EU Trade Mark Law to Cases Affecting the Origin Function' (2014) 36 EIPR 518.

6 Second Report of the British Parliament Select Committee on Health, para 4.

7 US Public Health Cigarette Smoking Act of 1969.

8 World Health Organization Framework Convention on Tobacco Control (Geneva 21 May 2003) 2302 UNTS 166, 42 ILM 518 (2003), entered into force 27 February 2005.

9 World Health Organisation, 'WHO Report on the Global Tobacco Epidemic 2021: Addressing New and Emerging Products' (2021), 81.

10 ibid 82.

11 ibid 83.

12 World Health Organisation, 'Global Strategy to Reduce the Harmful Use of Alcohol' (2010).

13 World Health Organisation, 'Global Action for the Prevention and Control of Noncommunicable Diseases 2013–2020' (2013).

14 World Health Organisation, 'Global Status Report on Alcohol and Health 2018 (2018), 105.

15 ibid 105.

16 World Health Organization, 'Set of recommendations on the marketing of foods and non-alcoholic beverages to children' (2010).

17 Quebec Consumer Protection Act, s 248.

18 Swedish Radio Act (1966:755) of 1 December 1991, s 11; Norwegian Broadcasting Act No 127 of 1992, s 3.1.

19 Abachizadeh K and others, 'Banning Advertising Unhealthy Products and Services in Iran: A One-Decade Experience' (2020) 13 Risk Management Healthcare Policy 965, 965–66.

20 UK Code of Broadcast Advertising (BCAP Code) for broadcast media, s 32.5; Code of Advertising Practice (CAP Code) for non-broadcast media, s 15.18.

21 Irish General Commercial Communications Code, s 16(10); Irish Children's Commercial Communications Code, s 11(4).

22 Chilean Decree No. 13 of 16 April 2015 amending Decree 977/1996 (Food Health Regulation), arts 110 bis and 110 ter.

23 Portuguese Law No. 30/2019, of 23 April adding, amongst others, art 20(A) to the Portuguese Advertising Act.

24 Taiwanese Regulations Governing Advertising and Promotion of Food Products Not Suitable for Long-Term Consumption by Children of 20 November 2014.

25 Lee Y and others, 'Effect of TV Food Advertising Restriction on Food Environment for Children in South Korea' (2017) 32 Health Promotion International 25, 26.

26 Mexican Regulation of 31 March 2014 informing of the nutritional and advertising criteria that advertisers of food and non-alcoholic beverages must observe to advertise their products on open and cable television, as well as in movie theatres, in accordance with the provisions of articles 22 Bis, 79(X) and 86(VI) of the General Health Law on Advertising, s 3(II).

27 Turkish By-law on the Procedures and Principles of Media Services (Radio and Television Supreme Council), art 9(7). See also Turkish Regulation regarding the commercial communication of foods not recommended for over-consumption (Radio and Television Supreme Council).

28 Arthur R, 'Singapore bans advertising for high-sugar beverages' (*Beverage Daily*, 14 October 2019) <https://www.beveragedaily.com/Article/2019/10/14/Singapore-bans-advertising-for-high-sugar-beverages> accessed 29 January 2023.

29 See jurisdictional table in Taillie LS and others, 'Governmental Policies to Reduce Unhealthy Food Marketing to Children' (2019) 77 Nutrition Reviews 787, 790–93.

30 *RJR-MacDonald Inc v Canada (Attorney General)* [1995] 3 S.C.R. 199 (Canada).

31 ibid 204.

32 ibid 207.

33 Canadian Tobacco Act of 1997.

34 *Canada (Attorney General) v JTI-Macdonald Corp* [2007] 2 SCR 610.

35 Directive 98/43/EC of the European Parliament and of the Council of 6 July 1998 on the approximation of the laws, regulations and administrative provisions of the Member States relating to the advertising and sponsorship of tobacco products OJ L 213, art 3.

36 *Case C-376/98 Germany v European Parliament* (2000) ECR I-8419.

37 ibid Opinion of AG Fennelly [162].

38 ibid [176].

39 *Lorillard Tobacco Co v Reilly* 121 S.Ct. 2404 (2001).

40 ibid 534–35.

41 ibid 554.

42 ibid 566–567 (2001). It is relevant to note that the Court did not reach the same conclusion in relation to sales restrictions that were also contained in the challenged measure.

43 US Cigarette Labelling and Advertising Act of 1965.

44 FCTC, art 11.1. (b)(v).

45 Canada Tobacco Products Information Regulation of 2000; Brazil Resolution RDC no. 104, of 31 May 31, 2001.
46 World Health Organisation, 'WHO Report on the Global Tobacco Epidemic 2021: Addressing New and Emerging Products' (2021), 22.
47 Canadian Cancer Society, 'Cigarette Package Health Warnings. International Status Report' (7th ed., 2021), 4.
48 Cunningham R, 'Canada publishes proposed regulations to require a health warning directly on every cigarette', (*Tobacco Control Blog*, 8 July 2022) <https://blogs.bmj.com/tc/2022/07/08/canada-publishes-proposed-regulations-to-require-a-health-warning-directly-on-every-cigarette/#:~:text=Rob%20Cunningham,period%2C%20ending%2025%20August%202022> accessed 29 January 2023.
49 Mexican General Health Law of 7 February 1984, art 218.
50 Colombian Law 30 of 1986, art 16.
51 US Alcoholic Beverage Labelling Act of 1988.
52 World Health Organisation, 'Global Strategy to Reduce the Harmful Use of Alcohol' (2010), 17 para 36(f).
53 World Health Organisation, 'Global Status Report on Alcohol and Health 2018' (2018), 112.
54 ibid 112.
55 International Alliance for Responsible Drinking, 'Health warning requirements' <https://iard.org/science-resources/detail/Health-Warning-Labeling-Requirements> accessed 29 January 2023.
56 ibid.
57 Pūras D, 'Statement by the UN Special Rapporteur on the right to health on the adoption of front-of-package warning labelling to tackle NCDs' (*Office of the United Nations High Commissioner for Human Rights*, 27 July 2020) <https://www.ohchr.org/en/statements/2020/07/statement-un-special-rapporteur-right-health-adoption-front-package-warning#_ednref4> accessed 29 January 2023.
58 Amendment to the Official Mexican Norm NOM-051-SCFI/SSA1-2010 of 26 March 2020, ss 4.5.3.4, 7.1.3 and 7.1.4.
59 Argentinian Law 27642 for the Promotion of Healthy Eating of 12 November 2021 (switching the 'Excess saturated fats' label for 'Excess total fats'), art 4.
60 Uruguayan Decree No. 272-018 of 29 August 2018, art 2 and Annex IV.
61 Chilean Decree No. 13 of 16 April 2015 amending Decree 977/1996 (Food Safety Regulation), art 120 bis.
62 Peruvian Law No. 30021 of 10 May 2013 (Law for the Promotion of Healthy Eating of Children and Teenagers), art 10.
63 Israeli Protection of Public Health Regulations (Food) (Nutritional Labelling) 5778-2017 of 25 December 2017, ss 5 and 9, and First Schedule.
64 Colombian Regulation 810 of 16 June 2021, art 32.
65 Brazilian Regulation 429 of 8 October 2020, art 18.
66 Tanni M, 'Singapore tightens regulations on sweet drinks to tackle diabetes' (*Nikkei Asia*, 27 December 2022) <https://asia.nikkei.com/Business/Food-Beverage/Singapore-tightens-regulations-on-sweet-drinks-to-tackle-diabetes#:~:text=Starting%20Dec.,rushing%20to%20take%20necessary%20measures> accessed 29 January 2023.
67 Canadian Regulations Amending the Food and Drug Regulations (Nutrition Symbols, Other Labelling Provisions, Vitamin D and Hydrogenated Fats or Oils): SOR/2022-168, 28 June 2022.
68 *RJR-MacDonald Inc. v. Canada (Attorney General)* (n xxviii).
69 ibid 208.
70 ibid 207–208.

71 *Canada (Attorney General) v. JTI-Macdonald Corp.* (n xxxii).
72 *RJ Reynolds Tobacco Company et al v Food & Drug Administration et al* 696 F.3d 1205 (D.C. Cir. 2012). But see *Discount Tobacco City & Lottery Inc v United States* 674 F.3d 509 (6th Cir. 2012), where tobacco manufacturers' facial challenge to the validity of the same Act was unsuccessful as regards, *inter alia*, the compatibility of the required pictorial health warnings with the First Amendment.
73 *RJ Reynolds Tobacco Company et al v Food & Drug Administration et al* (n lxx) 1211–12.
74 ibid 1219–1220.
75 *Cigar Association of America v FDA* 315 F. Supp.3d 143 (D.D.C., 2018).
76 ibid 153–154.
77 *Zauderer v Office of Disciplinary Counsel of Supreme Court of Ohio* 471 US 626 (1985) 651.
78 *Cigar Association of America v FDA* (n lxxiii) 166.
79 *Case C-547/14 Philip Morris Brands SARL et al v Secretary of State for Health* (2016) EU:C:2016:325.
80 ibid [209].
81 ibid Opinion of AG Kokott.
82 ibid [211].
83 ibid [233].
84 This has been acknowledged by, *inter alia*, the Dispute Settlement Body of the World Trade Organisation in its Panel Report upholding the validity of Australia's Tobacco Plain Packaging Act 2011: WTO, *Australia: Certain Measures Concerning Trademarks, Geographical Indications and Other Plain Packaging Requirements Applicable to Tobacco Products and Packaging - Panel Report* (28 June 2018) WT/DS435/R, WT/DS441/R, WT/DS458/R and WT/DS467/R [7.2563]-[7.2569].
85 This idea has also been discussed by Bonadio E, 'Bans and Restrictions on the Use of Trademarks and Consumers' Health' (2014) 4 IPQ 326, 339–40; and Ricketson S, 'Plain Packaging Legislation for Tobacco Products and Trade Marks in the High Court of Australia' (2013) 3(3) Queen Mary J IP L 224, 230.
86 WHO Framework Convention on Tobacco Control, Elaboration of Guidelines for Implementation of Article 11 of the Convention (August 21, 2008) FCTC/COP/3/7.
87 Australian Tobacco Plain Packaging Act 2011 (TPPA) and Tobacco Plain Packaging Regulations 2011.
88 WTO, *Australia: Certain Measures Concerning Trademarks, Geographical Indications and Other Plain Packaging Requirements Applicable to Tobacco Products and Packaging - Panel Report* (n lxxxii). This finding was later confirmed by the Appellate Body on appeal: WTO, *Australia: Certain Measures Concerning Trademarks, Geographical Indications and Other Plain Packaging Requirements Applicable to Tobacco Products and Packaging - Appellate Body Report* (9 June 2020) WT/DS435/R and WT/DS441/R.
89 Canadian Cancer Society, 'Cigarette Package Health Warnings. International Status Report' (6th Ed., 2018), 2.
90 Canadian Cancer Society, 'Cigarette Package Health Warnings. International Status Report' (7th Ed., 2021), 12.
91 ibid 12.
92 ibid 12.
93 World Trademark Review, "Indonesia considers alcohol plain packaging move" (31 August 2014) <https://www.worldtrademarkreview.com/article/indonesia-considers-alcohol-plain-packaging-move> accessed 29 January 2023.
94 Some examples include: Editorial, 'Alcohol and Cancer' (2017) 390 The Lancet 2215; Public Health England, 'The Public Health Burden of Alcohol and the

Effectiveness and Cost-Effectiveness of Alcohol Control Policies: An evidence review' (2016), 138; Moody O, 'Junk food easier to resist in plain packs' (*The Sunday Times*, 7 March 2017) <https://www.thetimes.co.uk/article/junk-food-easier-to-resist-in-plain-packs-63lljx3r0> accessed 6 January 2023.

95 In 2013, South Africa banned the use of images of babies or humanised figures on the labels of baby milk formula by virtue of the South African Regulations Relating to Foodstuffs for Infants and Young Children of 6 December 2012 GN R 991 in GG 35941, which entered into force on 6 December 2013. Some of the authors who categorized these measures as plain packaging include: Mills L, 'Formula For Plain (Bland) Packaging' (*The Anton Mostert Chair of Intellectual Property Blog*, 3 December 2013) <https://blogs.sun.ac.za/iplaw/2013/12/03/formula-for-plain-bland-packaging/> accessed 29 January 2023; Phillips J, 'Of principles and plain packaging: is infant formula different from tobacco?' (The IPKat Blog, 9 December 2013) <https://ipkitten.blogspot.com/2013/12/of-principles-and-plain-packaging-is.htmlhttps://blogs.sun.ac.za/iplaw/2013/12/03/formula-for-plain-bland-packaging/> accessed 29 January 2023.

96 Amendment to the Official Mexican Norm NOM-051-SCFI/SSA1-2010 of 26 March 2020, s 4.1.5(a).

97 This has been noted by the International Trademark Association, 'INTA News: INTA Raises Concerns About Proposed Brand Restrictions Legislation in Mexico' (*INTA*, 28 October 2020) <https://www.inta.org/news-and-press/inta-news/inta-raises-concerns-about-proposed-brand-restrictions-legislation-in-mexico/> accessed 29 January 2023.

98 *JT International SA et al v Commonwealth of Australia* [2012] HCA 43 (High Court of Australia).

99 ibid [42].

100 ibid [44].

101 *R (on the application of British American Tobacco (UK) Ltd) and Others v Secretary of State for Health* [2016] EWHC 1169 (Admin).

102 ibid [732].

103 ibid [749].

104 *R (on the application of British American Tobacco UK Ltd) v Secretary of State for Health* [2016] EWCA Civ 1182 (CA).

105 The WHO has produced useful guides reviewing the available evidence on the effectiveness of advertising bans, health warnings and plain packaging in reducing smoking prevalence, notably: World Health Organization, 'Evidence Brief: Tobacco Point-of-Sale Display Bans' (2017); World Health Organization, 'Plain Packaging of Tobacco Products: Evidence, Design and Implementation' (2016), 10–18; World Health Organization, 'Evidence Brief: How Large Pictorial Health Warnings on the Packaging of Tobacco Products Affect Knowledge and Behaviour' (2014).

106 Fagerström K, 'The Epidemiology of Smoking' (2002) 62 Drugs 1, 2.

107 Despite the growing body of research exploring the social costs of drinking in what is often termed 'passive drinking', these costs (which often have a negative impact on human health only indirectly) are not caused by a by-product of alcohol, but rather result from human behaviour induced by excessive alcohol intake. Donaldson L, '150 years of the annual report of the chief medical officer: on the state of public health 2008' (Department of Health 2009) <https://webarchive.nationalarchives.gov.uk/ukgwa/20130105021744/http://www.dh.gov.uk/en/Publicationsandstatistics/Publications/AnnualReports/DH_096206> accessed 24 March 2023. For a critical view on the coinage of 'passive drinking', see Burgess A, 'Commentary: The Politics of Health Risk Promotion. 'Passive Drinking': A 'Good Lie' Too Far?' (2009) 11 Health, Risk and Society 527.

108 O'Keefe JH and others, 'Alcohol and Cardiovascular Health: The Dose Makes the Poison … or the Remedy' (2014) 89 Mayo Clinic Proceedings 382.

Bibliography

Abachizadeh K and others, 'Banning Advertising Unhealthy Products and Services in Iran: A One-Decade Experience' [2020] 13 *Risk Management Healthcare Policy* 965.

Bonadio E, 'Bans and Restrictions on the Use of Trademarks and Consumers' Health' [2014] 4 *IPQ* 326.

Burgess A, 'Commentary: The Politics of Health Risk Promotion. 'Passive Drinking': A 'Good Lie' Too Far?' [2009] 11 *Health, Risk and Society* 527.

Davison M and Emerton P, 'Rights, Privileges, Legitimate Interests, and Justifiability: Article 20 of TRIPS and Plain Packaging of Tobacco' [2014] 29 *American University International Law Review* 505.

Editorial, 'Alcohol and Cancer' [2017] 390 *The Lancet* 2215.

Elsmore M, 'Trademarks, Tobacco, Health: Brokerage by Fundamental Rights?' in A. Alemanno and E. Bonadio (eds.), *The New Intellectual Property of Health Beyond Plain Packaging* (Edward Elgar 2016).

Fagerström K, 'The Epidemiology of Smoking' [2002] 62 *Drugs* 1.

Farley C and DeVaney K, 'Considering Trademark and Speech Rights through the Lens of Regulating Tobacco' [2015] 43 *AIPLA Quarterly Journal* 289.

Fernandez-Mora A, 'Trade Mark Functions in Business Practice: Mapping the Law Through the Search for Economic Content' [2021] 52 *IIC* 1370.

Fernandez-Mora A, 'A Counterintuitive Approach to the Interaction Between Trademarks and Freedom of Expression in the US and Europe: A Two-Way Relationship' [2021] 39 *Berkeley Journal of International Law* 293.

Harris D, 'TRIPS after Fifteen Years: Success or Failure, as Measured by Compulsory Licensing' [2011] 18 *Journal of Intellectual Property Law* 367.

Hestermeyer H, *Human Rights and the WTO: The Case of Patents and Access to Medicines* (OUP 2008).

Kur A, 'Trade Marks Function, Don't They? CJEU Jurisprudence and Unfair Competition Practices' [2014] 45 *IIC* 434.

Landes W and Posner R, 'Trademark Law: An Economic Perspective' [1987] 30 *Journal of Law and Economics* 265.

Lee Y and others, 'Effect of TV Food Advertising Restriction on Food Environment for Children in South Korea' [2017] 32 *Health Promotion International* 25.

O'Keefe JH and others, 'Alcohol and Cardiovascular Health: The Dose Makes the Poison … or the Remedy' [2014] 89 *Mayo Clinic Proceedings* 382.

Peacock A and others, 'Global Statistics on Alcohol, Tobacco and Illicit Drug Use: 2017 Status Report' [2018] 113 *Addiction* 1905.

Ricketson S, 'Plain Packaging Legislation for Tobacco Products and Trade Marks in the High Court of Australia' [2013] 3(3) *Queen Mary J IP L* 224.

Senftleben M, 'Function Theory and International Exhaustion: Why It Is Wise to Confine the Double Identity Rule in EU Trade Mark Law to Cases Affecting the Origin Function' [2014] 36 *EIPR* 518.

Taillie LS and others, 'Governmental Policies to Reduce Unhealthy Food Marketing to Children' [2019] 77 *Nutrition Reviews* 787.

PART III

Sexual Rights and Reproductive Justice

6

THE CAPABILITY APPROACH AND THE SEXUAL RIGHTS OF CHILDREN AND ADOLESCENTS

Gottfried Schweiger

6.1 Introduction

The philosophical literature on the rationale and content of children's and adolescents' sexual rights is very thin, especially in comparison to the social sciences and legal studies.[1] This is all the more regrettable because the debate about sexual rights is always also about moral rights, that is, about explicitly ethical questions. Legal sexual rights, especially those located at the level of human rights – and that is where sexual rights find their anchorage – also need to be discussed in terms of their ethical justification. This paper will attempt to spell out the sexual rights of children and adolescents, at least from the perspective of one ethical theory – namely, the capability approach – with a focus on differentiating between children and adolescents. This focus is justified and ethically interesting from two perspectives. First, the ethical discussion of the rights of children and adolescents is principally characterised by the fact that the differentiation of these two phases of life still receives too little consideration.[2] Second, this can also be seen at the level of the human rights of children and adolescents, namely, their foundation in the UN Convention on the Rights of the Child, where all people from birth to the age of 18 are subsumed under the subject "child" and the differentiation according to age and maturity is only superficial. Especially with regard to sexual rights – so an important thesis of this text – it is significant to work out the morally relevant differences and similarities between children and adolescents. The capability approach is a worthwhile ethical theoretical framework for doing so. On the one hand, it has already been used to explicate the rights of children (and adolescents),[3] but on the other hand, sexual rights have not yet been explicitly addressed.

DOI: 10.4324/9781003399933-10

The Capability Approach is also of interest to children's and adolescents' sexual rights because it is not only an ethical theory, but also a theory for determining well-being and, by extension, a theory for determining the best interests of children (and adolescents).[4] The capability approach is, therefore, particularly suitable for explicating the content of children's and adolescents' sexual rights as rights that protect children's and adolescents' (sexual) well-being. Whether the capability approach is also suitable for grounding children's sexual rights is another question. First of all, the capability approach is a theory of how to conceptualise (children's) well-being and is not yet a theory of moral rights or justice. In this respect, the capability approach is also compatible with a number of ethical theories. Mostly, the capability approach in political philosophy is combined with a theory of sufficiency, which argues that children are entitled to a sufficient degree of those important capabilities. That is also what I have defended in previous work.[5] Here, however, I will not deal with these issues. I will instead restrict myself to conceptual questions about how the content of children's sexual rights should be understood from the perspective of the capability approach.

This text is divided into three sections. In the first section, I will recapitulate the basics of the capability approach and its application to children and adolescents. I then turn to the sexual health of children and adolescents and describe it as a positive-impact set of capabilities.[6] Sexual health encompasses both physical and mental capabilities as well as capabilities such as agency and education. Such a positive understanding of sexual health does not reduce it to the absence of disease and illness or the protection against dangers and risks – although protection remains crucial – but includes the multiple positive effects of sexual health on the well-being of children and adolescents. Sexual rights, as I will argue in the second section, can be derived from the moral entitlement of children and adolescents to sexual health. Following a positive and broader understanding of sexual health, I will argue that sexual rights should not only be understood as protective rights – particularly against exploitation, violence, and abuse – but should also be understood to empower children and adolescents. In the third and final section, I discuss the relationship between autonomy and vulnerability with respect to sexual health, which are the two key characteristics for capturing the differences between children and adolescents and the rights corresponding to those differences.[7] While children are not yet able to be reflexive about their own sexuality and their focus is on the need for protection, the more mature adolescents become, the more they are to be recognised as agents and subjects. This, I will argue, corresponds to a change in vulnerability, which, however, by no means simply decreases gradually over the course of childhood and adolescence.[8] Rather, childhood and adolescent sexual vulnerability is dynamic, or so I will claim.

6.2 The Capability Approach and the Moral Rights of Children and Adolescents

The capability approach is many things: ethical theory, political philosophy, and social science research programme.[9] In this text, it is understood as an ethical theory, and specifically one that helps ground and flesh out the moral rights of children and adolescents. The capability approach was not developed with this goal in mind, and as it was originally developed – significantly by Martha Nussbaum and Amartya Sen – it is not transferable to children and adolescents without adaptation.[10] The capability approach is a liberal theory, in that it recognises and presupposes individual freedom as a central moral value: each person should be able to live a life according to his or her own idea of a good life. Capabilities are freedoms. Freedoms are understood as real possibilities to do things or achieve beings. For children, especially for younger children, this central focus on individual freedom cannot be implemented one-to-one because children (still) lack the capacity for autonomy. In the capability approach, mature, reflective preferences, and ideas of a good life are privileged. People should be enabled to form and realise these preferences and ideas. This claim misses the actual maturity and cognitive capabilities of children and, thus, also the needs and interests of children.

It is true that the capability approach in Nussbaum's version,[11] which privileges ten central capabilities that all people should be able to achieve to a sufficient degree, opens up an approach to asking which capabilities are particularly important for children. But here, too, the problem arises that children cannot reasonably select from this set of capabilities and that some central capabilities seem not to fit well with children (*e.g.*, the capability to seek employment). This leads to recognise that capabilities (freedoms) and functionings (beings and doings) play different normative roles for adults and children and adolescents. This can be illustrated by the oft-cited example of the difference between starving and fasting. The capability approach emphasises that all people should have the freedom not to go hungry, but they should also have the freedom to go hungry (fast) if they want to do so for well-considered reasons (*e.g.*, religious or health or political motives). Children clearly do not have the capacity of autonomy to make such a decision rationally and reflexively. Children should not be free to put themselves and their health at risk if they want to go hungry; they should be well nourished by those adults who are responsible for their well-being, and they should learn what healthy eating is and why it is important. It is only when children have developed a high degree of maturity – presumably this will typically be during adolescent years – that it makes any sense at all to talk about them being able to reflect on and make such decisions about their diet. Adolescents are no longer children and are distinct from them in terms of their capacity for autonomy.[12] Therefore, adolescents are also granted more rights than children and are already allowed and expected to make decisions for themselves to a greater extent. Nevertheless, adolescents are still developing and are more vulnerable than adults.

If the capability approach postulates that a good life consists of being able to freely exercise a minimum of valuable capabilities in order to be able to realise one's own life plans, then this cannot be transferred one-to-one to the question of the moral rights of children and adolescents. These do not consist primarily in freedoms (capabilities), but that their well-being is guaranteed and protected, even if this involves overriding the child's will. This means that functionings should be prioritised over capabilities during childhood, and possibly also during adolescence. It is only during childhood, and then especially in adolescence, that the capacity for autonomy is developed in order to be able to make independent and self-determined decisions. Thus, a dynamic of unfreedom and freedom emerges, and both poles must be balanced for good childhood and adolescents. Adolescents should always be given freedoms if they are able to make reflective decisions about them and if their decisions do not expose them and their well-being to sustained and severe danger. This also delineates the scope of moral rights of children and adolescents from the perspective of the capability approach. These rights protect all capabilities that are important for their well-being in the course of the development of their autonomy, the right to decide freely about more and more areas of their own actions and thereby realise their own idea of the subjectively good life. The capability approach thus describes an objective theory of the good life characterised by the attainment and disposition of important capabilities, and by emphasising the moral value of self-determination and freedom, gives place within this objective theory to the subjective choice of one's own conceptions of a good life. According to the capability approach, all children and adolescents have a moral entitlement to sufficient well-being and the capabilities to achieve it, but it is this very entitlement that also protects children and adolescents from developing and implementing their own conceptions of a subjectively good life according to their level of development, maturity, and autonomy.

6.3 Sexual Health of Children and Adolescents

From the point of view of the capability approach, the sexual rights of children and adolescents are to be understood from two perspectives: On the one hand, there is the question of what aspects of well-being or what capabilities these rights protect and enable; on the other hand, there is the question of how these rights reflect the developmental dynamics of child and adolescent autonomy. Finally, from the perspective of the capability approach, all moral rights of children and adolescents are there both to protect well-being and to promote and enable self-determination and freedom in appropriate ways and according to the development of the child and adolescent. Both aspects of sexual rights, well-being, and self-determination can be captured through the concept of sexual health. Sexual rights protect and enable sexual health, and sexual health encompasses both the dimensions of well-being and self-determination insofar as children and adolescents are able to do so.

Health and sexuality are also key capabilities in the capability approach, but their definition is controversial. In the capability approach, health can be understood as a positive-impact (or "fertile") capability. A capability is fertile if it positively influences the development and exercise of other capabilities.[13] Health, furthermore, is not a single capability but rather a bundle of capabilities.[14] The capability of health includes the capabilities of autonomy, agency, physical and mental well-being, physical integrity, and education. According to a prominent definition in the capability approach, a person is healthy when he or she is well enough physically and mentally to be able to do what he or she wants to do. Health thus enables self-determined actions. There are also problems associated with such a broad definition of health, since it must be delimited from people's wishes so that it does not become subjectively arbitrary. Here, too, objective criteria are needed to define the minimum capabilities that constitute health. This is particularly important for children and adolescents, since the focus here is on functioning, *i.e.,* the level of health that they should achieve. This is mainly a task of medicine, but also of other sciences that try to define health or what should be regarded as a disease. The fact that such a definition is not fixed, but changing, can be seen in the sometimes heated discussions about the inclusion of diseases in the International Classification of Diseases (ICD) and Health-Related Problems[15] or, in the field of mental health, in The Diagnostic and Statistical Manual of Mental Disorders (DSM).[16]

With such an understanding of health, which cannot be limited to a biological-medical normal state, it is also intended to make the social conditions of health visible.[17] By "social conditions" or "social determination of health," it is meant that health depends on a variety of social factors that affect the body and psyche. This is usually understood to include, in addition to learned behaviours, working conditions, social position (poverty, exclusion), environmental conditions, housing, place of residence, access to healthcare, or other relevant infrastructure (care, mobility, access to social services, and welfare). Research then shows that many health-related differences (*e.g.,* morbidity and mortality) are not based on natural differences but are socially determined.[18] Therefore, we can also speak of social inequalities here, which at least raise the question of justice. From the perspective of the capability approach, such findings are not surprising, since it assumes that all capabilities, including health, are based not only on the natural characteristics of people but also on social conditions, which function as conversion factors.

The WHO now advocates for a very broad definition of sexual health that encompasses not only the absence of disease and suffering but, more importantly, positive dimensions of well-being and self-determination in relation to sexuality. Such a broad definition aligns well with the normative and conceptual assumptions of the capability approach. This introduces a shift in perspective that no longer analyses sexual health primarily in terms of disease and risk.[19] This also carries over to the conceptualisation of sexual rights, which are then no longer limited to being protected from sexual diseases and being entitled to treatment if they occur. These considerations will now be applied to the sexual health of children and adolescents to develop a viable basis for articulating sexual rights.

First, it must be recognised that children and adolescents are sexual beings, and that sexual health matters to them at all. While this understanding has long been accepted in academia, the sexuality of children – and to some extent adolescents – is a taboo subject in society.[20] Children are imagined as asexual, with which is associated a construction of childlike innocence. Of course, this is not to say that child sexuality equals to that of adolescents and adults who have completed their physical sexual development.[21] Second, the sexual health of children and adolescents has an inherent developmental dimension. Thus, their sexual health describes not only a state but also developmental goals that they are expected to achieve. Healthy sexual development involves not only physical change but also multiple psychological processes, experimentation, and identity formation. Prevention and treatment of sexual diseases and developmental disorders is only one aspect of sexual health. Third, as a drastic process of change, puberty marks the transition from childhood to adolescence.[22] Thus, developmentally appropriate capabilities for children and adolescents to achieve sexual health must be determined in each case. This is primarily the responsibility of medicine and psychology, but it is not disconnected from social norms and practices. What is considered normal and healthy sexual behaviour for a child of a certain age always relates to extra-medical standards. Fourth, sexual health is not something that simply "happens" to children and adolescents. On the one hand, the conversion factors mentioned above play a role, that is, what resources, support, and social conditions children and adolescents need to be, become, and remain sexually healthy. On the other hand, children and adolescents are active sexual agents – again, it should be emphasised that for younger children this, of course, means something different than it does for adolescents and adults. That is, children and adolescents act sexually and influence their sexual health; they participate in achieving it. The influence of individual action must be differentiated. Serious diseases or developmental disorders are beyond the control of children and adolescents. However, positive aspects of sexual health that go beyond the absence of disease and suffering include an explicit action component, for example, dealing with one's own body, feelings, and sensations. Children and adolescents can also learn how to avoid risks, for example, by being informed about contraceptive methods. Fifth, sexual health also has a relational dimension. Emotional intelligence, adequate social behaviour, and the capability to form sustainable relationships are essential areas of sexual health.

Sexual health of children and adolescents is thus a bundle of capabilities that includes physical, mental, cognitive, and social dimensions. This includes healthy physical development, free from disease and disorder, as well as knowledge.[23] Knowledge about sexuality refers, for example, to biological processes as well as sexual functionality, to knowledge about the correct designation of body parts, to information about healthcare, legal basics, pregnancy and contraception, as well as relationship management. It also includes information about counselling centres and medical contact points for questions about sexual health. Healthy body awareness is also an essential part of sexual health, especially for children and adolescents who are going through profound development. The body and bodily awareness are the basis of children's and adolescent's sexual development. A positive relationship with the body is a prerequisite for an appreciative and protective relationship with one's own body as well as for positive contact with other people. Thus, the sexual health of children and adolescents should not be taboo; it should instead be taken seriously and recognised as part of health and well-being. In adolescents, the importance of developing an authentic sexual identity, reflecting on one's own sexuality, and self-determination and agency become more prominent. Dealing with one's own sexuality, both alone and with sexual partners, becomes an important part of sexual health because sexual curiosity and desire and the developmental processes of puberty represent significant changes compared to childhood sexuality. These developmental processes occur only roughly along statistically determinable age lines, so they are also culturally and historically variable.

6.4 Autonomy and Vulnerability in Child and Adolescent Sexuality

Sexual rights should now be understood as those rights that protect and enable sexual health. Central to the sexual rights of children and adolescents is the protection and enabling of their healthy sexual development, both physically and emotionally. The sexual health of children and adolescents is particularly vulnerable. This vulnerability is rooted in both the natural and social status of children and adolescents, and it should be understood dynamically.[24] Children are not yet able to care of themselves and protect themselves from risks and violations of their bodily integrity, risks which are heavily influenced by social norms and practices, for example, patriarchy and sexism.[25] Along with the concepts of vulnerability and autonomy, it is also possible to understand the difference between the sexual rights of children and adolescents, although this difference is not absolute, but based on typical differences between children and adolescents, both anthropologically and socially constructed. This is important to emphasise because the complexity of reality can only be approximated at the level of moral rights, which describe general political norms and rules.

For a long time, the discourse around sexual rights and sexual health focused mainly on two issues: on the one hand, the prevention of sexualised violence and violations of bodily integrity and sexual self-determination, especially of women; on the other hand, access to contraceptives to ensure reproductive autonomy and protection against sexually transmitted diseases. Only in recent years has the discourse been broadened to include positive aspects of sexuality such as pleasure, desire, lust, or satisfaction of sexual desires.[26]

Globally, children and adolescents, especially girls, are particularly vulnerable to sexual violence.[27] Their access to sex education and contraceptives is limited in many countries,[28] and they represent a large number of new HIV infections.[29] Their protection is therefore of particular importance. The vulnerability of children and adolescents is emphasised from different perspectives as an important differentiator from adults, and it is useful – at least from an ethical perspective – to distinguish different forms of vulnerability[30]: Children are more vulnerable physically and emotionally, in part because they are still developing. But they are also more vulnerable because they have a subordinate social status (especially in relation to adults in power or care relationships, whether in the family or in institutions). Children are more vulnerable because they cannot yet take care of themselves, nor can they protect themselves adequately against adults. All these reasons for being fundamentally more vulnerable also apply to their sexual health. In this context, children's sexual health and integrity can be both actively harmed and abused, but they can also be violated through neglect and lack of care. Now, one might think that vulnerability decreases during childhood and that adolescents are therefore less vulnerable. They are better able to defend themselves, less dependent on adults, and their social status (in public and in institutions) is higher. This reduction in vulnerability can be correlated with the increase in autonomy: the more autonomous children and adolescents become, the less vulnerable they are. However, the picture is more complex. Autonomy functions both as a trait that reduces and increases vulnerability. It can also be said that vulnerability is not primarily reduced but changed by the development and realisation of more and more capabilities during childhood, and that this is also the case in sexual health. Autonomy not only enables us to better protect ourselves, but also to put ourselves at risk, to take risks. The discourse of risk around sexual health, especially of girls, which brings sexually transmitted diseases or (unwanted) pregnancies to the fore, is also a discourse around the risks of active sexual acts. Of course, sexual abuse and violence play a role in these risks as well, but just not only. Adolescents, unlike children, can and do engage in sexual activity. This entails risks, which in turn are not equally distributed among all adolescents, according to social norms and practices and other factors.

However, children and adolescents, both boys and girls, should not only be positioned as victims and vulnerable objects in the discourse on sexual health and sexual rights, but the positive aspects of their sexuality and sexual development should be highlighted as well. Feminist researchers particularly emphasise that adolescent sexuality, again focusing on the long-neglected sexuality of girls, is important for adolescent well-being, self-esteem and self-confidence, and the formation of an authentic identity.[31] The state of the debate on sexual health can be summarised as including not only protection from sexual violence and sexually transmitted diseases, but also the opportunity to be sexually active in a self-determined way. Thus, without being able to elaborate on this here, a connection can also be made to the question of the quality of adolescent sexuality, their sexual acts, and relationships, *i.e.*, how adolescents can be supported in authentically developing and living their own sexual identity. This component of autonomy is, of course, dependent on anthropological conditions and developmental milestones: young children do not have the maturity and cognitive abilities to be labelled autonomous. Nevertheless, autonomy is not a natural trait that develops on its own. Autonomy is gradual on the one hand, so children and adolescents can be autonomous for certain domains of life, but not yet for others. It also depends on the complexity and scope of the decision to be made. This also applies to the area of sexual health, where decisions of varying scope are involved. On the other hand, autonomy, at least autonomy that involves rich choices and agency, is more than just a cognitive capacity. Autonomy and agency are intimately intertwined. Autonomy requires education and knowledge, as well as the resources to realise agency. An autonomous decision about a sexual act is only meaningfully possible if knowledge about human sexuality has been formed and if resources pertaining to that act are available (*e.g.*, contraceptives or private spaces). Knowledge about sexuality is as much a protective factor against sexual risk as are other positive attributes that can be fostered through sexual education (Huebner and Howell 2003). Thus, the relationship between protection and empowerment is complicated in this regard as well. Attempts to protect children and adolescents by negating their sexuality, prohibiting them from engaging in developmentally appropriate acts, or making such acts taboo have, contrary to the opinion of some parents or conservative policymakers, precisely the opposite effect.

What can be gained from this for a capability-based understanding of sexual rights of children and adolescents? Sexual rights are also rights of empowerment and self-determination, to the extent that children and adolescents are capable of doing so in their autonomy and maturity. Thus, protection from violation of their sexual health, whether by others, by lack of resources or structures, or by themselves, is only one aspect of sexual rights. The sexual developmental milestones – physical, cognitive, and emotional – that are important to child health are to be protected as functionings. That is, it is not about giving children freedoms (capabilities), but about ensuring their healthy development, which is then the basis for freedoms. This paternalism towards children becomes less justified as they mature, but it persists as a protective shield during adolescence. This means that while adolescent autonomy deserves respect and that adolescents are capable of making sexual and reproductive decisions, they should not yet be fully equated with adults in this regard either. Two key criteria for such paternalism are complexity of the decision and its consequences. Particularly in the case of life-saving and other serious medical decisions, it is pointed out that adolescents should not be allowed to decide alone here, even if their opinions should be heard. Monika Betzler also argues in this direction,[32] taking up the concept of "transitional paternalism,"[33] that parents have a right to decide, even against the will of an apparently autonomous adolescent, if the decision is particularly consequential (her example is that of a student who wants to drop out of school). Whether and which actions within the context of sexual rights are of such a nature as to warrant such paternalistic intervention remains to be clarified. One possible heuristic would weigh different factors against each other, including the severity of the consequences of an action, the likelihood of its occurrence, and the maturity of the child or adolescent. However, neither the dangers associated with adolescent sexuality should be overemphasised nor the adolescent capacity to make good autonomous decisions be underestimated. Again, it must be remembered that social norms and practices play a crucial role in how we frame the differences between children and adolescents. Girls as well as LBGTQIA+ adolescents are in a different position than boys and young men and they often face unjust prejudices, discrimination, and other obstacles.[34] Education, resources, communication opportunities, as well as friends, family, teachers, and confidants, *i.e.*, the conditions under which actions and decisions are made by children and adolescents, play a crucial role.

6.5 Conclusion

This chapter makes an attempt to describe the sexual rights of children and adolescents based on the capability approach. This is followed by further ethical and political issues to be addressed in detail at a later stage.

First, it should be mentioned that beyond what has been presented, many details are still open. I would like to mention, first and foremost, the question of the concrete specification of the capabilities that are to be protected by sexual rights. This can be understood as the question of content as well as of scope and thresholds. Differentiations in content are not only necessary with regard to the relevant differences between girls, boys, queer, or intersex children. It is clear that anthropology plays a role here, but not only. Access to and informed use of menstrual products is relevant only for those adolescents who menstruate. It must also be recognised that some sexual rights are more ethically (and socially and politically) disputed than others. For instance, adequate access to menstrual products is less controversial than the right to abortion for underage girls.

Not only is any relevant capability of sexual health yet to be determined, but also how much of that capability children and adolescents are entitled to as a moral right. In the context of health, the Convention on the Rights of the Child (CRC) speaks of a maximum that is legally secured, which does not seem plausible from the perspective of the capability approach.[35] At the very least, such a maximum would be that children and adolescents have a right to the maximum of sexual health; meaning that they have a right to the maximum of each of the capabilities that together constitute sexual health. Instead, without being able to elaborate here, I would argue for a threshold level to which every child and adolescents has a moral right.[36] They should all have *sufficient* sexual health. This would also mean that they should have sufficient, but not a maximum of, sexual autonomy. Such an approach to sufficiency would then have to set appropriate thresholds for each ability and come to terms with how to deal with inequalities realised above those thresholds. It can be doubted whether the capability approach is in itself capable of indicating how high these thresholds should be set and which capabilities should actually be considered morally valuable. It would go too far to present the various answers that have been given to this question.

Martha Nussbaum proposed in earlier versions to derive capabilities from an anthropological notion of human dignity, before later moving to a Rawls-inspired liberalism and now presenting her list of capabilities as the result of an overlapping consensus.[37] In this regard, Amartya Sen was primarily oriented towards democratic processes in which the relevant capabilities are selected. Ingrid Robeyns, who developed a list of capabilities specific to the issue of gender equity, proposed different criteria. Elsewhere, Gunter Graf and I have developed a methodology that draws on, among other things, the empirical work of Mario Biggeri on child well-being,[38] and argues from an objective list theory of the good life (*i.e.*, against theories of hedonism and preferences). We propose to develop the relevant capabilities of children from the concept of child well-being in close relation to the relevant sciences (including childhood studies, medicine, psychology, and pedagogy), which are both open to further modification and robust enough to specify the relevant capabilities. In the case of more mature children, their own views should also be given due consideration, as the CRC also suggests.[39] These can then also be clustered, as suggested by Jonathan Wolff and Avner de-Shalit,[40] to distinguish particularly important capabilities that have a positive impact on other capabilities. In any case, what seems central to me here is the insight that the capability approach is compatible with a range of ethical theories as well as methodologies, which should be taken as an advantage rather than a disadvantage. Thus, from the perspective of the capability approach, the content of those capabilities that are important for sexual health can also be generated in different ways.

Second, there is the question of responsibility for sexual rights and their concrete guarantee. This addresses the various agents in the lives of children and adolescents. The sexual health of children and adolescents requires protective measures as well as encouragement, support, and free space. The sexual rights of children and adolescents are violated by both active acts and neglect. At least three levels can be mentioned here: the level of individual interaction of children and adolescents both with each other and with adults and family embeddedness. This also addresses parental obligations to protect the sexual rights of their children. Still, the family is often the most dangerous place for children and adolescents to be exposed to sexual abuse and oppression. Many parents still lack the will or the ability to adequately accompany and support their children in their sexual development; instead, prejudice, taboos, and stigmatisation prevail. The next level is that of the organisations and institutions in which children and adolescents voluntarily or compulsorily find themselves. This institution or organisation is typically the school, which is both a social space and a space of learning. The lack of implementation of adequate sexuality education is still a major problem, even in the Global North, and is controversial for ideological reasons. Private as well as public institutions of medical care and social services, but also the workplace – after all, a significant part of children and adolescents worldwide work – are places where sexual rights are realised or violated. Finally, the social and political levels are addressed, which play a major role in the realisation of sexual rights. Here, the challenge is both to justify and implement concrete policies and legal regulations that promote and protect sexual rights. And to do so for all children and adolescents. This claim is important to emphasise because the violation of sexual rights – which also deserves its own ethical reflection – is linked to the violation of other rights as well as other injustices. The negative correlation of poverty and sexual rights should be mentioned here, as well as the violation of social rights in the context of flight and displacement. The social norms and practices that prevail in a society are partly influenced by legal regulations and partly lead a relatively stable life of their own. It is evident that cultural practices such as the circumcision of girls violate sexual rights. The fact that girls in patriarchal societies are exposed to higher risks is a global phenomenon. Which agents bear responsibility and whether the capability approach can make a contribution on this point remains to be clarified.[41]

The goals in this chapter were modest, but nonetheless important in developing an initial account of how the capability approach can better understand children and adolescents' sexual health and thus the content of their sexual rights. In doing so, it was possible to demonstrate that the capability approach can contribute to a central debate in the field of children's and adolescents' rights and that it has the tools to address key conceptual and related ethical-normative issues. While the capability approach's focus on freedom and agency is not unproblematic in its application to children and adolescents, it illustrates that sexual health is about more than just averting risk and that the goals of healthy development are also concerned with empowerment.

Notes

1 Brennan S, and Epp J, 'Children's Rights, Well-Being, and Sexual Agency' in A. Bagattini, and C. Macleod (eds.), *The Nature of Children's Well-Being*, vol 9 (1st edn., Springer 2015) <http://link.springer.com/10.1007/978-94-017-9252-3_14> accessed 9 February 2023; Helmer J and others, 'Improving Sexual Health for Young People: Making Sexuality Education a Priority' [2015] Sex Education 158.

2 Betzler M, 'The Moral Significance of Adolescence' [2021] 39(4) Journal of Applied Philosophy 547–61.

3 Dixon R, and Nussbaum M, 'Children's Rights and a Capabilities Approach: The Question of Special Priority' [2012] Cornell Law Review 549; Stoecklin D, and Bonvin J-M (eds.), *Children's Rights and the Capability Approach: Challenges and Prospects* (1st edn., Springer 2014).

4 Domínguez-Serrano M, del Moral-Espín L, and Gálvez Muñoz L, 'A Well-Being of Their Own: Children's Perspectives of Well-Being from the Capabilities Approach' [2018] 26(1) Childhood 22–38.

5 Schweiger G, and Graf G, *A Philosophical Examination of Social Justice and Child Poverty* (1st edn., Palgrave Macmillan 2015) <http://www.palgraveconnect.com/doifinder/10.1057/9781137426024> accessed 17 March 2023; Graf G, and Schweiger G, *Ethics and the Endangerment of Children's Bodies* (Palgrave Macmillan 2017).

6 Wolff J, and de-Shalit A, *Disadvantage* (1st edn., Oxford University Press 2007).

7 Giesinger J, 'Vulnerability and Autonomy – Children and Adults' [2019] Ethics and Social Welfare 216.

8 Schweiger G, and Graf G, 'Ethics and the Dynamic Vulnerability of Children' [2017] Les Ateliers de l'éthique/The Ethics Forum 243.

9 Robeyns I, 'The Capability Approach' in E. Zalta (ed.), *The Stanford Encyclopedia of Philosophy* (Summer 2011, 2011) <http://plato.stanford.edu/archives/sum2011/entries/capability-approach/>.

10 Biggeri M, Ballet J, and Comim F (eds.), *Children and the Capability Approach* (1st edn., Palgrave Macmillan 2011).

11 Nussbaum MC, *Creating Capabilities: The Human Development Approach* (1st edn., Belknap Press of Harvard University Press 2011).

12 Betzler (n 2); Franklin-Hall A, 'On Becoming an Adult: Autonomy and the Moral Relevance of Life's Stages' [2013] The Philosophical Quarterly 223.

13 Wolff and de-Shalit (n 6).

14 Venkatapuram S, *Health Justice: An Argument from the Capabilities Approach* (Polity Press 2011).

15 Uher R, and Rutter M, 'Classification of Feeding and Eating Disorders: Review of Evidence and Proposals for ICD-11' [2012] World Psychiatry 80; See also WHO, Classification of Diseases, available at https://www.who.int/classifications/classification-of-diseases

16 Striegel-Moore RH, and Franko DL, 'Should Binge Eating Disorder Be Included in the DSM-V? A Critical Review of the State of the Evidence' [2008] Annual Review of Clinical Psychology 305; See also Diagnostic and Statistical Manual of Mental Disorders, available at https://www.psychiatry.org/psychiatrists/practice/dsm

17 Braveman P, Egerter S, and Williams DR, 'The social determinants of health: coming of age' [2011] 32 Annu Rev Public Health 381–98.

18 Braveman P, and Gottlieb L, ‚The social determinants of health: it's time to consider the causes of the causes‘ [2014] 129 Suppl 2 Public Health Rep 19–31.

19 WHO, 'Defining Sexual Health: Report on Technical Consultation on Sexual Health' (WHO 2006) <http://www.who.int/reproductivehealth/publications/sexual_health/defining_sexual_health.pdf> accessed 10 March 2023.

20 Robinson K, *Innocence, Knowledge, and the Construction of Childhood: The Contradictory Nature of Sexuality and Censorship in Children's Contemporary Lives* (1st edn., Routledge 2013).

21 de Graaf H, and Rademakers J, 'Sexual Development of Prepubertal Children' [2006] Journal of Psychology & Human Sexuality 1.

22 Fortenberry JD, 'Sexual Development in Adolescents', *Handbook of Child and Adolescent Sexuality* (1st edn., Academic Press 2013) <http://linkinghub.elsevier.com/retrieve/pii/B9780123877598000076> accessed 11 March 2023.

23 Helmer and others (n 1); Tolman DL, Striepe MI, and Harmon T, 'Gender Matters: Constructing a Model of Adolescent Sexual Health' [2003] Journal of Sex Research 4.

24 Schweiger and Graf (n 8).

25 Cabezas M, and Schweiger G, 'Girlhood and Ethics' [2016] Girlhood Studies 37.

26 Ford JV, and others, 'Why Pleasure Matters: Its Global Relevance for Sexual Health, Sexual Rights and Wellbeing' [2019] International Journal of Sexual Health 217; Logie CH, 'Sexual Rights and Sexual Pleasure: Sustainable Development Goals and the Omitted Dimensions of the *Leave No One behind* Sexual Health Agenda' [2021] Global Public Health 1.

27 Veenema TG, Thornton CP, and Corley A, 'The public health crisis of child sexual abuse in low and middle income countries: an integrative review of the literature' [2015] 52(4) Int J Nurs Stud 864–81.

28 Chandra-Mouli V, and others, 'Contraception for Adolescents in Low and Middle Income Countries: Needs, Barriers, and Access' [2014] Reproductive Health 1.

29 Slogrove AL, and Sohn AH, 'The Global Epidemiology of Adolescents Living with HIV: Time for More Granular Data to Improve Adolescent Health Outcomes' [2018] Current Opinion in HIV and AIDS 170.

30 Andresen S, 'Childhood Vulnerability: Systematic, Structural, and Individual Dimensions' [2014] Child Indicators Research 699.

31 Halpern CT, 'Reframing Research on Adolescent Sexuality: Healthy Sexual Development as Part of the Life Course' [2010] Perspectives on Sexual and Reproductive Health 6; Lamb S, 'Toward a Healthy Sexuality for Girls and Young Women: A Critique of Desire' in E. L. Zurbriggen and T.-A. Roberts (eds.), *The sexualization of girls and girlhood* (1st edn., Oxford University Press 2013).

32 Betzler (n 2).

33 Tucker F, 'Developing Autonomy and Transitional Paternalism' [2016] Bioethics 759.

34 Egan RD, and Hawkes GL, 'Endangered Girls and Incendiary Objects: Unpacking the Discourse on Sexualization' [2008] Sexuality & Culture 291; Pampati S, and others, 'Sexual and Gender Minority Youth and Sexual Health Education: A Systematic Mapping Review of the Literature' [2021] Journal of Adolescent Health 1040.

35 "1. States Parties recognize the right of the child to the enjoyment of the highest attainable standard of health and to facilities for the treatment of illness and rehabilitation of health." Art. 24 of the CRC, https://www.unicef.org/child-rights-convention/convention-text

36 Schweiger and Graf (n 8).

37 Nussbaum (n 11).

38 Biggeri M, and Libanora R, 'From Valuing to Evaluating: Tools and Procedures to Operationalize the Capability Approach' in M. Biggeri, J. Ballet and F. Comim (eds.), *Children and the capability approach* (Palgrave Macmillan 2011).

39 Archard D, and Skivenes M, 'Balancing a Child's Best Interests and a Child's Views' [2009] The International Journal of Children's Rights 1.

40 Wolff and de-Shalit (n 6).

41 It is worth noting here, that the capability approach has dealt intensively with questions of gender justice as well Robeyns I, 'Sen's Capability Approach and Gender Inequality: Selecting Relevant Capabilities' [200] Feminist Economics 61., which are obviously important for sexual health and rights.

Bibliography

Andresen S, 'Childhood Vulnerability: Systematic, Structural, and Individual Dimensions' [2014] *Child Indicators Research* 699.

Archard D, and Skivenes M, 'Balancing a Child's Best Interests and a Child's Views' [2009] *The International Journal of Children's Rights* 1.

Betzler M, 'The Moral Significance of Adolescence' [2021] 39(4) *Journal of Applied Philosophy* 547–561.

Biggeri M, Ballet J, and Comim F (eds.), *Children and the Capability Approach* (1st edn., Palgrave Macmillan 2011).

Biggeri M, and Libanora R, 'From Valuing to Evaluating: Tools and Procedures to Operationalize the Capability Approach' in M. Biggeri, J. Ballet, and F. Comim (eds.), *Children and the Capability Approach* (Palgrave Macmillan 2011).

Braveman P, and Gottlieb L, 'The Social Determinants of Health: It's Time to Consider the Causes of the Causes' [2014] 129(Suppl 2) *Public Health Reports* 19–31.

Braveman P, Egerter S, and Williams DR, 'The Social Determinants of Health: Coming of Age' [2011] 32 *The Annual Review of Public Health* 381–398.

Brennan S, and Epp J, 'Children's Rights, Well-Being, and Sexual Agency' in A. Bagattini, and C. Macleod (eds.), *The Nature of Children's Well-Being*, vol 9

(1st edn., Springer 2015). <http://link.springer.com/10.1007/978-94-017-9252-3_14> accessed 9 February 2023.

Cabezas M, and Schweiger G, 'Girlhood and Ethics' [2016] *Girlhood Studies* 37.

Chandra-Mouli V. and others, 'Contraception for Adolescents in Low and Middle Income Countries: Needs, Barriers, and Access' [2014] *Reproductive Health* 1.

de Graaf H, and Rademakers J, 'Sexual Development of Prepubertal Children' [2006] *Journal of Psychology & Human Sexuality* 1.

Dixon R, and Nussbaum M, 'Children's Rights and a Capabilities Approach: The Question of Special Priority' [2012] *Cornell Law Review* 549.

Domínguez-Serrano M, del Moral-Espín L, and Gálvez Muñoz L, 'A Well-Being of Their Own: Children's Perspectives of Well-Being from the Capabilities Approach' [2018] 26(1) *Childhood* 22–38.

Egan RD, and Hawkes GL, 'Endangered Girls and Incendiary Objects: Unpacking the Discourse on Sexualization' [2008] *Sexuality & Culture* 291.

Ford JV and others, 'Why Pleasure Matters: Its Global Relevance for Sexual Health, Sexual Rights and Wellbeing' [2019] *International Journal of Sexual Health* 217.

Fortenberry JD, 'Sexual Development in Adolescents', *Handbook of Child and Adolescent Sexuality* (1st edn., Academic Press 2013).

Franklin-Hall A, 'On Becoming an Adult: Autonomy and the Moral Relevance of Life's Stages' [2013] *The Philosophical Quarterly* 223.

Giesinger J, 'Vulnerability and Autonomy – Children and Adults' [2019] *Ethics and Social Welfare* 216.

Graf G, and Schweiger G, *Ethics and the Endangerment of Children's Bodies* (Palgrave Macmillan 2017).

Halpern CT, 'Reframing Research on Adolescent Sexuality: Healthy Sexual Development as Part of the Life Course' [2010] *Perspectives on Sexual and Reproductive Health* 6.

Helmer J, and others, 'Improving Sexual Health for Young People: Making Sexuality Education a Priority' [2015] *Sex Education* 158.

Huebner, AJ, & Howell, LW (2003). Examining the relationship between adolescent sexual Risk-Taking and perceptions of monitoring, communication, and parenting styles. *Journal of Adolescent Health*, 33, 71–78. 10.1016/s1054-139x(03)00141-1

Lamb S, 'Toward a Healthy Sexuality for Girls and Young Women: A Critique of Desire' in E. L. Zurbriggen and T.-A. Roberts (eds.), *The Sexualization of Girls and Girlhood* (1st edn., Oxford University Press 2013).

Logie CH, 'Sexual Rights and Sexual Pleasure: Sustainable Development Goals and the Omitted Dimensions of the *Leave No One behind* Sexual Health Agenda' [2021] *Global Public Health* 1.

Nussbaum MC, *Creating Capabilities: The Human Development Approach* (1st edn., Belknap Press of Harvard University Press 2011).

Pampati S, and others, 'Sexual and Gender Minority Youth and Sexual Health Education: A Systematic Mapping Review of the Literature' [2021] *Journal of Adolescent Health* 1040.

Robeyns I, 'Sen's Capability Approach and Gender Inequality: Selecting Relevant Capabilities' [2003] *Feminist Economics* 61.

Robeyns I, 'The Capability Approach' in E. Zalta (ed.), *The Stanford Encyclopedia of Philosophy* (Summer 2011, 2011). <http://plato.stanford.edu/archives/sum2011/entries/capability-approach/>

Robinson K, *Innocence, Knowledge, and the Construction of Childhood: The Contradictory Nature of Sexuality and Censorship in Children's Contemporary Lives* (1st edn., Routledge 2013).

Schweiger G, and Graf G, *A Philosophical Examination of Social Justice and Child Poverty* (1st edn., Palgrave Macmillan 2015).

Schweiger G, and Graf G, 'Ethics and the Dynamic Vulnerability of Children' [2017] *Les Ateliers de l'éthique/The Ethics Forum* 243.

Slogrove AL, and Sohn AH, 'The Global Epidemiology of Adolescents Living with HIV: Time for More Granular Data to Improve Adolescent Health Outcomes' [2018] *Current Opinion in HIV and AIDS* 170.

Stoecklin D, and Bonvin J-M (eds.), *Children's Rights and the Capability Approach: Challenges and Prospects* (1st edn., Springer 2014).

Striegel-Moore RH, and Franko DL, 'Should Binge Eating Disorder Be Included in the DSM-V? A Critical Review of the State of the Evidence' [2008] *Annual Review of Clinical Psychology* 305.

Tolman DL, Striepe MI, and Harmon T, 'Gender Matters: Constructing a Model of Adolescent Sexual Health' [2003] *Journal of Sex Research* 4.

Tucker F, 'Developing Autonomy and Transitional Paternalism' [2016] *Bioethics* 759.

Uher R, and Rutter M, 'Classification of Feeding and Eating Disorders: Review of Evidence and Proposals for ICD-11' [2012] *World Psychiatry* 80.

Veenema TG, Thornton CP, and Corley A, 'The public health crisis of child sexual abuse in low and middle income countries: an integrative review of the literature' [2015] 52(4) *The International Journal of Nursing Studies* 864–881.

Venkatapuram S, *Health Justice: An Argument from the Capabilities Approach* (Polity Press 2011).

WHO, 'Defining Sexual Health: Report on Technical Consultation on Sexual Health' (WHO 2006). <http://www.who.int/reproductivehealth/publications/sexual_health/defining_sexual_health.pdf> accessed 10 March 2023.

Wolff J, and de-Shalit A, *Disadvantage* (1st edn., Oxford University Press 2007).

7

REPRODUCTIVE JUSTICE AND ETHICS OF CONSENT IN ASSISTED LIVING FACILITIES FOR DISABLED PEOPLE

A Critical Reflection for Socio-Legal Policies on Long-Term Care in India

Keerty Nakray

7.1 Introduction

Disability denotes a complex health and social problem, which reflects, at individual levels, the experiences of various morbidities and their social consequences. At collective levels, the experiences of groups of people with various health morbidities impair their participation in social activities, unlike those without these morbidities. Often, an individual's physical and intellectual disability (ID) leads to non-conformity to societal notions of an ideal body. A disabled body triggers societal discomfort, which manifests in stigma, discrimination, and social exclusion. Social movements have highlighted this, which led to shifts in social-legal policies to bring about more inclusion, at least, on the surface. From an ethical perspective, if society creates enabling conditions for disabled people, they will have equal opportunities. But it is easier said than done. Women with disabilities face added barriers in accessing their reproductive rights, for instance, through poor access to healthcare facilities and information, lackadaisical attitudes of healthcare workers, and the overall infantilisation and invisibilisation of women with disabilities. Among many other reasons, it is the systemic prejudice and discrimination against women with disabilities that results in numerous severe waves of abuse of their sexual and reproductive rights. Some of the abusive practices include coerced sterilisation, forced contraception, and/or limited or no contraceptive choices, suppression of menstruation, poorly managed pregnancy and birth, forced abortion, termination of parental rights, denial of/or forced marriage, and other forms of torture and violence, including gender-based violence.[1]

DOI: 10.4324/9781003399933-11

The World Health Organisation (WHO) states that disability refers to the interaction between individuals with a health condition (e.g., cerebral palsy, down syndrome, and depression) and personal and environmental factors (e.g., negative attitudes, inaccessible transportation, public buildings, and limited social supports).[2] An estimated 1 billion people experience disability, around 15% of the world's population, with almost 190 million (3.8%) aged 15 years and older with complications requiring health services.[3] With changing demographics and social patterns worldwide, the population with disabilities is increasing due to risk determinants such as ageing, climate change, pollution, and abuse. During the 2012 United Nations Conference on Sustainable Development, Rio and 20 other member states agreed to launch a process to develop sustainable development goals (SDGs) to succeed in the Millennium Development Goals (MDGs-2015). SDGs have included disabilities: Goal 4 addresses equal education opportunities and improving education facilities to include women, persons with disabilities (PWDs), and equal pay for work of equal value; Goal 10 addresses inequality and encourages inclusion for people, including PWDs; Goal 11 aims to create inclusive cities and create accessible public spaces, particularly for PWDs. Goal 17 focuses on collecting timely and reliable data disaggregated by disability.[4]

India is the focus of this chapter because it was one of the first few countries to formulate legal and policy frameworks ensuring access to abortion and contraception. However, safe abortion is still unobtainable for many women, and the overall protection of the reproductive rights of disabled people residing in assisted living facilities is still poor.[5] Moreover, long-term social care remains poorly understood and governed in India.

The main aim of the chapter is to examine the notions of network consent amongst high-risk individuals with high levels of severely intellectually disabled living in assisted living facilities. Based on critical disability studies (CDS), Section 7.2 discusses erotic segregation and theorises stigma and discrimination prevalent in social policies and laws.[6] Section 7.3 examines the notions of network consent in assisted living facilities.[7] It also explores shared decision-making as a collaborative process between families and healthcare providers to evaluate the life choices available to intellectually impaired people and negotiate consent[8]. Section 7.4 summarises some statutes and case law that deal with informed consent of disabled people in India. Finally, the chapter concludes with implications for long-term social care policies in India.

7.1.1 Background

The Indian census of 2011 defines a person with 'mental retardation' as one who either lacks understanding/comprehension as compared to her/his age group; or is unable to communicate her/his needs compared to other persons of her/his age group; or has difficulty in doing daily activities; or has difficulty in understanding routine instructions; or has extreme difficulty in making decisions, remembering things or solving problems.[9] By this definition, India estimates having around 1.5 million persons with mental retardation, of which 0.9 million are males and 0.6 million are females. ID is an underexplored area of research in India, and Indian children have the highest ID risk due to developmental delays and social conditions.[10] Based on National Sample Survey Organisation (NSSO) data, Lakhan et al. estimated that India has a prevalence of 10.5/1,000 in ID, and the urban population has a slightly higher rate (11/1,000) than the rural.[11] Community-based surveys conducted during the past two decades in India showed that the total prevalence of psychiatric disorders was around 5.8%. In contrast, a recent NSSO report revealed a prevalence of as little as 0.2%.[12]

Care dependence is defined as the need for frequent human help or care beyond that habitually required by a healthy adult.[13] In India, informal caregivers include spouses, adult offspring, and other relatives or friends, with most primary caregivers being women[14] who bear the economic, social, and psychological costs of caring.[15] In India, under sub-section (d) of Section 2 of the Rights of Persons with Disabilities Act, 2016, a caregiver is "any person, including parents and other family members who, with or without payment, provides care, support or assistance to a person with disability." According to the estimates of the 76th round of the NSSO of PWDs from 2018, around 37.72% PWDs did not require the services of a caregiver, while 0.26% said that they required the services of a caregiver but could not access them. A large section (62.02%) of PWDs said that they had been using the services of a caregiver. According to the NSSO survey, spouse provides around 30.74% of the caregiving services to PWDs, mothers 26.47%, daughters-in-law 10.54%, sons 9.49%, daughters 4.16%, hired caregivers 0.60%, and institutional caregivers 0.36%.[16]

Long-term social care is at a nascent stage in India. Informal long-term care within families is primarily neglected within government policies, with caring for disabled people and ill-being almost invisible. With a lack of support systems, the informal carers are likely to experience burnouts and either quit or face emotional and physical consequences. Formal long-term care facilities provide a variety of services, both medical and personal, to people who are unable to live independently.[17] Assisted living facilities are emerging for the aged and disabled, often set up by parents of disabled adults, such as Autism Residential Community in Vellore (set up by the parent of a son with autism). Similarly, in Chennai, the Special Child Assistance Network (SCAN), a 600-member organisation, plans to create gated communities for disabled adults.[18] Despite the slow emergence of long-term social care and living facilities, India needs reforms to create multi-sectoral systems for supporting and incentivising caregiving within families, communities, and organisations.

7.2 Newgenics and Politics of Social Reproduction

CDS is an intellectual endeavour to comprehend the lived experiences of disabled individuals in the real world. From a theoretical standpoint, it seeks a departure from medical and social notions of ability and disability and bases itself on mainstream discourses on civil, political, and human rights discourses to expand rights to all human beings.[19] As a field of study, it encompasses humanities, social sciences, and medicine to bring about a shift from individualised experiences of self and life to more societal conditions that produce and reproduce these experiences at individual and collective levels.[20] Critical disability theorists have also associated themselves with activism to impact policy and society. Minich argues that critical disability theory involves the scrutiny of normative ideologies [that] should occur not for its own sake but to produce knowledge in support of justice for people with stigmatised bodies and minds.[21] CDS has similar intellectual roots as race, feminist, caste, or ethnicity studies. However, feminists, people of colour, and *Dalits* can directly express their voice, which is often lacking with disabled people such as the intellectually impaired who are often represented by carers.

The era marked by the post-industrial revolution, world wars, medical technological advancements, and social movements led to the shift in comprehending disability from individual impairment to a societal problem.[22] In 1973, the Union of the Physically Impaired Against Segregation (UPIAS) established the 'social model of disability' to reject the WHO's usage of medicalised notions of impairment/disability/handicap.[23] It sought to address social inadequacies to create inclusion for disabled people instead of individual failure. As Shakespeare notes that the social model of disability is limited in its scope, though it is an advocacy tool for activists, it undermines the significance of the medical model for disabled people.[24] Disability is primarily a health condition requiring medical interventions and social care. The social model of disability tends to oversimplify 'disability'; however, what is needed is a dynamic understanding of social and medical models of disability.[25]

Within disability studies, physical access has been the centre point of advocacy. However, these debates have diversified in developed countries to include reproductive and social rights. The questions of reproductive ethics and justice evoke a range of social and legal controversies. The concerns that emerge include assisting fertility (assisted reproduction, surrogacy, and genetic manipulation of offspring), restricting fertility (contraception and sterilisation), terminating a pregnancy (abortion), and concerns that are more general over maternal and foetal best interests.[26] Nevertheless, as argued by disabled anthropologist Robert Murphy:

> The sexual problems of the disabled are aggravated by a widespread view that [disabled people] are either malignantly sexual, like libidinous dwarfs or, more commonly, completely asexual, an attribute frequently applied to the elderly as well.[27]

Reproductive justice has been a difficult terrain, even within progressive politics. Malacrida described the constraints on disabled people's reproductive choices and overall treatment as a case of "newgenics."[28] Traditionally, eugenic policies often segregate people into institutional care, preventing them from social interactions and reproduction to limit the birth of "flawed human beings."[29] In Canada and the United States, for example, some institutions for disabled people either funnelled their residents into the eugenic system or, in some cases, even performed sterilisations in-house on residents in the hope of improving the stock of the general population; others offered "voluntary" sterilisation as a condition of discharge or as a means of avoiding internment.[30]

Along the same lines, the American disabled feminist Anne Finger also emphasises that "[s]exuality is often the source of our deepest oppression; it is also often the source of our deepest pain. It is easier for us to talk about – and formulate strategies for changing – discrimination in employment, education, and housing than to talk about our exclusion from sexuality and reproduction."[31] Like children, the disabled are infantilised and desexualised as devoid of any need for sexual intimacy. They are subjected to *erotic segregation* from fears of erotophobia, which Patton defined as "the terrifying, irrational reaction to the erotic which makes individuals and society vulnerable to psychological and social control in cultures where pleasure is strictly categorised and regulated."[32] Post-human disability studies, like DisHuman and DisSexual studies, provide the necessary paradigm shifts towards understanding intimate citizenship. Liddiard, for example, argues that a DisHuman analysis:

> ... allows us to claim (normative) citizenship (associated with choice, a sense of autonomy, being part of a loving family, the chance to labour, love and consume) while simultaneously drawing on disability to trouble, re-shape and re-fashion liberal citizenship, ultimately, then, to invoke alternative kinds of citizenship and ways of being in the world.[33]

Similarly, dis-sexuality questions the binaries associated with sexual ableism: Normalised/Other, crip/queer, rejected/desired, natural/technologised, autonomous/collaborative, intimate/commodified, private/exposed, orgasmic/non-orgasmic, as well as the liminal spaces in between. Historically, eugenic scientists created categories of normal and abnormal groups based on statistical norms, which became dominant ways of thinking about acceptable moral standards for human beings and life.[34]

Rainey's book *Love, Sex and Disability: The Pleasures of Care* discusses the multi-faceted nature of care, sexuality, and intimacy. As a primary carer to her husband suffering from multiple sclerosis, sexuality assumed plural forms of care and intimacy. Care is often viewed as exploitative and draining, but Rainey sees it as a form of love and selfhood in her work.[35] She contextualises her work wherein the couple is involved in a mutually reinforcing relationship based on reciprocity. She writes, "while I helped with toileting, we talked about the boundaries of the body, privacy, and body image. The dressing could generate a conversation about the role of touch in the moral agency; shaving could lead to a discussion of gender performativity."[36] As evident from Rainey's first-person account, both partners exist in reciprocity to complete each other, with touch being an essential mode of intimate connection. It draws us into a complex understanding of self, personhood, care, and love. Care and love form the normative foundation for that relationship between couples and societies.

Disabled people have a greater need for care and support, which often entails the transgression of physical privacy associated with individual autonomy. Regarding gender dynamics, hegemonic ideas of masculinity on men's independence are undermined when they depend on carers for their daily needs. Similarly, women's femininity is transgressed when they are not the primary carers but care recipients. Beyond these social expectations are individualised ideas of self, relationships, and belonging. Care becomes essential to establishing intimacy and universality through a loving relationship (albeit the disability). Caring and love are vital links between selfhood, inter-relationship with others, and broader social connection. Our existence depends on our capability to connect with others. The questions of ability and disability do not arise if we connect with others with a sense of universal humanness. Often disabled bodies are targets of hatred as a deviation from the imaginary understanding of the perfect human body, marking their incomplete selfhood. This thinking paradigm shifts away from modernist constructs of a perfect body and mind.[37]

The stigma and discrimination in society shape the institutional biases against the intellectually impaired. Here, it becomes necessary to mention three significant misconceptions about the intellectually impaired, which make these laws and regulations discriminatory and the overall conduct of the state towards disabled people arbitrary. First, it is a common but mistaken assumption that if someone is disabled, they would also be sexually inactive and have no sexual or reproductive interests.[38] The second mistaken assumption is about parental unfitness of PWDs, which encourages disinclination to give fertility services to them and discourages referrals for fertility therapy.[39] Even after growing awareness about heritability, people still fear that children of disabled people will be disabled and further push women into a guilt trap by calling them selfish for their pregnancy. A study in Mexico suggested that women with disabilities were regarded as irresponsible and careless for wanting to have children because their disability would be passed on or they would be "bad mothers," often leading them to go for an abortion or give up the child for adoption.[40] Lastly, the prominence of the misleading belief about the inability of disabled people to make their decisions or that a disability will impact a person's competence. For instance, in cases where a patient has an intellectual or developmental disability, healthcare professionals may ignore the idea of obtaining in-formed consent by improperly associating their disability with the inability to comprehend or communicate.[41]

7.3 Network Consent in Long-Term Social Care Policies in Assisted Living

Policies and laws for disabled people are based on regressive social norms, which perceive them as asexual and lacking in a legal capacity. In fact, "legislation on the capacity to consent to sex can be a barrier to intimate relationships for people with intellectual disabilities."[42] Article 12(3) of the Convention on Rights of Persons with Disabilities (CRPD) requires state parties to provide PWDs access to the support needed in exercising their legal capacity.[43] This is to ensure that the rights, will, and preferences of PWDs are enjoyed on an equal basis with others. Moreover, the Committee on the Rights of Persons with Disabilities has clarified that supported decision-making must replace substitute decision-making arrangements as these are discriminatory and deny equal enjoyment of the right to exercise legal capacity for persons.[44]

The laws governing the reproductive health and rights of PWDs world-wide are flagrantly prejudiced. Women with minor physical disabilities in India are denied reproductive health services because it is assumed that it is not likely that they will ever get married.[45] Also, in China, the Maternal and Infant Health Care Law requires doctors to suggest abortion to pregnant women whose prenatal tests show that their foetus has a "serious hereditary disease" or "serious deformity."[46] On the one hand, this law aims to obtain consent for abortion from women. However, on the other hand, it also asserts that the couple "should" follow the physician's recommendation of abortion. A law in Russia ultimately robs the patient's decision-making power by allowing for medical intervention without consent if the patient is mentally disabled.[47] Similar to this is the contentious system in Japan called the *hogo-sha* system, which gives authority to a guardian to intervene and make decisions, also involving healthcare on behalf of someone with a mental disability.[48] In Canada, in a case of a 10-year-old disabled girl, it was ruled by the Court of Appeal of British Columbia that a physician would perform a hysterectomy if her parents had consented to it.[49] In Australia, 1045 disabled girls under 18 were forced and sterilised between 1992 and 1997.[50] Sterilisation was performed even on 9-year-old girls to eliminate menstruation and avoid pregnancy.[51]

7.3.1 Long-Term Social Care in Assisted Living Communities

Long-term care is a residential home where people with intellectual and physical impairments live with others, wherein formal carers rather than familial members fulfil their needs for care and relationships. It is a complex care environment where even end-of-life decisions are undertaken[52] (including the execution of the wills of primary carers in favour of their adult children). In developed countries, 'assisted living' (AL) is an umbrella term for non-medical residential care settings that provide 24-hour oversight, meals, assistance with daily living activities, and medications.[53] It draws on social care rather than medical care and provides a home to the severely intellectually disabled, especially if their families cannot care for them. Within these settings, the PWDs exercise their capabilities to live with relative levels of autonomy and freedom,[54] unlike nursing homes which might house aged PWDs with higher levels of physical frailty and those who require enhanced monitoring.[55] It requires a certain level of economic capacity to choose AL, as resources are required to properly care for PWDs. ALs can be small care residences with five residents or larger ones. Some might be corporate-owned and operate out of modern buildings that accommodate over 250 older residents. Others might be standalone buildings or part of nursing homes or campuses. Some might be aesthetically appealing, whereas others are plain and minimal.[56] In India, long-term care in traditional assisted living homes is a new phenomenon, meant to meet the needs of the intellectually challenged people whose families cannot care for them in their homes. But it leads to complex moral and ethical decision-making involving residents and their carers.

One of the aspects of ethics in assisted living is seeking consent. The process of consent is challenging for the intellectually impaired due to their intellectual limitations. They do not communicate or express themselves in standard ways. In these scenarios, proxy consent often denotes a person's legal rights to consent on behalf of a minor or a ward. However, this right is not absolute and is conditional, meaning that even though the concerned person has the right to consent, the concerned person must be medically and legally competent to consent, and the concerned person should be a legally and medically competent adult. The two types of proxy consent include (i) a power of attorney to consent for medical care provided by the patient in conditions of temporary incompetence by the medical care, and (ii) the living will.[57] In both circumstances, the right of consent is delegated to a legally and medically competent authority.

In social care settings, consent requires considerably more deliberations. According to Wetle, "determining the capacity to make decisions is an inexact [58] Often 'decisional capacity' recognises that persons with intellectual impairment may have varying abilities in decision-making in different scenarios. No valid, standardised method exists to determine decisional capacity.[59] Regarding sexual freedom, there are contradictions as expectations of asexuality from the residents mark assisted living. Assisted living enforces a regimented way of life with limited surveillance and curtails autonomy for this vulnerable population.[60]

Boni-Saenz outlines two possible supplements to the current legal framework for capacity to consent.[61] For those individuals with acquired cognitive impairments such as dementia, "advance consent" means that an individual develops a sexual advance directive for periods of cognitive impairment while residing in long-term care institutions. For individuals with lifelong cognitive impairments, such as Down syndrome, "network consent" would rely on the assistance of a supportive network to realise the legal capacity to consent to sex.[62] It derives its name from a recognition that some individuals achieve sexual decision-making capacity through the assistance of a decision-making support network.

The test for network consent should proceed in three general steps. The first step is to gauge whether the individual has the threshold capacity to express volition to a sexual decision. This volition is traditionally expressed as verbally saying "yes" to sex. People with intellectual impairments, however, may have difficulty with standard communication. Alternatively, it might require an interpretation of cues by someone familiar with the person's communication methods, including non-verbal signals or facial expressions. If one is incapable of even this basic level of communication of volition, then one cannot proceed to be a sexual agent. If one meets this requirement, then one has sexual consent capacity without the need for assistance. Suppose a person with persistent intellectual impairments does not have the mental capacity to reason about a specific sexual decision and its consequences. In that case, the Court must proceed to the third step and broaden the inquiry to determine whether an adequate decision-making support system is in place and participated in making the relevant sexual decision. This support system can take many forms, including friends, family, or institutional staff. The system will often include people who have been legally appointed to make decisions for a person with intellectual impairments, such as a guardian or attorney-in-fact. However, legal authorisation to act as a surrogate decision maker is insufficient to establish a valid decision-making support system. In other words, a decision-making support system does not exist to make a sexual decision as a surrogate for persons with intellectual impairments, it exists to facilitate their wishes and desires. It is possible that there will be many individuals who are potential members of the decision-making support system, and they might disagree on how best to actualise the sexual desires of a person with intellectual impairments.

Long-term care institutions are not ideally suited to perform these tasks; many institutions are substandard. As discussed above, advance directives will work best in a quality long-term care system, and many institutions may not be prepared to implement them yet. Facilitating the sexual lives of residents is possible only if long-term care institutions are cognisant of the need for sexual expression among residents and adopt policies that facilitate sexual environments with sexual choice and freedom from sexual abuse. Unlike medical settings, which involve relatively formally regulated institutional settings often monitored by a team of healthcare professionals, the care in assisted living varies.[63] Even within developed contexts, social care ethics in long-term care settings is complicated and depends on morality rather than clearly defined rules and regulations. Most decisions are driven by values, principles, and methods for identifying and resolving ethical conflicts. The bioethical principles as laid out by Beauchamp and Childress[64] can be applied to such decisions, they identify:

a *Autonomy focuses on identifying and supporting the capacity for residents to* exercise self-determination and authenticity regarding care, activities, and preferences.
b *Beneficence* promotes the resident's best interests while avoiding harm, particularly when resident's capacity is compromised due to an illness such as dementia.
c *Nonmaleficence* is crucial in that care workers, administrators, and care communities should avoid actions and regulations that are likely to cause harm to residents.
d *Justice* is the idea of giving each their due by providing equal access, fair allocation of benefits and burdens, and ensuring procedural fairness throughout the entire community of stakeholders.

Long-term care requires ethical decision-making in the everyday lives of people who do not have the same cognitive capacities to decide for themselves.[65] At the heart of all ethical decision-making is respect for human dignity. Decision-making with cognitive deficits limits comprehension and the capacity to assess risks for short- and long-term implications for one's lives. For instance, a study showed that patients with mild intellectual impairment could express choice but had impaired appreciation, reasoning, and understanding.[66] Therefore, carers are essential mediators of decision-making. Generally, consent is defined as voluntary and informed, and the person consenting must be able to make the decision.[67] This is well-understood in medical settings (such as through Gillick Competence which recognises the autonomy of children in giving consent for medical treatment),[68] but long-term care settings are more challenging. Doctors are assumed to have superior knowledge; they are expected to share this information with the patient to enable consensual decision-making.[69] In long-term care, intellectually impaired adults might live without a carer in a formal setting. Often the adults might have been abandoned by their families due to stigma and discrimination, which means that their biologically related carers are not involved in decision-making. Critical life decisions are left to the formal carers. All these issues with consent in long-term care institutions need to be understood alongside the legal framework of a given context, which is what I will describe next.

7.4 Indian Laws Dealing with Consent of Disabled People

In India, the following statutes provide the legal framework for informed consent of disabled people:

1 The Rights of Persons with Disabilities Act, 2016
2 The National Trust for the Welfare of Persons with Autism, Cerebral Palsy, Mental Retardation and Multiple Disabilities Act, 1999
3 The Mental Healthcare Act (MHCA), 2017.

(1) *The Rights of Persons with Disabilities Act, 2016*: The United Nations Convention on the Rights of Persons with Disabilities (CRPD), 2006 was adopted by UN General Assembly on December 13, 2006. India signed CRPD in 2007 and it came into force in 2008. CRPD obliges states to harmonise domestic laws with the Convention.[70] The Rights of Persons with Disabilities Act, 2016 (RPWD Act) is the disability legislation passed by the Indian Parliament to fulfil its obligations under CRPD. On reproductive rights, Section 10 of the RPWD Act assures that the appropriate Government shall ensure that PWDs will have access to appropriate reproductive and family planning information. It also protects PWDs informed consent in stating that no person with a disability shall be subject to any medical procedure which leads to infertility without his or her free and informed consent. Section 13 of the Act provides assurance for legal capacity by conferring the right on PWDs to (equally with others) own or inherit property, movable or immovable, control their financial affairs and access bank loans, mortgages, and other forms of financial credit. The section also provides safeguards by demanding that any person providing support to a person with a disability shall not exercise undue influence and

shall respect his or her autonomy, dignity, and privacy. Section 14 provides further support for PWDs with limited decision-making capacity. It states that if a district court or any designated authority finds that a PWD, who had been provided adequate and appropriate support but is unable to take legally binding decisions, may be provided further support of a limited guardian to take legally binding decisions on his behalf in consultation with such person.[71]

(2) *The National Trust for Welfare of Persons with Autism, Cerebral Palsy, Mental Retardation and Multiple Disabilities Act, 1999*[72] (further amended in 2015): This is arguably the most comprehensive statute for the intellectually impaired who have limited decision-making capacity. Section 14 of the Act covers guardianship, it states that a parent of a PWD or his relative may make an application to the local level committee for appointment of any person of his choice to act as a guardian of the PWD or any registered organisation may make an application in the prescribed form to the local level committee for appointment of a guardian for a PWD.[73] Section 17 provides for removal of guardian in situations of abuse and misappropriation of property.[74]

(3) *The Mental Healthcare Act (MHCA), 2017*: MHCA tends to prioritise informed consent the most among statutes that deal with the informed consent of disabled people in India. It emphasises capacity and consent, and greater responsibility is put on the psychiatrist to seek comprehensive informed consent. Seeking explicit informed consent is meant to be helpful for the patients, and adopting it in regular psychiatric practice, including its documentation, is also meant to safeguard the practitioners from potential litigations.[75] Section 2(i) of the MHCA defines informed consent as "consent given for a specific intervention, without any force, undue influence, fraud, threat, mistake or misrepresentation, and obtained after disclosing to person adequate information, including risks and benefits of, and alternatives to, the specific intervention in a language and manner understood by the person." Chapter II, Section 4 of MHCA states that every person, including a person with mental illness, shall be deemed to have capacity to make decisions regarding their mental healthcare or treatment. But to ensure that a PWD, especially one with an ID, has such capacity, capacity assessments must be carried out. Since capacity assessments are central to all care- or treatment-related decisions for independent and supported admissions, it would be reasonable to argue that capacity assessments should be done by an independent psychiatrist, other than the one treating the patient to ensure objectivity. From the patient's perspective, this might also ensure protection of their autonomy and warranted care when their capacity is lost.

Chapter III of MHCA lays down requirements for an advance directive (AD). Any person who is not a minor has the right to prepare an AD, a legal document developed by the patient which includes a description of how the person wants to be cared for and treated for their mental illness when they lose the capacity to decide on treatment or care. In addition, the person can also specify how they do not want to be cared for or treated. As caring for a person with mental illness can be demanding, the MHCA recognises the need for involving family members by providing a framework for this while ensuring the individual rights of the person with mental illness. The AD is one such provision in the Act that ensures that the person with mental illness understands their rights, the need to plan future treatment, and take precautionary measures.[76] MHCA also makes informed consent mandatory for admission, electroconvulsive therapy, discharge planning, and psychosurgery. It requires that permission should be taken from the Mental Health Review Board for ablative procedures. The Act allows for a nominated representative who can provide consent when the person with mental illness cannot do so.

In addition to these statutes, the consent to reproductive procedures in India is dealt under the Medical Termination of Pregnancy Act, 1971 (MTPA), which prohibits the medical termination of a pregnancy of a mentally ill person, "except with the consent in writing of her guardian."[77] In other words, MTPA pushes women with mental illness into the trap of guardianship since it does not define a mentally ill person, resulting in ambiguity about the ambit of the Act. This allows healthcare providers to protect their interests by requesting the guardian's consent and simultaneously breaching the privacy of women with disability.[78] This was reflected in the landmark case of *Suchita Srivastava* in 2009.[79] In this case, the Chandigarh Administration was the guardian of a woman with an ID, and it petitioned the Punjab and Haryana High Court for an abortion after the woman was raped while living in a government welfare institution.[80] Although the woman had explicitly stated her intention of continuing with the pregnancy, a Division Bench of the High Court of Punjab and Haryana held that it was in the best interests of the mentally disabled woman to undergo an abortion. The woman had become pregnant because of an alleged rape while she was an inmate at a government-run welfare institution in Chandigarh. Along with being mentally ill, she was also an orphan who did not have any parent or guardian to look after her or her prospective child. In its order, the High Court directed the termination of pregnancy despite an Expert Body's findings which showed that the victim had expressed her willingness to bear a child. At the time of the appeal, the woman was 19 weeks into her pregnancy, and MTPA (unamended in 1971) only permitted abortion up to 20 weeks gestation under Section 3. However, the Supreme Court overturned the High Court's decision by citing Article 21 of the Indian Constitution,[81] which considers women's reproductive autonomy intrinsic to their rights to personal liberty.[82]

But even after this judgement, there have been reports of forced abortions on women with mental disabilities.[83]

Another case that demonstrates the archaic treatment of women with disabilities in relation to reproductive consent is *Anand Manharlal Brahmbhatt* v. *the State of Gujarat*.[84] In this case, a woman by the name of Sunitaben was referred to Aadhar Mental Health Helpline by a person who reported a mentally retarded woman aimlessly walking around. The Helpline Team reached out to the woman and conducted a medical examination, which included a Urine Pregnancy Test (UPT). The test came back positive. Sunitaben, who was subsequently discovered to be 14 weeks pregnant, was apprehended by Gujarat police. On the advice of a healthcare staff that included a gynaecologist and a psychiatrist, the Chief Metropolitan Magistrate ordered the pregnancy to be terminated at a government hospital. The Gujarat High Court affirmed the decision, ruling that the woman's mental state made it unsafe to carry the pregnancy to term. The court cited the case of *Suchita Srivastava* and noted that, unlike the case before them, Suchita had "mild retardation." As Sunitaben was diagnosed with schizophrenia, which the court considered "a severe mental illness," it was decided that she would not have been capable of looking after her child or taking any decision in that regard.[85]

The MTPA was amended in 2021, but the amendments ignored landmark decisions such as the *Puttuswamy* ruling.[86] In *Puttuswamy,* the Supreme Court, in declaring privacy a fundamental right, reaffirmed that a woman's freedom to make reproductive decisions is essential to her right to privacy, dignity, and bodily integrity, and thus a constitutional right. It is noteworthy that the Vienna Declaration and Programme of Action of 1993 states that "special attention" must be provided to guarantee of "non-discrimination, and the equal enjoyment of all human rights and fundamental freedoms by disabled persons, including their active participation in all aspects of society."[87] Therefore, reproductive freedom of all women, including PWDs, also includes rights to marry, familial life, access to family planning and reproductive health services, the right to give informed consent to all medical procedures, including sterilisation and abortion, and freedom from sexual abuse and exploitation.[88] That PWDs in India do not have such reproductive freedom is a severe socio-legal problem.

In 2016, the Indian Supreme Court issued a judgement in the case *Devika Biswas* v. *Union of India & Others*[89] that moved beyond the reproductive health framework to recognise women's autonomy and gender equality as core elements of women's constitutionally protected reproductive rights. In this case, the Supreme Court established that state policies and programmes leading to sterilisation violate women's fundamental and human rights. The Court recognised reproductive rights as both parts of the right to health and an aspect of personal liberty under Article 21 of the Constitution. It defined such rights as the right to "access a range of reproductive health information, goods, facilities and services to enable individuals to make informed, free, and responsible decisions about their reproductive behaviour."[90] This definition should extend to all women in India, including PWDs, but reports suggest that it has not been the case thus far.[91]

This section aims to show that the corpus of laws dealing with consent of disabled people in India is varied, and medical and legal professionals enjoy high levels of discretion in such matters. The existing laws tend to reinforce the bureaucratic structures with a limited understanding of the autonomy of the severely disabled, which is why consent and reproductive rights should be negotiated as dynamic domains to push the boundaries of social care for PWDs.

7.5 Conclusion

Long-term social care in residential settings is a novel concept in India. Traditionally, it was presumed that the families would care for the disabled, elderly, and infirm. With changing society, nuclear families need to rely on formal support systems. An essential concern for elderly parents is arranging care for their adult children once they pass away.[92] Though long-term social care and assisted living is emerging in India, there is little information on these facilities. Moreover, there is no information on the governance structures in these institutions. The poor development of a multi-sectoral response from public health institutions and community-based institutions places adults with disabilities in a vulnerable situation. Non-availability of evidence-based facts, lack of coordination between the government and NGOs, the absence of a coherent community-level strategy, limited competence and capacity of decentralising services, and limited models of good practices are the other lacunas in the system.[93]

CDS and network consent, as argued in the chapter, provide the necessary intellectual foundations for recognising the liberties that should be enjoyed by the severely intellectually impaired people in India. The continued stigma and discrimination of the severely intellectually disabled can be explained in terms of erotic segregation and eugenics, and their implications for social reproduction. The dominant ideas of normalcy pervade parenting and regulate social reproduction, these ideas are based on the presumption that everyday parenting is equal to perfect families and upbringing. Prejudices are replete in our everyday practices in care institutions. The notion of 'network consent' creates opportunities for new social justice paradigms. We must push our boundaries to the notions of personhood and move beyond 'eugenics' to accept diversity as a way of life.

Also, we must engage deeply with stakeholders on questions of consent with dynamism within assisted living homes. Various stakeholders include formal and informal carers and health and social care professionals. Essential laws in the field of disability do recognise the autonomy of the severely intellectually disabled. Ethical frameworks draw extensively from medical sciences that stress on autonomy and informed consent. However, as discussed in the section on Indian laws, practices are varied, and decisions are often left to the discretion of medical and legal professionals. The existing laws reinforce the bureaucratic structures with a limited understanding of the autonomy of the severely disabled. Network consent provides us with the necessary template that can be incorporated in the context of long-term care as an iterative process wherein the principles of autonomy and authenticity, beneficence, nonmaleficence, and justice are respected. As modern society progresses to push the parameters of social justice, we need to expand social care policies to include and protect the rights of the severely intellectually impaired, especially after their primary carers, such as parents, die, or bequeath their wealth to their offspring in care homes.

Acknowledgements

I am very grateful to the Editors, Drs Himani Bhakuni and Lucas Miotto Lopes and the participants of the Justice in Global Health Workshop Series. Their comments helped me think through my chapter. I am also grateful to Mr Janadharan and students of Spandana Vocational Rehabilitation Centre, Karnataka for spending time with me.

Notes

1 Frohmader C, 'Dehumanised: The Forced Sterilisation of Women and Girls with Disabilities in Australia' Women with Disabilities Australia (WWDA) (2013), <Publications – Women With Disabilities Australia (wwda.org.au)> Accessed 27 March 2023; Ortoleva S and Lewis H, 'Forgotten Sisters – A Report on Violence Against Women with Disabilities: An Overview of its Nature, Scope, Causes and Consequences' (2012) North-eastern University School of Law Research Paper No. 104–2012. At: <http://ssrn.com/abstract=2133332>, Accessed 24 March 2023.
2 World Health Organisation 'Disability'(2023), <Disability and health (who.int)> Accessed 24 March 2023.
3 ibid.
4 United Nations, 'Sustainable Development Goals (SDGs) and Disability' (2015) <Sustainable Development Goals (SDGs) and Disability | United Nations Enable>, Accessed on 24 March 2023.
5 Centre for Reproductive Rights, 'Reproductive Rights in Indian Courts' (2017) Reproductive-Rights-In-Indian-Courts.pdf (reproductiverights.org) (reproductiverights.org), Accessed on 24 March 2023.
6 Hillman J, Sexual Consent Capacity: Ethical Issues and Challenges in Long-Term Care, Clinical Gerontologist, (2017) 40(1) Clinical Gerontologist 43–50.

7 Black B and others, 'Predictors of Providing Informed Consent or Assent for Research Participation in Assisted Living Residents (2008) 16(1) The American Journal of Geriatric Psychiatry 83–91.
8 Shah P and others, 'Informed Consent' in StatPearls [Internet]. Treasure Island (FL): StatPearls Publishing; 2023 Jan. https://www.ncbi.nlm.nih.gov/books/NBK430827/ Accessed on 24 March 2023.
9 Census of India 'Census of India 2011 Data on Disability'2011. Census of India 2011 Data on Disability (un.org), Accessed on 24 March 2023.
10 Lakhan R, Ekúndayò O, and Shahbazi, M, 'An Estimation of the Prevalence of Intellectual Disabilities and Its Association with Age in Rural and Urban Populations in India' Oct–Dec (2015) 6(4) J Neurosci Rural Pract 523–528.
11 ibid.
12 Kumar S and others, 'Prevalence and Pattern of Mental Disability Using Indian Disability Evaluation Assessment Scale in A Rural Community of Karnataka Jan (2008) 50(1) Indian Journal Psychiatry 21–23.
13 World Health Organisation, 'Evidence profile: caregiver support', 2017 WHO-MCA-17.06.01-eng.pdf Accessed on 24 March 2023.
14 Pot A and others, 'iSupport: A WHO global online intervention for informal caregivers of people with dementia' (2019) 18 World Psychiatry 365–366.
15 World Health Organisation (2017) Evidence profile: caregiver support WHO-MCA-17.06.01-eng.pdf Accessed on 24 March 2023.
16 Baruah P and Wankhar D, 'The care-giving conundrum: How to look after the disabled' (2021)
    The care-giving conundrum: How to look after the disabled (down-toearth.org.in), Accessed on 24 March 2023.
17 Centre for Disease Control, Nursing Homes and Assisted Living (2021) (Long-Term Care Facilities) Long-term Care Facilities | CDC, Accessed on 24 March 2023.
18 Mathai K, When Assisted Living Takes an Inclusive Turn, (2021) <http://timesofindia.indiatimes.com/articleshow/81337759.cms?utm_source=contento-finterest&utm_medium=text&utm_campaign=cppst> Accessed on 24 March 2023.
19 Stanford Encyclopaedia of Philosophy, 'Critical Disability Theory' (2019) Critical Disability Theory (Stanford Encyclopedia of Philosophy), Accessed on 24 March 2023.
20 Goodley D and others, 'Provocations for Critical Disability Studies' (2019) 34(6) Disability & Society 972–997.
21 Minich J, 'Enabling Whom? Critical Disability Studies Now' (2016) 5(1) Lateral, doi:10.25158/L5.1.9.
22 Titchkosky T, 'Disability Studies: The Old and the New' (2000) 25(2) The Canadian Journal of Sociology 197–224.
23 Ingstad B and Whyte S., Disability and Culture (First edn., Berkeley: University of California Press 1995); Wendell, S., 1996. The Rejected Body: Feminist Philosophical Reflections on Disability (New York and London: Psychology Press 1996).
24 Shakespeare T, Disability: The Basics (First edn., London: Routledge 2018).
25 ibid.
26 Centre for Bioethics and Social Justice, 'What is Bioethics' (2023) What Is Bioethics? <msu.edu>, Accessed 25 March 2023.
27 Murphy RF, The Damaged Self, in Brown P and Closser S, Understanding and Applying Medical Anthropology (London and New York: Routledge 2016).
28 Malacrida C, 'Mothering and Disability: From Eugenics and Newgenics' in Watson N, Alan Roulstone A and Thomas C, Routledge Handbook of Disability Studies (Routledge London 2019), 467–479.

29 ibid.
30 Stalker K, 'Theorising the Position of People with Learning Difficulties Within Disability Studies' in Watson N, Alan Roulstone A and Thomas C, *Routledge Handbook of Disability Studies* (Routledge London 2019)
31 Finger A, 'Forbidden fruit' (1992) 233 New Int 8-10; Wilkerson A, 'Disability, Sex Radicalism, and Political Agency' (2002) 14 NWSA Journal 33–57.
32 Patton C, Sex & Germs: The Politics of AIDS (Black Rose Books 1986).
33 Liddiard K, 'Theorising disabled people's sexual, intimate and erotic lives: Current Theories for Disability and Sexuality' in Shuttleworth R. and Mona L (eds.) *The Routledge Handbook of Disability and Sexuality* (First edn. Routledge, 2021).
34 Feely M, 'Thinking Differently with Deluze about the sexual capacities of bodies and the case of infertility amongst men with Down Syndrome' in Shuttleworth R. and Mona L (eds.) *The Routledge Handbook of Disability and Sexuality* (First edn, Routledge 2021).
35 Rainey S, *Love, Sex and Disability: The Pleasures of Care,* Boulder (Colorado: Lynne Rienner Publishers 2014).
36 Noddings N, *Caring: A Relational Approach to Ethics and Moral Education* (Berkeley: University of California Press 1986).
37 Shildrick M, *Dangerous Discourses of Disability, Subjectivity and Sexuality* (London: Palgrave Macmillan, 2009)
38 Acharya K and Lantos JD, 'Considering Decision-Making and Sexuality in Menstrual Suppression of Teens and Young Adults with Intellectual Disabilities' (2016) 18(4) AMA J Ethics 365-72.
39 Silvers A, Francis L, and Badesch B, 'Reproductive Rights and Access to Reproductive Services for Women with Disabilities', (2016) 18(4) AMA J Ethics 430–437.
40 Rodriguez PTV, 'Twice Violated – Abuse and Denial of Sexual and Reproductive Health Rights of Women with Psychosocial Disabilities in Mexico' (2015) Disability Rights International, Colectivo Chuhcan. Mexico-report-English-web.pdf (driadvocacy.org), Accessed 27 March 2023.
41 Corey S and Bulova P, 'Is Proxy Consent for an Invasive Procedure on a Patient with Intellectual Disabilities Ethically Sufficient? Commentary' (2016) 18 (4) AMA J Ethics 373–378.
42 Arstein-Kerslake A, 'Understanding sex: the right to legal capacity to consent to sex' (2015) 30(10) Disability and Society 1459–1473.
43 Sarkar T, 'Guardianship and Alternatives: Decision-Making Options' in: Rubin IL and others (Eds.), *Health Care for People with Intellectual and Developmental Disabilities across the Lifespan* (Springer 2016).
44 Scholten M, Gather J, and Vollmann J, 'Das kombinierte Modell der Entscheidungsassistenz: Ein Mittel zur ethisch vertretbaren Umsetzung von Artikel 12 der UN-Behindertenrechtskonvention in der Psychiatrie [The Combined Supported Decision Making Model: A Template for An Ethically Justifiable Implementation of Article 12 of the UN Convention on the Rights of Persons with Disabilities in psychiatry] 19 September (2022) Nervenarzt. German. doi: 10.1007/s00115-022-01384-1. Epub ahead of print. PMID: 36121451.
45 See Best K, 'Disabled Have Many Needs for Contraception, Network', (1999) 19(2) Res Triangle Park N C Winter 16-8, quoting Meenu Sikand of the Canadian Association of Independent Living Centres' International Committee.
46 See People's Republic of China Passes "Eugenics" Law, (1994) Reproductive Freedom News (CRLP, New York, N.Y.), Dec. 2, 1994.
47 See Law on Fundamentals of Russian Federation Legislation on Public Health Care (Law No. 5487-1) (passed on July 23, 1993, published on August 18, 1993,

in Ross. Gazeta) translated in Joint Publications Research Service, Document No. JPRS-UST-94-002, 33, item 1318, Ch. 6, art. 34.

48 See Pamela Schwartz Cohen, Psychiatric Commitment in Japan: International Concern and Domestic Reform, 14 UCLA Pac. Basin L.J. 28, 39–40 (1995).

49 See In re K. v. Public Trustee 4 W.W.W. 724 (1985).

50 See Hastings E, 'Burning Issues for People with Disabilities' available at <http://www.wwda.org.au/hasting.htm> Accessed 24 March 2023.

51 Centre for Reproductive Rights, 'Reproductive Rights and Women with Disabilities A Human Rights Framework' (2002) <https://www.reproductiverights.org/sites/default/files/documents/pub_bp_disabilities.pdf> Accessed 28 March 2023.

52 Kemp CL and others, 'The Ethics in Long-Term Care Model: Everyday Ethics and the Unseen Moral Landscape of Assisted Living' (2022) 41(4) J Appl Gerontol, 1143–1152.

53 Carder P, O'Keeffe J, and O'Keeffe C, Compendium of Residential Care and Assisted Living Regulation and Policy: 2015 Edition (2015) Washington, DC: U.S. Department of Health & Human Services, Office of the Assistant Secretary for Planning and Evaluation.

54 Harris-Kojetin L and others, 'Long-term Care Providers and Services Users in the United States', (2019) National Center for Health Statistics 3(43) Vital Health Stat.

55 Silver BC and others, 'Increasing Prevalence of Assisted Living as A Substitute for Private-pay Long-term Nursing Care', (2018) 53(6) Health Serv Res 4906–20.

56 Golant S, 'Defending Assisted Living As a Long Term Care Option, (2019) Available from: Defending Assisted Living As a Long Term Care Option | Newgeography.com Accessed 25 March 2023.

57 Law and Physician Homepage, PROXY CONSENT <lsu.edu> Accessed 26 March 2023.

58 Wetle T, 'Ethical issues and value conflicts facing case managers of frail elderly people living at home' in McCullough LB and Wilson NL (eds), *Long-term Care Decisions: Ethical and Conceptual Dimensions* (The Johns Hopkins University Press, Baltimore, 1995).

59 ibid.

60 Barmon C and others, 'Understanding Sexual Freedom and Autonomy in Assisted Living: Discourse of Residents' Rights Among Staff and Administrators', (2017) 72(3) J Gerontol B Psychol Sci Soc Sci 457–467.

61 Boni-Saenz A, 'Advanced Consent and Network Consent' in Shuttleworth R and Mona L (eds.), *The Routledge Handbook of Disability and Sexuality* (1st edn, Routledge 2021).

62 ibid.

63 Holmes AL, Bugeja L, and Ibrahim JE, 'Role of a Clinical Ethics Committee in Residential Aged Long-Term Care Settings: A Systematic Review' (2020) 21(12) J Am Med Directors Assoc 1852–1861.

64 Beauchamp T, and Childress J, *Principles of Biomedical Ethics* (5th edn., New York: Oxford University Press, 2001).

65 Kemp and others (n 52).

66 Feinberg LF and Whitlatch CJ, 'Are Persons With Cognitive Impairment Able to State Consistent Choices?' (2001) 41(3) *Gerontolo* 374–382.

67 Alderson P and others, 'Children's Informed Signified and Voluntary Consent to Heart Surgery: Professionals' (2022) 29(4) Nurs Ethics 1078–1090.

68 Griffith R, 'What is Gillick competence?' (2016) 12(1) Human Vaccines & Immunotherapeutics, 244–247. The right of a child under 16 to consent to medical examination and treatment, including immunization was decided by the House of Lords in *Gillick v West Norfolk and Wisbech AHA* [1986] where a

mother of girls under 16 objected to Department of Health advice that allowed doctors to give contraceptive advice and treatment to children without parental consent. Their Lordships held that a child under 16 had the legal competence to consent to medical examination and treatment if they had sufficient maturity and intelligence to understand the nature and implications of that treatment.

69 Dalal PK, 'Consent in Psychiatry – Concept, Application & Implications' (2020) 151(1) Indian J Med Res 6–9.
70 Government of India, Department of Empowerment of Persons with Disabilities Acts | Department of Empowerment of Persons with Disabilities | MSJE | Government of India (disabilityaffairs.gov.in) Accessed on 26 March 2023.
71 Ministry of Social Justice and Empowerment (2016) The Rights of Persons with Disabilities Act, 2016A2016-49_1.pdf (legislative.gov.in) Accessed on 26 March 2023.
72 The National Trust Empowering Abilities, Creating Trust Trained Caregivers | Ministry of Social Justice and Empowerment (MSJE) (thenationaltrust.gov.in) 2023: National Trust for the Welfare of Persons with Autism, Cerebral Palsy, Mental Retardation and Multiple Disabilities (Amendment) Rules, 2015 notified on 04.02.2015. Available at https://upload.indiacode.nic.in/showfile?actid=AC_CEN_25_35_00004_199944_1517807323315&type=rule&filename=Feb,%202015.pdf Accessed on 26 March 2023.
73 Section 13(2) of The National Trust for Welfare of Persons with Autism, Cerebral Palsy, Mental Retardation and Multiple Disabilities Act, 1999 states that "A local level committee shall consist of –

   a An officer of the civil service of the Union or of the State, not below the rank of a District Magistrate or a District Commissioner of a district; (a) an officer of the civil service of the Union or of the State, not below the rank of a District Magistrate or a District Commissioner of a district;
   b A representative of a registered organisation; and (b) a representative of a registered organisation; and
   c A person with disability as defined in clause (t) of section 2 of the Persons with Disabilities (Equal Opportunities, Protection of Rights and Full Participation) Act, 1995 (1 of 1996). (c) a person with disability as defined in clause (t) of section 2 of the Persons with Disabilities (Equal Opportunities, Protection of Rights and Full Participation) Act, 1995 (1 of 1996)."

74 The National Trust for Welfare of Persons with Autism, cerebral palsy, Mental Retardation and Multiple Disabilities Act, 1999.
75 Harbishettar V, Enara A, and Gowda, M, 'Making the most of Mental Healthcare Act 2017: Practitioners' perspective' (2019) 61(Suppl 4) Indian Journal of Psychiatry S645–S649.
76 ibid.; Duffy R and Kelly B, *India's Mental Healthcare Act*, 2017 (Springer 2020).
77 The Medical Termination of Pregnancy Act, 1971 ACT NO. 34 OF 1971 Microsoft Word – A1971-34.docx (indiacode.nic.in) Accessed on 25 March 2023
78 Raman S, 'India's Laws Fail To Uphold Abortion Rights Of Women With Disabilities, (2021) BehanBox. Available at <India's Laws Fail To Uphold Abortion Rights Of Women With Disabilities - BehanBox>
79 Suchita Srivastava & Anr v. Chandigarh Administration, (2009) 14 SCR 989. Available at
   Suchita Srivastava & Anr vs Chandigarh Administration on 28 August 2009 (indiankanoon.org) Accessed on 25 March 2023.
80 ibid.
81 Article 21, Constitution of India, 1949 states that "No person shall be deprived of his life or personal liberty except according to procedure established by law".
82 ibid.

83 Raman (n 78).
84 Anand Manharlal Brahmbhatt v. State of Gujarat, 28 July 2015 (Special Crim. App. No. 4204/2015). Available at Anand Manharlal Brahmbhatt vs State Of Gujarat & 2 on 28 July 2015 (indiankanoon.org) Accessed 29 March 2023.
85 Anand Manharlal Brahmbhatt v. State of Gujarat, 28 July 2015 (Special Crim. App. No. 4204/2015). Available at Anand Manharlal Brahmbhatt vs State Of Gujarat & 2 on 28 July 2015 (indiankanoon.org) Accessed 29 March 2023.
86 Justice K.S.Puttaswamy (Retd) v. Union Of India, (2017) 10 SCC 1. Available at https://main.sci.gov.in/supremecourt/2012/35071/35071_2012_Judgement_24-Aug-2017.pdf Accessed 29th March 2023. Accessed on 25 March 2023.
87 United Nations Office of Human Rights, 'Vienna Declaration and Programme of Action', 1993 <https://www.ohchr.org/en/professionalinterest/pages/vienna.aspx> Accessed 29 March 2023.
88 Centre for Reproductive Rights (n 51).
89 Devika Biswas v. Union of India, AIR 2016 SC 4405.
90 ibid.
91 Raman (n 78).
92 "A number of parents are getting old and are clueless as to what their children will do without them. Our effort is to try and create an environment where they can become self-sufficient," said Singh. Chhakchhuak R, 'Long way to go for care of autistic adults' (April 23, 2013) Deccan Herald. Available at: https://www.deccanherald.com/content/328123/long-way-go-care-autistic.html Accessed 29 March 2023.
93 Kumar S, Roy G, and Kar S, 'Disability and Rehabilitation Services in India: Issues and Challenges' (2012) 1(1) J Family Med Prim Care 69–73.

Bibliography

Acharya K and Lantos JD, 'Considering Decision-Making and Sexuality in Menstrual Suppression of Teens and Young Adults with Intellectual Disabilities' [2016] 18(4) *The AMA Journal of Ethics* 365–372.
Alderson P and others, 'Children's Informed Signified and Voluntary Consent to Heart Surgery: Professionals' [2022] 29(4) *Nurs Ethics* 1078–1090.
Anand Manharlal Brahmbhatt v. *State of Gujarat*, 28 July 2015 (Special Crim. App. No. 4204/2015).
Arstein-Kerslake A, 'Understanding Sex: The Right to Legal Capacity to Consent to Sex' [2015] 30(10) *Disability and Society* 1459–1473.
Article 21, Constitution of India, 1949 states that "No person shall be deprived of his life or personal liberty except according to procedure established by law".
Barmon C and others, 'Understanding Sexual Freedom and Autonomy in Assisted Living: Discourse of Residents' Rights Among Staff and Administrators' [2017] 72(3) *The Journals of Gerontology. Series B, Psychological Sciences and Social Sciences* 457–467.
Baruah P and Wankhar D, 'The care-giving conundrum: How to look after the disabled' [2021].
Beauchamp T, and Childress J, *Principles of Biomedical Ethics* (5th edn, New York: Oxford University Press, 2001).
Black B and others, 'Predictors of Providing Informed Consent or Assent for Research Participation in Assisted Living Residents' [2008] 16(1) *The American Journal of Geriatric Psychiatry* 83–91.

Boni-Saenz A, 'Advanced Consent and Network Consent' in R. Shuttleworth and L. Mona (eds.), *The Routledge Handbook of Disability and Sexuality* (1st edn, Routledge 2021).

Carder P, O'Keeffe J, and O'Keeffe C, Compendium of Residential Care and Assisted Living Regulation and Policy: 2015 Edition (2015) Washington, DC: U.S. Department of Health & Human Services, Office of the Assistant Secretary for Planning and Evaluation.

Census of India 'Census of India 2011 Data on Disability'2011. CENSUS OF INDIA 2011 DATA ON DISABILITY (un.org) (Accessed on 24 March 2023).

Centre for Bioethics and Social Justice, 'What is Bioethics' (2023) What Is Bioethics? <msu.edu> (Accessed 25 March 2023).

Centre for Disease Control, Nursing Homes and Assisted Living (2021) (Long-Term Care Facilities) Long-term Care Facilities I CDC (Accessed on 24 March 2023).

Centre for Reproductive Rights, 'Reproductive Rights in Indian Courts' [2017] Reproductive-Rights-In-Indian-Courts.pdf (reproductiverights.org) (reproductiverights.org), Accessed on 24 March 2023).

Centre for Reproductive Rights, 'Reproductive Rights and Women with Disabilities A Human Rights Framework' [2002] <https://www.reproductiverights.org/sites/default/files/documents/pub_bp_disabilities.pdf> (Accessed 28 March 2023).

Cohen PS, 'Psychiatric Commitment in Japan: International Concern and Domestic Reform' [1995] 14 *UCLA Pac. Basin L.J.* 28, 39–40 .

Corey S and Bulova P, 'Is Proxy Consent for an Invasive Procedure on a Patient with Intellectual Disabilities Ethically Sufficient? Commentary' [2016] 18(4) *The AMA Journal of Ethics* 373–378.

Dalal PK, 'Consent in Psychiatry – Concept, Application & Implications' [2020] 151(1) *Indian Journal of Medical Research* 6–9.

Devika Biswas v. Union of India, AIR 2016 SC 4405.

Duffy R and Kelly B, *India's Mental Healthcare Act, 2017* (Springer 2020).

Feely M, 'Thinking Differently with Deluze about the Sexual Capacities of Bodies and the Case of Infertility Amongst Men with Down Syndrome' in R. Shuttleworth and L. Mona (eds.), *The Routledge Handbook of Disability and Sexuality* (First edn, Routledge 2021).

Feinberg LF and Whitlatch CJ, 'Are Persons With Cognitive Impairment Able to State Consistent Choices?' [2001] 41(3) *Gerontology* 374–382.

Finger A, 'Forbidden fruit' (1992) 233 New Int 8–10; Wilkerson A, 'Disability, Sex Radicalism, and Political Agency' [2002] 14 *NWSA Journal* 33–57.

Frohmader C, 'Dehumanised: The Forced Sterilisation of Women and Girls with Disabilities in Australia' Women with Disabilities Australia (WWDA) (2013), <Publications – Women With Disabilities Australia (wwda.org.au)> (Accessed 27 March 2023).

Golant S, 'Defending Assisted Living As a Long Term Care Option' [2019] Available from: Defending Assisted Living As a Long Term Care Option I Newgeography.com (Accessed 25 March 2023).

Goodley D and others, 'Provocations for Critical Disability Studies' [2019] 34(6) *Disability & Society* 972–997.

Government of India, Department of Empowerment of Persons with Disabilities Acts I Department of Empowerment of Persons with Disabilities I MSJE I Government of India (disabilityaffairs.gov.in) (Accessed on 26 March 2023).

Griffith R, 'What is Gillick competence?' [2016] 12(1) *Human Vaccines & Immunotherapeutics* 244–247.

Harbishettar V, Enara A, and Gowda, M, 'Making the most of Mental Healthcare Act 2017: Practitioners' perspective' [2019] 61(Suppl 4) *Indian Journal of Psychiatry* S645–S649.

Harris-Kojetin L and others, 'Long-term Care Providers and Services Users in the United States' (2019) *National Center for Health Statistics* 3(43) *Vital Health Stat.*

Hastings E, 'Burning Issues for People with Disabilities' available at <http://www.wwda.org.au/hasting.htm> (Accessed 24 March 2023).

Hillman J, 'Sexual Consent Capacity: Ethical Issues and Challenges in Long-Term Care, Clinical Gerontologist' [2017] 40(1) *Clinical Gerontologist* 43–50.

Holmes AL, Bugeja L, and Ibrahim JE, 'Role of a Clinical Ethics Committee in Residential Aged Long-Term Care Settings: A Systematic Review' [2020] 21(12) *J Am Med Directors Assoc* 1852–1861.

In re K. v. Public Trustee 4 W.W.W. 724 (1985).

Ingstad B and Whyte S, *Disability and Culture* (First edn, Berkeley: University of California Press 1995); Wendell, S., 1996. The Rejected Body: Feminist Philosophical Reflections on Disability (New York and London: Psychology Press 1996).

Justice KS *Puttaswamy (Retd)* v. *Union Of India*, (2017) 10 SCC 1.

Kemp CL and others, 'The Ethics in Long-Term Care Model: Everyday Ethics and the Unseen Moral Landscape of Assisted Living' [2022] 41(4) *Journal of Applied Gerontology* 1143–1152.

Kumar S and others, 'Prevalence and Pattern of Mental Disability Using Indian Disability Evaluation Assessment Scale in A Rural Community of Karnataka Jan' [2008] 50(1) *Indian Journal Psychiatry* 21–23.

Kumar S, Roy G, and Kar S, 'Disability and Rehabilitation Services in India: Issues and Challenges' [2012] 1(1) *Journal of Family Medicine and Primary Care,* 69–73.

Lakhan R, Ekúndayò O, and Shahbazi, M, 'An Estimation of the Prevalence of Intellectual Disabilities and Its Association with Age in Rural and Urban Populations in India' [Oct-Dec 2015] 6(4) *The Journal of Neurosciences in Rural Practice* 523–528.

Law and Physician Homepage, PROXY CONSENT <lsu.edu> Accessed 26 March 2023.

Law on Fundamentals of Russian Federation Legislation on Public Health Care (Law No. 5487-1) (passed on July 23, 1993, published on August 18, 1993, in Ross. Gazeta) translated in Joint Publications Research Service, Document No. JPRS-UST-94-002, 33, item 1318, Ch. 6, art. 34.

Liddiard K, 'Theorising disabled people's sexual, intimate and erotic lives: Current Theories for Disability and Sexuality' in R. Shuttleworth and L. Mona (eds.), *The Routledge Handbook of Disability and Sexuality* (First edn. Routledge 2021).

Malacrida C, 'Mothering and Disability: From Eugenics and Newgenics' in N. Watson, A. Alan Roulstone and C. Thomas (eds), *Routledge Handbook of Disability Studies* (Routledge London 2019), 467–479.

Mathai K, *When Assisted Living Takes an Inclusive Turn* [2021] <http://timesofindia.indiatimes.com/articleshow/81337759.cms?utm_source=contentofinterest&utm_medium=text&utm_campaign=cppst> (Accessed on 24 March 2023).

Minich J, 'Enabling Whom? Critical Disability Studies Now' [2016] 5(1) *Lateral*, doi:10.25158/L5.1.9

Ministry of Social Justice and Empowerment (2016) THE RIGHTS OF PERSONS WITH DISABILITIES ACT, 2016A2016-49_1.pdf (legislative.gov.in) (Accessed on 26 March 2023).

Murphy RF, 'The Damaged Self', in P. Brown and S. Closser (eds), *Understanding and Applying Medical Anthropology* (London and New York: Routledge 2016).

Noddings N, *Caring: A Relational Approach to Ethics and Moral Education* (Berkeley: University of California Press 1986).

Ortoleva S and Lewis H, 'Forgotten Sisters – A Report on Violence Against Women with Disabilities: An Overview of its Nature, Scope, Causes and Consequences' [2012] *North-eastern University School of Law Research* Paper No. 104–2012. At: <http://ssrn.com/abstract=2133332> (Accessed 24 March 2023).

Patton C, *Sex & Germs: The Politics of AIDS* (Black Rose Books 1986).

People's Republic of China Passes "Eugenics" Law, (1994) Reproductive Freedom News (CRLP, New York, N.Y.), Dec. 2, 1994.

Pot A and others, 'iSupport: A WHO global online intervention for informal care-givers of people with dementia' [2019] 18 *World Psychiatry* 365–366.

Rainey S, *Love, Sex and Disability: The Pleasures of Care, Boulder* (Colorado: Lynne Rienner Publishers 2014).

Raman S, 'India's Laws Fail To Uphold Abortion Rights Of Women With Disabilities' [2021] *BehanBox*. Available at <India's Laws Fail To Uphold Abortion Rights Of Women With Disabilities – BehanBox>

Rodriguez PTV, 'Twice Violated – Abuse and Denial of Sexual and Reproductive Health Rights of Women with Psychosocial Disabilities in Mexico' [2015] Disability Rights International, Colectivo Chuhcan. Mexico-report-English-web.pdf (driadvocacy.org), Accessed 27 March 2023.

Sarkar T, 'Guardianship and Alternatives: Decision-Making Options' in I. L. Rubin and others (Eds.), *Health Care for People with Intellectual and Developmental Disabilities across the Lifespan* (Springer 2016).

Scholten M, Gather J, and Vollmann J, 'Das kombinierte Modell der Entscheidungsassistenz: Ein Mittel zur ethisch vertretbaren Umsetzung von Artikel 12 der UN-Behindertenrechtskonvention in der Psychiatrie' [The Combined Supported Decision Making Model: A Template for An Ethically Justifiable Implementation of Article 12 of the UN Convention on the Rights of Persons with Disabilities in psychiatry] 19 September (2022) Nervenarzt. German. doi: 10.1007/s00115-022-01384-1. Epub ahead of print. PMID: 36121451.

See Best K, 'Disabled Have Many Needs for Contraception, Network' [1999] 19(2) *Res Triangle Park N C Winter 16-8, quoting Meenu Sikand of the Canadian Association of Independent Living Centres' International Committee.*

Shah P and others, 'Informed Consent' in StatPearls [Internet]. Treasure Island (FL): StatPearls Publishing; 2023 Jan-. https://www.ncbi.nlm.nih.gov/books/NBK430827/ (Accessed on 24 March 2023).

Shakespeare T, *Disability: The Basics* (First edn, London: Routledge 2018).

Shildrick M, *Dangerous Discourses of Disability, Subjectivity and Sexuality* (London: Palgrave Macmillan, 2009)

Silver BC and others, 'Increasing Prevalence of Assisted Living as A Substitute for Private-pay Long-term Nursing Care' [2018] 53(6) *Health Services Research* 4906–4920.

Silvers A, Francis L, and Badesch B, 'Reproductive Rights and Access to Reproductive Services for Women with Disabilities' [2016] 18(4) *The AMA Journal of Ethics* 430–437.

Stalker K, 'Theorising the Position of People with Learning Difficulties Within Disability Studies' in N. Watson, A. Alan Roulstone and C. Thomas (eds), *Thomas, Routledge Handbook of Disability Studies* (Routledge London 2019)

Stanford Encyclopaedia of Philosophy, 'Critical Disability Theory', *Critical Disability Theory* (Stanford Encyclopedia of Philosophy 2019), Accessed on 24 March 2023.

Suchita Srivastava & Anr v. Chandigarh Administration, (2009) 14 SCR 989.

Suchita Srivastava & Anr vs Chandigarh Administration on 28 August 2009 (indiankanoon.org) (Accessed on 25 March 2023)

The care-giving conundrum: How to look after the disabled (downtoearth.org.in), Accessed on 24 March 2023.

The Medical Termination Of Pregnancy Act, 1971 ACT NO. 34 OF 1971 Microsoft Word – A1971-34.docx (indiacode.nic.in) (Accessed on 25 March 2023)

The National Trust Empowering Abilities, Creating Trust Trained Caregivers | Ministry of Social Justice and Empowerment (MSJE) (thenationaltrust.gov.in) 2023: National Trust for the Welfare of Persons with Autism, Cerebral Palsy, Mental Retardation and Multiple Disabilities (Amendment) Rules, 2015 notified on 04.02.2015.

The National Trust for Welfare of Persons with Autism, Cerebral Palsy, Mental Retardation and Multiple Disabilities Act, 1999.

Titchkosky T, 'Disability Studies: The Old and the New' [2000] 25(2) *The Canadian Journal of Sociology* 197–224.

United Nations Office of Human Rights, 'Vienna Declaration and Programme of Action', 1993

United Nations, 'Sustainable Development Goals (SDGs) and Disability' [2015] <Sustainable Development Goals (SDGs) and Disability | United Nations Enable> (Accessed on 24 March 2023).

Wetle T, 'Ethical issues and value conflicts facing case managers of frail elderly people living at home' in McCullough LB and Wilson NL (eds), *Long-term Care Decisions: Ethical and Conceptual Dimensions* (Baltimore: The Johns Hopkins University Press 1995).

World Health Organisation, 'Disability' [2023], <Disability and health (who.int)> (Accessed 24 March 2023).

World Health Organisation (2017) Evidence profile: caregiver support WHO-MCA-17.06.01-eng.pdf (Accessed on 24 March 2023).

World Health Organisation, 'Evidence profile: caregiver support' [2017] WHO-MCA-17.06.01-eng.pdf (Accessed on 24 March 2023).

PART IV

Health Governance, Security, and Transitions

8

JUSTICE IN GLOBAL HEALTH GOVERNANCE

The Role of Enforcement[1]

Daniel Elliot Weissglass

8.1 Introduction

The governance of global health systems falls chiefly on the World Health Organization (WHO), a United Nations body charged with promoting global health. The WHO provides guidance, directs resources, and is the source of several legally binding documents which direct global health efforts. Chief among these documents is the International Health Regulations (IHR), which binds its signatories to policies designed "[...] to prevent, protect against, control and provide a public health response to the international spread of disease in ways that are commensurate with and restricted to public health risks, and which avoids unnecessary interference with international traffic and trade"[2] where disease is construed broadly to include any "[...] illness or medical condition, irrespective of origin or source, that presents or could present significant harm to humans".[3]

The IHR, due to its broad scope and central mission, can be reasonably considered as the central document of global health law. Its scope runs considerably broader than the WHO's other legal instruments – the Framework Convention for Tobacco Control (FCTC) and the Pandemic Influenza Preparedness Framework (PIP) – which focus, respectively, on the control of tobacco products and the sharing of samples of novel influenzas.[4] Because of its breadth, the IHR creates a wide range of binding obligations for signatory parties, obligations including the development of health system capacities, the notification to the WHO of certain health events, the recognition of the WHO's authority to declare emergencies of international concern, the restriction of public health measures

DOI: 10.4324/9781003399933-13

to those minimally restrictive of international trade and travel, and standards for the resolution of disputes between parties about the interpretation of the IHR and its provisions. Despite some gaps in the underlying framework of the IHR, like the failure to embrace the close connection between human, animal, and environmental health,[5] it is the most significant effort yet made to establish a comprehensive system of global health governance.

The IHR is undermined, however, by a fundamentally political problem: noncompliance. Frequent noncompliance with the IHR, taken broadly to include all failures to fulfil the obligations specified therein, is a chief cause of the practical failures of the IHR.[6] While some noncompliance may be excusable, due to resource limitations, disaster, or states of emergency, no noncompliance is safe for the global community. While the way we will need to address noncompliance will likely differ based on the conditions that have brought it about, the elimination of all forms of noncompliance is a critical step to protecting global health.

The practical consequences of noncompliance are well-recognised, but the political consequences have been comparatively overlooked. In this chapter, I will explore these political consequences, focusing on the complex relationships between noncompliance and the normative foundations of the IHR, demonstrating that noncompliance erodes and is promoted by the erosion of noncompliance, and arguing that this cycle of noncompliance and normative erosion creates a practical and political necessity for systems of enforcement in future revisions of the IHR. First, I review some of the key provisions of the IHR and establish a pattern of pervasive noncompliance with those provisions. Then, I argue that this noncompliance creates not only practical, but political problems in virtue of it creating an environment for the perpetuation of both substantive and procedural injustices. Finally, I present a more rigorous model for ensuring compliance with global health law, which – through the use of limited enforcement powers – may serve to support and protect the normative foundations of the IHR.

8.2 The International Health Regulations: Provisions and Practice

The IHR creates a number of obligations for state parties, which can be roughly placed into three categories: health system development, notification to the WHO, and limits on public health measures. Each of these sets of provisions plays a critical role in preparing the global community to prevent the international spread of disease, and parties have committed to compliance with them – save for a few reservations made at the time the regulations were adopted.[7] However, as we will see, noncompliance with these provisions is well-known and commonplace, in some cases being more common than compliance.

8.2.1 Health System Development

Well-developed health system capacities are a critical piece of the prevention of the international spread of disease. Without appropriate surveillance, control, and care systems in place, the global system is unable to detect or respond to health events as they unfold. Accordingly, the IHR establishes a set of minimal health system capacities which all parties are required to develop. These standards, described at length in Annex 1 of the IHR, include surveillance systems capable of detecting potential health risks, systems to report detected threats, the ability to plan and implement emergency responses, and communication systems to coordinate these capacities.[8]

It was decided at the 61st World Health Assembly that state parties would submit annual evaluations of their compliance with these provisions.[9] Since 2015, these evaluations have been conducted using the State Party Self-Assessment Annual Report (SPAR), a tool which asks parties to assess their implementation of required capacities on a scale from 1 (critically under-developed) to 5 (developed). The SPAR includes 15 metrics, ranging across political and legal support, financing, laboratory systems, health surveillance, human resources, community engagement, etc. As the name suggests, this data is the product of state self-assessment, not external review. However, these data may be supplemented – at the request of a member state – by those drawn from several alternative sources: joint external evaluations (JEE) of a state party's health system development jointly undertaken by the state party and the WHO at the request of the state party, after-action reviews, and simulation exercises.[10]

An early warning of the current, and rather grim, state of noncompliance was the repeated extension of deadlines for the implementation of essential health capacities. The initial implementation deadline was 2012, with nations being permitted to apply for a two-year extension of this deadline by demonstrating both a need for the time and a plan to bring about implementation. A further two-year extension is permitted, but only under 'exceptional circumstances'.[11] However, the World Health Assembly granted them to all 81 states requesting them – making such an extension far from exceptional.[12]

Even with this extraordinarily permissive attitude, one which categorises the circumstances of more than a third of state parties as 'exceptional', the final deadline for capacity development should have been 2016. However, as of 2021, five years past this deadline, the WHO reported that the average regional implementation rate of all capacities is only 65%. At present, no WHO region reports complete compliance – with reported implementation rates ranging from 49% (AFRO) to 74% (EURO).[13] That is, even by state parties' self-assessment, noncompliance with requirements of health system capacity is commonplace.

The reality, in fact, is likely worse than it appears. Comparisons of the results of state self-assessments – then conducted with the International Health Regulations Monitoring Tool (IHRMT), a precursor to the SPAR – to those of JEE have shown that national self-assessments tend to over-estimate preparedness on each indicator by one step on the 1–5 scale.[14] Given the voluntary nature of the JEE, participation in this process is itself an indicator of good faith effort to meet capacity goals, and so we should be worried that not only is there widespread exaggeration of the sort indicated here, but that this exaggeration is – in general – probably even greater than the data suggest. On top of that, some state parties make no report what-soever, with 12 state parties having provided no report in 2021.[15] It is probable, given that this itself is a form of noncompliance, that states electing to make no report are worse-off than average. The clear indication is that noncompliance with provisions relating to the development of health system capacity is common and significant.

8.2.2 Notification to the WHO

The IHR requires member states to report any health threat which might qualify as a public health emergency of international concern, as well as any measures taken in response to that threat, within 24 hours of its detection. Annex 2 of the IHR provides a decision tool, which divides health threats into three categories. The first category includes particularly severe and rare diseases – such as smallpox, wild poliomyelitis, novel influenzas, severe acute respiratory syndrome (SARS), etc. – that must be reported if they are 'unusual or unexpected and may have serious public health impact'. The second and third categories – consisting of those posing somewhat less severe global threat (cholera, viral haemorrhagic fevers, West Nile, etc.) and of all other conditions that may significantly impact international public health – provide somewhat more discretion in the form of asking member states to assess whether the potential public health impact is serious, whether the threat is unusual, whether it might spread internationally, and whether there is a risk of trade restrictions. A case which is serious and unexpected, unexpected with the potential to spread, or with a significant risk of spread and a significant risk of international travel or trade restrictions must then be reported to the WHO.[16]

Beyond these cases, states may seek out the consultation of the WHO in support of their own disease control efforts. This voluntary practice allows a state to remain in communication with the WHO regarding unfolding health events and receive support on developing disease control measures. The WHO may also gather information through other channels, including reports from media or other unofficial sources. Likewise, state parties are expected to notify the WHO within 24 hours if they detect a potential threat in another country through the presence of imported or exported infected or contaminated humans, vectors, or goods. The WHO may then request verification from a state party, who should respond withing within 24 hours to acknowledge the request, provide available information, and conduct an assessment using the decision tool described in Annex 2 of the IHR.[17]

Noncompliance with these provisions may be somewhat harder to detect than noncompliance with others, as we only become aware of noncompliance through post-hoc investigations in cases where disease does, in fact, spread internationally. Cases of noncompliance where a legitimate threat was unreported, but never spread internationally, may not ever be discovered. Despite this, however, some investigations have shown significant instances of noncompliance. Significant delays in notification have been observed during outbreaks of SARS in 2003, novel influenza (H1N1) in 2009, Ebola in 2014, and COVID-19 in 2019. These delays come from a range of sources, indicating a wide range of failures in the notification system.[18]

Among the more innocent failures are those relating to limited surveillance capacity. During the H1N1 outbreak, the Mexican government reported cases quickly and responsively – once they were detected. The detection of this outbreak, however, was delayed by a lack of effective health surveillance systems. While an important demonstration of the interconnection of the provisions of the IHR, and the fundamental role of health system development in protecting global health, we can understand state parties in these circumstances as compliant with notification provisions, but not with developmental requirements.[19]

A similar sort of notification failure can result from complexities of state political systems. This is especially the case in federal governments, in which considerable power may sit with provincial or state governments rather than the national government. The limitations of federal systems were raised by the United States in its response to the IHR, where it indicated that the implementation of health systems would be left to the authority – state or federal – deemed appropriate by its laws. Iran, notably, indicated that it considered such reservations as fundamentally incompatible with the demands of the IHR – and an attempt to "[...] evade its due responsibilities and obligations".[20] The limits that federalism placed on state power to comply with the IHR were demonstrated in the 2005 SARS outbreak, when the Canadian federal government was unable to quickly collect data from the Province of Ontario due to the powers retained by provincial governments in the Canadian system. The WHO then issued a quasi-quarantine order for the city of Toronto to control the spread of SARS.[21] These problems, however, can also exist in unitary states – though in such cases often less due to the *de jure* powers of subnational governments, but as a product of limits in the structure of the public health system. This seems to have been a limitation in China's ability to respond to SARS, with it taking over a month for case reports to reach the national government – in part due to a complex chain through which such information had to be passed. China then redesigned its surveillance system significantly, with guidance from the WHO, to be less affected by these problems.[22] These cases, I think, are ambiguous between noncompliance with developmental provisions or notification provisions, depending largely on how one construes the scope of such agreements to apply to federalised or otherwise localised states.

In less innocent cases, however, failures of notification are the result of direct obstruction by local or national government. During the 2014 Ebola outbreak, Guinean authorities did not notify the WHO until more than two months after the first identifiable case of Ebola, neglected to report large number of deaths from a then-unknown disease on the border with Sierra Leone, and repeatedly downplayed the severity of the outbreak. Likewise, Sierra Leonean officials allowed only deaths confirmed by laboratory testing to be reported, a high standard which slowed reporting speed, and refused to share data with Médecins Sans Frontières (MSF), though they were responding to the outbreak.[23] In such cases, we have a clear indication of noncompliance with notification requirements per se.

8.2.3 Limited Public Health Measures

As an expression of its commitment to respecting the freedom of movement and limiting harm to international travel and trade, the IHR prohibits state parties from implementing public health measures which entail unnecessary imposition upon international travel and trade. These limits cite and express commitment to the importance of protecting principles of informed consent, respecting the concerns of travellers, providing appropriate accommodation for travellers, the protection of personal data, and more broadly respecting the dignity and protecting the rights of all people.[24]

These limitations generally prohibit invasive measures – including mandatory examination or vaccination – except when strictly necessary and require scientific evidence in support of both the efficacy and necessity of such measures when they are implemented. More broadly, state parties are required to implement only those health measures which are justifiable in virtue of the available scientific evidence. WHO recommendations are presumed to be based on such evidence, and therefore any measures recommended by the WHO are permitted. This includes any temporary recommendations pertaining to a public health emergency of international concern (PHEIC), a state of emergency which can be declared by the Director-General of the WHO, thereby enabling the WHO to make temporary recommendations regarding public health measures.[25]

State parties that elect to apply health measures that go beyond those implemented by the WHO and have significant impact on international traffic, where a 'significant impact' is considered as anything causing a delay of 24 hours or greater for travellers or goods, should provide the justification for such practices to the WHO within 48 hours. The WHO may then assess the implemented measure and may request the nation to abandon that measure. Other states impacted by the measure may also ask to consult the state which implements it.[26]

Despite these requirements, excessively restrictive or damaging public health measures are frequently implemented in response to global health events. After the H1N1 outbreak was declared a PHEIC, many nations implemented excessively severe restrictions of travel and trade – including quarantining travellers originating from Mexico, the United States, and Canada, quarantining citizens of those countries regardless of potential exposure, and the ban of certain imports. These practices continued despite the Director-General of the WHO urgently reminding nations of their obligations not to implement such measures. No state implementing these measures complied with the requirement that state parties submit public health measures in excess of WHO recommendations to the WHO with a justification of those measures. When the Ebola outbreak was declared a PHEIC, over 40 countries similarly exceeded recommended control, and only a few of those doing so reported the excessive measures.[27] This trend has continued to the present, and many members of the international community rapidly embraced destructive and illegal measures aimed to protect the health of their own population at the cost of significant harm to the well-being and rights of the international community, especially during the early days of the COVID-19 pandemic.[28] In fact, the severity and scale of these control measures seem comparatively greater than in the past, indicating that global compliance with public health measure limitations is decreasing over time.[29]

8.3 Noncompliance, Injustice, and the Normative Erosion of the IHR

We have seen that there is good evidence for relatively widespread noncompliance with the core provisions of the IHR. This pervasive pattern of noncompliance undermines the ability of the IHR to create a global health system suited to prevent the international spread of disease and severely limits the ability of the IHR to achieve its practical goals.[30] The COVID-19 pandemic has vividly demonstrated the consequence of noncompliance for the world; failures to develop capacity prevented state parties from identifying and responding to the emergence of COVID-19 appropriately, failures of notification left the globe slow to respond, and excessive public health measures catastrophically damaged the global economy, undermined global cooperation, and unduly restricted basic human freedoms while simultaneously diverting resources from more effective health control measures.[31] In no small part due to these failures, the costs of the pandemic were extraordinary. In terms of its economic cost, the world economy shrank by 3%, the output of 90% of countries was reduced, and the overall reduction in output was greater than in the Great Depression or either World Wars.[32] The human costs have been similarly horrific: the WHO has recorded over 700 million cases, and nearly 7 million deaths.[33] And, of course, these costs increase as the pandemic continues to unfold.

The problem of noncompliance, however, is not merely a practical one – it creates problematic political consequences in virtue of its perpetuation of pervasive injustice in the global health system. These injustices, in turn, undermine not just the practical success of the IHR – but its very normative foundation. Achieving compliance with the IHR is then not only important in improving global health outcomes, but also in bringing about a more just global health system and – critically – in maintaining the legitimacy of the global health system.

That the global health system is unjust is a near triviality, and even a passing review of the global health system reveals deep and impactful disparities that seem almost impossible to justify. Huge differences in health outcomes result from disparities in the social determinants of health, social factors – including healthcare access, education, availability of safe food and water, the design of public spaces, wealth, and others – that significantly impact health outcomes. Child mortality, for instance, is closely correlated with extreme poverty, rurality, female illiteracy, lower per-capita healthcare expenditures, fewer outpatient visits, limited access to safe water, poor sanitation systems, and low immunisation rates. As a result, children born in the worst-off regions of the world are roughly ten times more likely to die before the age of five than those born in the best-off regions of the world.[34] These disparities are both correctable and the results of forces well beyond the control of the individuals affected by them, so that it is implausible to justify them through appeals to the futility of intervention, failures of personal responsibility, or the making of poor choices. This is most vividly clarified by the disproportionate burden of these disparities on young children, who cannot be meaningfully expected to bear the consequences of global systems – nor to make and enact choices that would allow them to escape these consequences.[35] The (neo)colonial histories and presents of the global system demonstrate further that these circumstances should not be considered the responsibility of those suffering from them, and importance of these practices to the wealth of high-income countries (HICs) suggests a more appropriate locus of responsibility may be found. These practices – maintained in the modern context in the form of extractive loans and the purchase of natural resources which enrich kleptocratic and despotic leaders at the cost of the general public, policies which enable those leaders to embezzle their wealth and evade taxes, 'brain drain' through which low- and middle-income country (LMIC) health professionals are recruited by HICs, the enforcement of a global intellectual property regime which disadvantages LMICs, etc. – provide a clear indication that the responsibility for addressing global health disparity falls on the global community.[36]

In context of the urgent inequalities of the global health system, it is worth noting that accomplishing the practical goals of the IHR will both require and result in an improvement of global health justice. A key challenge for the implementation of the IHR is relative weak spots in the global health system which are not prepared to surveil the health of the local populace, provide care sufficient to promote their health, or implement public health measures to prevent further spread of disease. Such weak spots create the conditions for the emergence and spread of novel disease, create safe havens for diseases to mutate and evolve so as to bypass existing control measures, and make vulnerable the global economic and political system through creating pockets of unpredictable potential collapse. Accomplishing the goals of the IHR will require the expansion of health surveillance, healthcare, and public health systems to parts of the world currently doing without – this is the only way these weak spots might be strengthened Strengthening the global health system in this way will disproportionately benefit the worst-off, and thereby improve global health justice, in two ways.

First, fulfilling the capacity requirements of the IHR will directly require making substantial improvements to the access that the 'worst-off' have to health systems – from surveillance to care – by bringing the systems that cover those populations into compliance with the IHR's standards. This is, in effect, a sufficientarian precondition for the IHR's success; the IHR can only be successful if state health systems are brought up to a minimum standard of quality – which will in turn improve the actual circumstances of those subject to those systems. Building the global capacities required by the IHR will thereby significantly improve the situation of many of the worst-off.

Second, the effect of health capacities on reducing the international spread of disease will be most felt by the worst-off, as they are the most likely to suffer the consequences when disease spreads. During outbreaks, the health resources that are already difficult for the worst-off to access become even less accessible as health systems are overburdened and goods may be hoarded by those better-off. This is especially acute in market-based health systems, where goods are rationed according to one's ability to pay for them. Likewise, the worst-off are especially vulnerable to infection in the first place – poor living conditions, overcrowding, reliance on public transport, etc. make the worst-off both more likely to get ill and more likely to suffer serious effects. As a result, the health consequences of outbreaks will almost always fall disproportionately on the shoulders of those already worst-off.[37]

The worst-off are also at disproportionate risk of suffering the economic harms of outbreaks, as demonstrated during the COVID-19 pandemic, during which job insecurity and income loss were concentrated among members of vulnerable groups, within- and between- country inequality has also grown, and global poverty has increased for the first time this generation. Outbreaks both worsen existing inequalities and create new ones, and preventing them will both ameliorate existing injustices and protect against their worsening.[38] To the degree that compliance with the IHR is a path towards improving global health justice, noncompliance perpetuates an unjust global health system. At the very least, we can understand noncompliance as a sort of obstruction of justice, whereby noncompliant states prevent the global system from performing functions essential to its due efforts to carry our justice.

This obstruction, however, does not exhaust the injustices caused by noncompliance, and a second sort of injustice is brought about by the promise-breaking of parties to the IHR. Promise-keeping, at least those made under appropriate conditions, can be understood as a fundamental principle of justice – called by Rawls the 'principle of fidelity'. The principle of fidelity is an application of the principle of fairness – which states that each person is required to do their part as defined by just institutions in which they freely participate – to the act of promising. The act of promising is taken, by Rawls, to be governed by social rules, constituting an institution, which requires that one does what one promises unless certain, excusing conditions obtain. Accordingly, the principle of fairness requires that we complete those actions which we freely promise to undertake, so long as that institution of promising is just, the promise is made freely, and no excusing conditions obtain.[39]

Whatever else it may be, the IHR is, at least, a set of promises made by signing parties to one another. The signing of the IHR was voluntary, and – while there are many injustices in the global system – it seems unlikely that the practice of promising through the voluntary signing of treaties or other such documents will be found to be fundamentally unjust.[40] I'll presume, then, in the following, that compliance with the provisions of the IHR is required at least a matter of justice by the principle of fidelity, except when excusing conditions obtain. While excusing conditions do likely obtain in at least some cases – such as the inability of resource-limited nations to rapidly develop their health system capacities – the bulk of noncompliance is hard to see in this way, and the failure of states capable of meeting their obligations to do so seems a clear violation of the principle of fidelity. Importantly, the nature of the IHR and the scope of its agreements prevent us from taking a number of possible excusing conditions as being such. For instance, we cannot take the risk of the international spread of disease to excuse noncompliance with limits on public health measures, as that promise is specifically conditioned on in that context.

Understood as consisting of just promises, the failure of parties to comply with their promises under unexceptional circumstances represents a significant violation of the normative obligations of those parties. As such, it is appropriate to consider unexcused noncompliance a violation of justice. This would be the case even if no harm came as a result of this noncompliance, but noncompliance is rarely harmless. At the very least, complying states take on the costs of compliance with the presumption that other states will do so as well, creating a system of mutual benefit. When that presumption is violated, they end up the victim of a sort of fraud – by which they contribute to a purportedly common project while others free-ride, perhaps devoting resources owed to developing global health capacities towards outcompeting compliant states in other arenas. When such presumption is violated in a way that directly harms, or places at risk of harm, compliant nations – through non-notification or the imposition of unduly restrictive public health measures against reporting states – the injustice of such cases seems especially pronounced. As compliance may not always be in the best interest of an individual actor, it can be understood as a sort of premium that states pay, meant to be repaid by guarantees of compliance on the behalf of other state parties. When these guarantees fail, and other state parties are noncompliant, the compliant state has been harmfully misled.

Noncompliance with the IHR, then, contributes to substantive injustices – unfairness in the outcomes of the global health system – by perpetuating health disparities, as well as procedural injustice – unfairness in the processes of global health governance – through failures of promise-keeping. These injustices do not merely result in a global health system which is unfair, but they erode critical components of the normative justification for demanding compliance. We can understand this erosion as happening through at least three mechanisms: that systems which do not adequately consider the wellbeing of parties lose normative standing with respect to the neglected parties, that promises made to comply are conditioned on the compliance of others, and that a lack of consistent enforcement results in any enforcement being problematically inconsistent.

Generally, parties seem answerable to only the laws of communities which sufficiently include them – where such inclusion requires the ability to meaningfully participate in political functions, being treated with appropriate respect, and a fair opportunity to acquire wealth.[41] While we may have other important normative reasons for complying with a given law, political exclusion seems to undermine the normativity of law per se – and so the status of something as the law of a community which excludes us seems to have no clear normative implication for us. The international political order, it seems, importantly fails to include LMICs across many measures, but perhaps most vividly in its failure to allow a fair opportunity to develop wealth. The same colonial histories and neo-colonial presents discussed above make economic development unduly challenging for LMICs, and the special connection of the lack of inclusion in the ability to develop wealth and the substantive injustices of the global health system make this connection particularly potent. This gives good reason for LMICs to consider global health law itself as having little normative authority over their actions over their actions in context of widespread noncompliance which obstructs efforts made to remedy these injustices, such that unexcused noncompliance, in particular, can be taken as a continuing failure of the global community to appropriately include LMICs and their interests.

Likewise, the promises of the IHR can be plausibly understood as being conditional – implying obligation only if the circumstances upon which they are conditioned obtains. If, for instance, I promise to help a neighbour move so long as they move on a Saturday, I would not seem bound to help them move were they to move on any other day. We can understand promises of compliance to the IHR to be conditioned on the presumed compliance of others. That is, when state parties voluntarily consent to the terms of international law, as they do when signing a document like the IHR, they are committing themselves to the described exercise or limitation of their powers only insofar as other signees comply with the terms of that law. Sufficient violation of the presumption of general compliance may constitute an excusing condition sufficient to free parties from the obligations that they took on in virtue of their agreement to do so. This means that the regular violation of a mutual promise by some parties may therefore liberate other parties of the obligation to keep the promise made. The presumption of general compliance is most obviously apt when the noncompliance of others would require compliant parties to take on greater costs than reasonably expected – as would be the case were a party to comply with notification requirements in a context where other parties will not comply with limits on public health measures. In fact, fear of the economic and political costs of notification is often cited as a motivation for noncompliance with notification requirements.[42] The role of preconditions in determining obligations for promise-keeping suggests that this fear, given that much of those costs will result from noncompliant actions on the part of other parties, may be a potent normative, as well as practical, justification for noncompliance with notification.

Finally, while the consistent nonapplication of a set of obligations might at least seem superficially fair, the possibility of inconsistent application raises considerable concerns about procedural justice. Beyond patterns of noncompliance, we can see the irregular application of the IHR demonstrated by the WHO's practice in declaring PHEICs. The standards for deciding whether something is a PHEIC remain vague and have been inconsistently applied. In some cases, as for H1N1, the declaration of a PHEIC was extremely quick. In other cases, such as the 2014 Ebola outbreak, for which a

PHEIC was declared four months after confirming the state of the outbreak, it seems to have taken far too long.[43] Such irregularity is compounded by the relative lack of transparency in the PHEIC decision-making process, a lack of clear criteria, and the likelihood of state lobbying to influence the process given the significant economic and political consequences of such declarations.[44] The irregular application of the provisions of the IHR suggests deep procedural problems which undermine the trustworthiness of the procedure itself. This, in turn, may undermine the normative strength of demands to comply with the terms of the IHR. This is especially the case when provisions are applied in a way which is clearly inconsistent, preferential, and/or discriminatory. In such cases, parties – especially those harmed by this inconsistency – would seem to have a legitimate grievance and could, in extreme cases, be justified in considering the IHR no longer binding – at least as applied in practice.

This multifaceted erosion of the normative force of the IHR as a result of noncompliance may itself contribute to further noncompliance. There is good empirical evidence to suggest that the belief that both the perception of a system as being procedurally just and it being believed to be legitimate predicts compliance, at least for individuals.[45] Some have argued, similarly, that legitimacy, and the resulting internalisation of relevant norms, has been noted as a driver of state compliance with international law.[46] If this is right, then we should expect that state parties will be more likely to comply with the dictates of the IHR when those dictates involve appropriate procedures and legitimate authority. If noncompliance, in fact, erodes the normative force of the IHR as I have suggested, this means that the obligations of parties to comply become weaker. If the perception of normative force tracks this, then we should expect that noncompliance results in weaker perceived obligation.

This vicious cycle through which noncompliance erodes normativity and eroding normativity increases noncompliance, is a powerful case against the possibility of ensuring general compliance with the IHR merely through widespread normative assent – as this very assent is vulnerable to noncompliance. This relationship helps to explain a puzzling question: why should so many parties be noncompliant with the terms of an agreement that they have, in virtue of their signing it, claimed to take as normatively binding? As some noncompliance is unavoidable, emerging naturally from practical and normative conflicts between competing interests which demand the use of limited resources, it is hard to prevent the beginning of this process of erosion. We can imagine this as a sort of tragedy of the commons, a circumstance where the self-interested behaviour of the actors sharing a resource or benefit will, over time, erode that resource. Such circumstances make governance by conscience difficult, due to the powerful considerations of self-interest in favour of free riding.[47]

Key to note, however, is that it is not just the global health system – but the legitimacy of the global health system – which is our commons. Parties, then, need not be considered insensitive to normativity for our tragedy to occur – because the commons being eroded by noncompliance includes that normativity itself.

This peculiarly normative tragedy of the commons is especially dangerous and indicates that hopes for an effective model of global health governance chiefly through shared normative commitments[48] are not likely to succeed. To protect the commons that is the normative value of global health law, we need to alter the incentives of actors so that compliance is typically less costly than noncompliance. We need, that is, a system of enforcement. In doing so, we might replace the vicious cycle with a virtuous one, through which both the normative force of the IHR and compliance with it might be protected. That is, enforcement can not only stem the erosive force of noncompliance, but can repair the normative assessment of the IHR itself. In the final section of this chapter, I will explore paths towards enhancing the ability of the IHR to enforce its provisions.

8.4 Enforcement, Compliance, and Justice

The problem of noncompliance presents both practical and political problems for the IHR and the WHO and is frequently cited as a key obstacles to the success of the global health system.[49] Practically, the terms of the IHR being subject to widespread noncompliance has caused significant harm to the global community. Politically, this same noncompliance has created serious injustice in the global health system – in large part by creating what might be reasonably considered as excusing conditions for further noncompliance. This effect, undermining the normative fabric of the IHR itself, creates serious problems for some approaches which aim to prevent noncompliance – especially those operating chiefly through legitimacy and/or normativity. This, in turn, creates a need for enforcement powers sufficient to enforce promise-keeping not only to reduce noncompliance through enforcement but also to maintain the normative value of the IHR itself.[50]

The IHR's mechanism for enforcement is the dispute resolution process outlined in Article 56 of the IHR. The dispute resolution process is designed to help reach a consensus among state parties with conflicting views about how the provisions of the IHR should be understood or implemented. There are roughly three paths laid out in the IHR for dispute resolution. First, in the case of disputes between state parties who have committed beforehand to be subject to binding arbitration, the matter is referred to arbitration according to the Permanent Court of Arbitration Optional Rules for Arbitrating Disputes between Two States. Second, in the case of disputes between state parties, where at least one disputing party has not committed to binding arbitration, the resolution of dispute is left as a matter of negotiation – which may be carried out directly between disputing parties or with the involvement of the Director-General as mediator. Finally, in the case of disputes between the state parties and the WHO itself, the matter is referred to the World Health Assembly.[51]

The IHR dispute resolution mechanism leaves a lot to be desired as a tool of enforcement. Chiefly, this model of dispute resolution is voluntary, non-binding, and reduces the process to little more than political negotiation. While states are obligated by the IHR to seek dispute resolution, they are not obligated to actually resolve disputes. Likewise, use of arbitration and mediation is entirely voluntary. Though states may elect to submit to binding arbitration, this is also voluntary and – at least as recently as 2014 – no member state has so elected. Finally, both the direct negotiation between state parties and the referral of conflicts between the WHO and a state party to the WHA – a fundamentally 'majority rules' system – results in a system governed chiefly by political power and influence rather than legislation and/or scientific expertise.[52]

The fundamental failure of this approach to dispute resolution has been demonstrated in large-scale breakdowns of the global system during times of dispute. A key example of the consequence of the lack of substantive dispute resolution is given by the Indonesian government's 2006 with-holding of samples of a novel strain of influenza (H5N1) that had ex-hibited pandemic potential. The Indonesian government correctly noted that such samples might be used to create a vaccine for the strain of influenza, which would then be prohibitively expensive for LMICs – precisely those countries which would be expected to suffer most seriously from the outbreak. The resulting dispute was eventually resolved with the development of the PIP – a system for creating contracts between those sharing disease samples and those using them to create vaccines, meant to ensure that sample sharing is adequately incentivized. While a likely a step forward for international health law, despite the limitations of the PIP, resolving this dispute took over six years. Such a delay during a pandemic threat could have extraordinarily severe consequences.[53] Similarly, the threatened, though reversed, withdrawal of the United States from the WHO during the COVID-19 pandemic was claimed to be motivated by a US dispute with the WHO about the implementation of key provisions of the IHR – especially those relating to the declaration of PHEIC – in response to COVID-19. As a result of this unresolved dispute, the WHO nearly lost the support of one of its largest funders and a key source of technical support.[54] In both cases, disputes about the implications and implementations of global health law threatened to undermine the ability of the global health community to respond to health events.

This suggests that the IHR dispute resolution mechanisms need to be revised. A reasonable set of criteria for a successful revision is that we require the dispute resolution system to[55]:

1 Guarantee that a resolution is made;
2 Be able to react quickly in emergency situations;
3 Decide transparently and fairly;
4 Ensure the acceptance of and compliance with the decisions made;
5 Maintain friendly relations between involved parties;
6 Be realistically implementable.

Accomplishing these standards collectively would considerably improve the ability of the WHO to ensure compliance with the IHR.

A promising start towards such a proposal is a three-tiered system which begins with an initial legal opinion which might be appealed to an advisory body, the findings of which might then be further appealed to an adjudicative body.[56] An initial legal opinion can be provided quickly by a relevant expert – such as the Chief Legal Officer of the WHO, for disputes solely between state parties, or the Chief Legal Officer of the UN, for disputes including the WHO itself. This initial opinion could serve to give rapid guidance of a kind essential to the often time-sensitive concerns of the IHR, simultaneously serving to inform parties about the terms of compliance with the IHR and to expedite any further disputes about those terms. When parties wish to appeal an initial legal opinion, this appeal can be adjudicated by similar to that laid out in the current IHR, but strengthened through required referral to an advisory body, which might be an existing body (i.e., the UN Mediation Standby Team) or something tailor-made to handle disputes in the IHR. These advisory bodies are well-suited to allow parties to develop their own solutions to disputes and provide flexible problem-solving possibilities. If, after the decision of the advisory board, some party or parties remain dissatisfied, the issue may be appealed to an adjudicative body. As with the advisory board, adjudication may be referred to existing entities outside of the WHO – like the ICJ, though this would require some modification to permit the WHO to stand before the ICJ – or a WHO internal entity might be created for this purpose. Such an adjudicative body could serve to provide final, binding opinions.[57]

This proposal considerably develops the structure of the IHR's dispute resolution process, but should be expanded in several ways to achieve its goals. First, it is not clear that this proposal would address a problematic lack of transparency in the dispute resolution system of the IHR. Were we to generalise the existing rules for binding arbitration, based on the Permanent Court of Arbitration Optional Rules for Arbitrating Disputes between Two States, the proposed mechanism would inherit a confidentiality clause which would prohibit the findings of the arbitration from being shared without consent of all parties.[58] This constitutes a problematic confidentiality which prevents public findings except with the express agreement of the disputing states. This makes findings non-transparent, in turn preventing the development of something like case law – a defined, public consensus about the interpretation of the IHR honed through successive iterations of dispute resolution. Second, the ability of the WHO to enforce the findings of its adjudicative body remains unclear. As it is, the ability to make 'binding' solutions is significant, but the lack of enforcement powers means that the state parties may nonetheless have little reason to comply. Noncompliance with these findings would risk erosion of the legitimacy of the dispute resolution process, as described above.

Non-transparency and resulting concerns of lack of consistency are rather easily addressed. By requiring all stages of the process to be recorded and made openly available, parties to the IHR – and the international community at large – will be able to review the findings of the process. As both lack of transparency and inconsistency in application can constitute significant threats to procedural justice, this will help to ensure the just functioning of the global health system. Furthermore, by providing a process of progressive interpretation, this will reduce the space for future disputes in the interpretation of the IHR – as previous rulings will be available for reference and will serve as a kind of default initial legal opinion.

The creation of substantial enforcement powers is considerably more complex. A first step towards enforcement of the IHR might be accomplished already through the maintenance of a transparent dispute resolution – enforcement through public 'naming-and-shaming' of noncompliant states may serve to incentivize compliance through soft power and the diplomatic costs of being seen as a bad member of the international community. To bring this to full effect, however, the dispute resolution system will need to be active – not passive – and the WHO will need to work regularly to assess the compliance of state parties with the IHR. We can take these assessments to take the form of initial legal opinions in the broader framework, and parties wishing to contest their inclusion on such a list might do so through the appeals process described above.

Naming-and-shaming, however, isn't likely to be sufficient for enforcement purposes, given its dependence on informal incentives. A more substantial approach to enforcement could be had through conditional support – where certain kinds of support from the WHO are available only to members complying with the IHR and its regulations. One of the most common recommendations in the literature is of this kind: that the WHO should provide designated funds for the development of health systems in states with severe need, but that the receipt of those funds should be contingent on WHO oversight or the accomplishment of key developmental goals.[59] We could also make access to proposed insurance funds designed to reimburse nations for the costs resulting from compliance with notification conditional. These funds would reduce the incentive to not comply with notification provisions, hopefully improving compliance rates.[60] We might make access to these funds contingent on engaging in proper notification practices, refraining from punitive public health measures, etc.

There are good reasons to endorse conditional support as a useful tool for the WHO, but it is likely not sufficient for all purposes. Conditional support has two advantages as a model of enforcement. First, it provides support to nations in need – those lacking necessary resources for development and those suffering the consequences of their good global citizenship, in the cases given above. This actively incentivizes compliance. Second, it provides a real sense of consequence for noncompliant states, through lack of access to the relevant support. This, in turn, actively disincentivizes noncompliance. However, conditional support has one serious failing – it seems to provide weighty enforcement for LMICs that are dealing with scarcity, but would be much less compelling for HICs. This has problematic practical and political implications. Practically, such a strategy would be unlikely to significantly counteract HIC noncompliance. Politically, the result is a system which is disproportionately coercive on LMICs, raising concerns of politically inequity.

The relative immunity of HICs to enforcement through conditional support mechanisms can be partly addressed through the use of a stronger sort of conditionality, called 'outcasting'. The core idea of outcasting is that rules might be enforced by excluding those not complying with them from benefiting from certain cooperative enterprises.[61] While many aspects of the IHR – such as the right to request WHO aid in dealing with public health emergencies – are probably not the sort of thing that we would want to exclude even noncompliant states from, especially given that doing so would put the global community at greater risk of the international spread of disease, there are some provisions which might be effectively enforced this way. In particular, it may be advisable, under some conditions, to take non-notification and/or excessively limiting public health measures to exclude a party from protections against limiting public health measures implemented by other parties. This would provide a clear economic incentive to comply and would make non-notification for fear of the implementation of such policies much less appealing – as the costs of failure to notify may be much greater.

Outcasting is a powerful tool, and likely to be the most powerful that could be regularly deployed without disrupting the global health system more broadly. However, we might consider – in rare cases – that there could be value in a broader range of sanctions. Sanctions might range from fines placed on nations by the WHO, economic or political penalties enforced by the general membership of the WHO, etc. The type and extent of these sanctions would need to be carefully considered, however, given that sanctions have – at best – a mixed record and may worsen economic inequalities which underpin significant challenges in the global health system.[62] It is nonetheless possible that some sanctions, perhaps tightly targeted and widely supported, could be effective for specific cases. In general, however, we should aim to use the least disruptive measures possible to ensure enforcement – which will rarely include sanctions.

A possible structure for the enforcement process is to begin with naming-and-shaming noncompliant states through public announcements which identify their noncompliance, the actions that need to be taken to achieve compliance, deadlines for achieving benchmarks of compliance, and an indication of the enforcement actions to be taken if those deadlines are not met. Enforcement actions should, presumably, begin with the least coercive measures – likely exclusion from conditional support and/or less damaging forms of outcasting. If noncompliance persists, escalation to more severe outcasting may be appropriate. In rare cases, where the harm caused is exceptionally severe, other methods have failed, and sanctions appear likely to be successful, then these may be considered. Again, we should begin with the least severe and least coercive sanctions, and escalate only if necessary and justifiable. States could, of course, appeal their identification as noncompliant, the deadlines given to them to become compliant, the penalties threatened for continued noncompliance, or other terms of the enforcement process through the dispute resolution process described above.

Creating a stronger regime for global health law – one which is able to function when it is most at need – is a significant challenge. Widespread patterns of noncompliance demonstrate the failure of the IHR to do just this. While normative endorsement is a powerful driver of compliance, we cannot expect it to be enough in the case of global health law – evidenced, directly, by the existence of those patterns of noncompliance. Instead, a better-structured system of enforcement is required. This chapter has presented one possible model for such enforcement. That said, more fundamental than the particular model is the recognition that noncompliance erodes normative systems themselves, and therefore the normativity of global health law must be protected through some sort of enforcement action.

Notes

1 This chapter is the product of a long period of work and revision, beginning with a conference and ending with a number of fruitful exchanges with the editors of this volume. I want to thank the participants of the Justice in Global Health Workshop Series, and, in particular Himani Bhakuni and Lucas Miotto, the editors of this volume, for a wide range of helpful feedback and guidance – as well as for their patience with my sometimes painfully slow revisions.

2 World Health Organization, *International Health Regulations (2005)* (World Health Organization 2005) 10.
3 Ibid., 7.
4 Gostin LO, DeBartolo MC and Katz R, 'The global health law trilogy: towards a safer, healthier, and fairer world' (2017) 390 The Lancet 1918.
5 Ibid.
6 Ibid. See also Hoffman SJ, 'Making the International Health Regulations Matter' in Simon Rushton and Jeremy Youde (eds), *Routledge Handbook of Global Health Security* (Routledge 2014); Habibi R and others, 'Do not violate the International Health Regulations during the COVID-19 outbreak' (2020) 395 The Lancet 664.
7 World Health Organization, *Reservations to the International Health Regulations, 1969, 1970*).
8 World Health Organization, *International Health Regulations (2005)*.
9 World Health Organization, *Sixty-First World Health Assembly: Resolutions and Decisions, Annexes* (2008).
10 World Health Organization, *International Health Regulations (2005)*; World Health Organization, *Guidance Document for the State Party Self-Assessment Annual Reporting Tool* (2018); World Health Organization, 'e-SPAR: State Party Annual Report' 2021) <https://extranet.who.int/e-spar> accessed; World Health Organization, *Joint External Evaluation Tool: International Health Regulations (2005)*, 2022).
11 World Health Organization, *International Health Regulations* (2005).
12 Gostin LO and Katz R, 'The International Health Regulations: The Governing Framework for Global Health Security' (2016) 94 The Milbank Quarterly 264.
13 World Health Organization, 'e-SPAR: State Party Annual Report'.
14 Tsai F-J and Turbat B, 'Is countries' transparency associated with gaps between countries' self and external evaluations for IHR core capacity?' (2020) 16 Globalization and Health 1.
15 World Health Organization, 'e-SPAR: State Party Annual Report'.
16 World Health Organization, *International Health Regulations* (2005).
17 Ibid.
18 Burkle FM, 'Global Health Security Demands a Strong International Health Regulations Treaty and Leadership from a Highly Resourced World Health Organization' (2015) 9 Disaster Medicine and Public Health Preparedness 568; Ottersen T, Hoffman SJ and Groux G, 'Ebola again shows the international health regulations are broken: What can be done differently to prepare for the next epidemic?' (2016) 42 American Journal of Law and Medicine 356; Gostin LO, Habibi R and Meier BM, 'Has Global Health Law Risen to Meet the COVID-19 Challenge? Revisiting the International Health Regulations to Prepare for Future Threats' (2020) 48 Journal of Law, Medicine & Ethics 376; Aavitsland P and others, 'Functioning of the International Health Regulations during the COVID-19 pandemic' (2021) 398 The Lancet 1283.
19 Ottersen T, Hoffman SJ and Groux G, 'Ebola again shows the international health regulations are broken: What can be done differently to prepare for the next epidemic?'.
20 World Health Organization, *International Health Regulations (2005)* 61–62.
21 Burkle FM, 'Global Health Security Demands a Strong International Health Regulations Treaty and Leadership from a Highly Resourced World Health Organization'.
22 Ibid.
23 Ottersen T, Hoffman SJ and Groux G, 'Ebola again shows the international health regulations are broken: What can be done differently to prepare for the next epidemic?'.

24 World Health Organization, *International Health Regulations* (2005).
25 Ibid.
26 Ibid
27 Ottersen T, Hoffman SJ and Groux G, 'Ebola again shows the international health regulations are broken: What can be done differently to prepare for the next epidemic?'.
28 Habibi R and others, 'Do not violate the International Health Regulations during the COVID-19 outbreak'.
29 Gostin LO, Habibi R and Meier BM, 'Has Global Health Law Risen to Meet the COVID-19 Challenge? Revisiting the International Health Regulations to Prepare for Future Threats'.
30 Hoffman SJ, 'Making the International Health Regulations Matter'Gostin LO, DeBartolo MC and Katz R, 'The global health law trilogy: towards a safer, healthier, and fairer world'.
31 Aavitsland P and others, 'Functioning of the International Health Regulations during the COVID-19 pandemic'Gostin LO, Habibi R and Meier BM, 'Has Global Health Law Risen to Meet the COVID-19 Challenge? Revisiting the International Health Regulations to Prepare for Future Threats'Habibi R and others, 'Do not violate the International Health Regulations during the COVID-19 outbreak'.
32 International Bank for Reconstruction and Development/The World Bank, *Finance for an Equitable Recovery*, 2022).
33 World Health Organization, 'WHO Coronavirus (COVID-19) Dashboard' n.d.) <https://covid19.who.int/>.
34 Ruger JP and Kim H-J, 'Global health inequalities: An international comparison' (2006) 60 Journal of Epidemiology and Community Health 928.
35 Weissglass DE, 'Contextual bias, the democratization of healthcare, and medical artificial intelligence in low- and middle-income countries' (2021) Bioethics Bhalotra S and Pogge T, 'Ethical and Economic Perspectives on Global Health Interventions' in Garret W. Brown, Gavin Yamey and Sarah Wamala (eds), *The Handbook of Global Health Policy* (John Wiley & Sons, Ltd. 2012).
36 Bhalotra S and Pogge T, 'Ethical and Economic Perspectives on Global Health Interventions'Kirigia JM and others, 'The cost of health professionals' brain drain in Kenya' (2006) 6 BMC Health Services Research 1Benatar SR, Gill S and Bakker I, 'Global health and the global economic crisis.' (2011) 101 American Journal of Public Health 646.
37 Oxfam, *Pandemic of Greed: A wake-up call for vaccine equity at a grim milestone* (2022)Bhalotra S and Pogge T, 'Ethical and Economic Perspectives on Global Health Interventions'.
38 International Bank for Reconstruction and Development/The World Bank, *Finance for an Equitable Recovery*Blundell R and others, 'COVID-19 and Inequalities' (2020) 41 Fiscal Studies 291.
39 Rawls J, *A Theory of Justice* (Revised edn, The Belknap Press of Harvard University Press 1999).
40 This is an important feature of the IHR, and protection against concerns that the demands of the IHR – in its current form, or if granted the enforcement powers that I will suggest at the end of this chapter – might constitute a violation of sovereignty. One power of sovereign states seems to be the ability to bind themselves to agreements, just as autonomous individuals might sign a contract. Enforcing such an agreement, especially in ways defined by that agreement itself, seems unlikely to substantially impose on state sovereignty. That there might be concerns here about sovereignty was brought to my attention by Himani Bhakuni, an editor of this volume.

41 Duff RA, *Punishment, Communication, and Community* (Studies in Crime and Policy, Oxford University Press 2000).
42 Ottersen T, Hoffman SJ and Groux G, 'Ebola again shows the international health regulations are broken: What can be done differently to prepare for the next epidemic?'.
43 Ibid.
44 Gostin LO, DeBartolo MC and Katz R, 'The global health law trilogy: towards a safer, healthier, and fairer world'Gostin LO and Katz R, 'The International Health Regulations: The Governing Framework for Global Health Security'.
45 Walters GD and Bolger PC, 'Procedural justice perceptions, legitimacy beliefs, and compliance with the law: a meta-analysis' (2019) 15 Journal of Experimental Criminology 341.
46 Koh HH, 'Why Do Nations Obey International Law?' (1997) 106 Yale Law Journal 2599
47 Hardin G, 'The Tragedy of the Commons' (1968) 162 Science.
48 Ruger JP, 'Normative foundations of global health law' (2008) 96 Georgetown Law Journal 423Ruger JP, 'Global health governance as shared health governance' (2012) 66 J Epidemiol Community Health 653.
49 Ottersen T, Hoffman SJ and Groux G, 'Ebola again shows the international health regulations are broken: What can be done differently to prepare for the next epidemic?'Gostin LO, DeBartolo MC and Katz R, 'The global health law trilogy: towards a safer, healthier, and fairer world'Gostin LO, Habibi R and Meier BM, 'Has Global Health Law Risen to Meet the COVID-19 Challenge? Revisiting the International Health Regulations to Prepare for Future Threats'Gostin LO and Katz R, 'The International Health Regulations: The Governing Framework for Global Health Security'Hoffman SJ, 'Making the International Health Regulations Matter'.
50 A reasonable concern here is that enforcement may 'crowd out' other motivations, reducing any intrinsic motivation to comply with the policies of the IHR and hurting compliance overall. I am not certain as to whether 'crowding out' is a reasonable concern at the level of states, as I am not sure how meaningful it is to talk about their 'intrinsic motivation' is given their different 'psychology'. That said, whether crowding out would occur is an empirical question, and I would take the demonstration of its occurrence to be a serious consideration in opposition of my proposal. I owe my awareness of this concern to Lucas Miotto, an editor of this volume.
51 World Health Organization, *International Health Regulations* (2005).
52 Hoffman SJ, 'Making the International Health Regulations Matter'.
53 Ibid.
54 Maxmen A, 'What US exit from the WHO means for global health: Experts forsee troubles ahead as Donald Trump ends US relationships with the agency.' (2020) 582 Nature Gostin LO and others, 'US withdrawal from WHO is unlawful and threatens global and US health and security' (2020) 396 The Lancet 293.
55 Hoffman SJ, 'Making the International Health Regulations Matter'.
56 Ibid.
57 Ibid.
58 Permanent Court of Arbitration, *Permanent Court of Arbitration Optional rules for Arbitrating Disputes between Two States* (1992).
59 Gostin LO, DeBartolo MC and Katz R, 'The global health law trilogy: towards a safer, healthier, and fairer world'.
60 Ottersen T, Hoffman SJ and Groux G, 'Ebola again shows the international health regulations are broken: What can be done differently to prepare for the next epidemic?'.

61 Hathaway O and Shapiro SJ, 'Outcasting: Enforcement in domestic and international law' (2011) The Yale Law Journal.
62 Afesorgbor SK and Mahadevan R, 'The Impact of Economic Sanctions on Income Inequality of Target States' (2016) 83 World Development 1Haas RN, 'Economic Sanctions: Too Much of a bad Thing' (*Brookings*, 1998) <https://www.brookings. edu/research/economic-sanctions-too-much-of-a-bad-thing/> (Accessed 3 March 2023).

Bibliography

Aavitsland P and others, 'Functioning of the International Health Regulations during the COVID-19 Pandemic' [2021] 398 *The Lancet* 1283.

Afesorgbor SK and Mahadevan R, 'The Impact of Economic Sanctions on Income Inequality of Target States' [2016] 83 *World Development* 1.

Benatar SR, Gill S and Bakker I, 'Global Health and the Global Economic Crisis' [2011] 101 *American Journal of Public Health* 646.

Bhalotra S and Pogge T, 'Ethical and Economic Perspectives on Global Health Interventions' in G. W. Brown, G. Yamey and S. Wamala (eds), *The Handbook of Global Health Policy* (John Wiley & Sons, Ltd. 2012).

Blundell R and others, 'COVID-19 and Inequalities' [2020] 41 *Fiscal Studies* 291.

Burkle FM, 'Global Health Security Demands a Strong International Health Regulations Treaty and Leadership from a Highly Resourced World Health Organization' [2015] 9 *Disaster Medicine and Public Health Preparedness* 568.

Duff RA, *Punishment, Communication, and Community* (Studies in Crime and Policy, Oxford University Press 2000).

Gostin LO and others, 'US Withdrawal from who is Unlawful and Threatens Global and US Health And Security' [2020] 396 *The Lancet* 293.

Gostin LO, DeBartolo MC and Katz R, 'The Global Health Law Trilogy: Towards a Safer, Healthier, and Fairer World' [2017] 390 *The Lancet* 1918.

Gostin LO, Habibi R and Meier BM, 'Has Global Health Law Risen to Meet the COVID-19 Challenge? Revisiting the International Health Regulations to Prepare for Future Threats' [2020] 48 *Journal of Law, Medicine & Ethics* 376.

Gostin LO and Katz R, 'The International Health Regulations: The Governing Framework for Global Health Security' [2016] 94 *The Milbank Quarterly* 264.

Haas RN, 'Economic Sanctions: Too Much of a bad Thing' (Brookings 1998) <https://www.brookings.edu/research/economic-sanctions-too-much-of-a-bad-thing/>

Habibi R and others, 'Do not violate the International Health Regulations during the COVID-19 outbreak' (2020) 395 *The Lancet* 664.

Hardin G, 'The Tragedy of the Commons' [1968] 162 *Science*.

Hathaway O and Shapiro SJ, 'Outcasting: Enforcement in Domestic and International Law' [2011] *The Yale Law Journal*

Hoffman SJ, 'Making the International Health Regulations Matter' in S. Rushton and J. Youde (eds), *Routledge Handbook of Global Health Security* (Routledge 2014).

International Bank for Reconstruction and Development/The World Bank, *Finance for an Equitable Recovery*, (2022).

Kirigia JM and others, 'The Cost of Health Professionals' Brain Drain in Kenya' [2006] 6 *BMC Health Services Research* 1.

Koh HH, 'Why Do Nations Obey International Law?' [1997] 106 *Yale Law Journal* 2599.

Maxmen A, 'What US exit from the WHO means for Global Health: Experts Forsee Troubles Ahead as Donald Trump ends US Relationships with the Agency' [2020] 582 *Nature*

Ottersen T, Hoffman SJ and Groux G, 'Ebola again shows the International Health Regulations are Broken: What can be done Differently to Prepare for the Next Epidemic?' [2016] 42 *American Journal of Law and Medicine* 356.

Oxfam, *Pandemic of Greed: A wake-up call for vAccine Equity at a Grim Milestone* (2022).

Permanent Court of Arbitration, *Permanent Court of Arbitration Optional rules for Arbitrating Disputes between Two States* (1992).

Rawls J, *A Theory of Justice* (Revised edn, The Belknap Press of Harvard University Press 1999).

Ruger JP, 'Normative Foundations of Global Health Law' [2008] 96 *Georgetown Law Journal* 423.

Ruger JP, 'Global Health Governance as Shared Health Governance' [2012] 66 *Journal of Epidemiology and Community Health* 653.

Ruger JP and Kim H-J, 'Global Health Inequalities: An International Comparison' [2006] 60 *Journal of Epidemiology and Community Health* 928.

Tsai F-J and Turbat B, 'Is Countries' Transparency Associated With Gaps Between Countries' Self and External Evaluations for IHR Core Capacity?' [2020] 16 *Globalization and Health* 1.

Walters GD and Bolger PC, 'Procedural Justice Perceptions, Legitimacy Beliefs, and Compliance with the Law: A Meta-analysis' [2019] 15 *Journal of Experimental Criminology* 341.

Weissglass DE, 'Contextual Bias, the Democratization of Healthcare, and Medical Artificial Intelligence in Low- and Middle-income Countries' [2021] *Bioethics*.

World Health Organization, *Sixty-First World Health Assembly: Resolutions and Decisions, Annexes* (2008).

World Health Organization, *Guidance Document for the State Party Self-Assessment Annual Reporting Tool* (2018).

World Health Organization, *International Health Regulations (2005)* (World Health Organization 2005).

World Health Organization, *Reservations to the International Health Regulations, 1969,* (1970).

World Health Organization, *Joint External Evaluation Tool: International Health Regulations (2005),* (2022).

World Health Organization, 'e-SPAR: State Party Annual Report' [2021] <https://extranet.who.int/e-spar>

World Health Organization, 'WHO Coronavirus (COVID-19) Dashboard' (n.d.) https://covid19.who.int/

9

THE ETHICAL ISSUES RAISED BY THE SECURITISATION OF HEALTH

Ryoa Chung and Joanne Liu

9.1 Introduction

This chapter will discuss the contemporary phenomenon of the securitisation of health, which raises ethical issues that global health justice researchers and advocates must address. The concept, which sometimes overlaps with the notion of global public health security, is at the heart of burgeoning literature in international relations theory but is little discussed in philosophical terms. The contribution of this chapter is to shed philosophical light on the ethical issues raised by this phenomenon and to place them within the fields of international ethics and global health justice. This interdisciplinary exchange will also benefit political scientists, international lawyers, and global public health scholars.

The chapter is divided into two parts. The first part (Section 9.2) focuses on the intuitive relationship between *human security* and the *human right to health*. However, it is crucial to clarify the conceptual distinction between the latter and *securitisation of health*. In light of these distinctions, we can better identify the problematic tensions that the language of security introduces. The second part (Section 9.3) deals with the concept and phenomenon of securitisation of health. The securitisation of health is understood to protect national interests against health risks and gives rise to a form of health nationalism. We aim to clarify the terms and identify the slippery slopes to which the nexus of "health, peace, and security" can lead if we are not careful to defend the human right to health unconditionally.

DOI: 10.4324/9781003399933-14

9.2 Human Security and the Right to Health

First, it is essential to understand the primacy of the *human right to health* as a fundamental component of *human security*. We do not claim that health is the exclusive or even the most important dimension of human security but that the primacy of the human right to health must always prevail over the political language and considerations of security.

The international recognition of the right to health is enshrined in the founding Constitution of the World Health Organisation (WHO) of 1946. Health is described as "a state of complete physical, mental and social well-being and not merely the absence of disease and infirmity."[1] The mere notion of health gives rise today to substantial philosophical discussions concerning the distinction between the concepts of health and well-being (that the WHO Constitution does not establish) and the very polysemy of the concept of health.[2] However, according to the WHO definition: "The enjoyment of the highest attainable standard of health is one of the fundamental rights of every human being without distinction of race, religion, political belief, economic or social condition."[3] When included in Article 25 of the Universal Declaration of Human Rights, the right to health is embedded in a broader social conception of the minimum conditions for a decent human life and, more specifically, access to health care.[4] The Article states:

> Everyone has the right to a standard of living adequate for the health and well-being of himself and of his family, including food, clothing, housing and medical care and necessary social services, and the right to security in the event of unemployment, sickness, disability, widowhood, old age or other lack of livelihood in circumstances beyond his control.[5]

From the wording of Article 25, the relationship between health and security seems intuitively obvious. However, it was not until the 1990s that the notion of human security emerged within the United Nations (UN) community, following the publication of the 1994 Human Development Report, to designate the set of fundamental capacities that every person should be able to exercise and the primary resources everyone should be able to access to enjoy basic material security.[6] The UN definition of human security involves seven sectors, including health security interconnected with economic, food, environmental, personal, community, and political security.

The United Nations Development Programme developed the human security model to emphasise the fundamental interests of individuals and populations that ground the principles of international cooperation and solidarity. In many regards, this model was developed to counterbalance the notion of national security, especially when the perceived interests of states lead to the sacrifice of human rights, either of their nationals or non-nationals. When the *raison d'état* dictates the primacy of national interests in contexts of economic competition, political tensions, armed conflict, competition for scarce resources, or global health crises, among other scenarios, states will claim their right to national security to justify non-cooperation. However, some observers believe that integrating health issues into the security discourse helps elevate them to the level of high politics, where the survival of states is at stake, to capture the attention of governments.[7] If this is the case, it is necessary to take note of the perverse consequences that can arise from the securitisation of health, as we will try to illustrate in the following sections.

Analysing the conceptual genesis of the human right to health enables us to uncover the philosophical dimension. Numerous multidisciplinary analyses of the historical and political context of the post-World War II period shed light on the ethical aspirations, according to some, or the political negotiations of the new balance of power, according to others, which gave rise to the formation of the UN and its branches, including the WHO, the Bretton Woods institutions, and the Universal Declaration of Human Rights. Space does not permit us to go into detail on these historical considerations and their evolution, which is beyond our scope. However, significant philosophical work justifying a human right to health appeared in the late 20th and early 21st centuries. In the sphere of contemporary Anglo-American political philosophy, we can identify at least three major perspectives for thinking about the right to health: 1) a Rawlsian defence of access to health resources according to Norman Daniels; 2) a capability approach according to the economist Amartya Sen; and 3) a theory of basic rights according to Henry Shue.

A conventional reading of the Western history of ideas links the philosophical genesis of human rights to Kantian notions of dignity, of the intrinsic worth of every person who deserves respect for their moral status. In the aftermath of the Holocaust and amidst the still smouldering ruins of World War II, the preamble of the Universal Declaration of Human Rights used the vocabulary of Kant's practical philosophy and Enlightenment liberalism to express the inalienable nature of human dignity. However, in these times of decolonisation shaking all disciplines, with Western philosophy upfront, it is necessary to reveal the darkness that the Enlightenment overshadowed concerning misogynistic, racist, ableist biases that profoundly influenced the evolution of modern colonial medicine.[8] Nevertheless, for all the legitimate criticism that the UN paradigm and the Western liberal human rights tradition may raise, the recognition of a human right to health does not yet have a more successful alternative to channel the ethical aspiration to which it tends, and which can be translated, we believe, in all cultural contexts. Although we lack the means to engage in it ourselves in the space of this chapter, a broader intercultural dialogue on these fundamental issues is deeply needed.

In Western philosophical terms, several approaches converge on the idea that recognising a right to health can yield universal consensus. A first approach stems from the work of the philosopher Norman Daniels who, in the wake of the publication of John Rawls' *Theory of Justice*[9] and the debate on the need for public health care in the United States, has argued that the *right to health* means the *right to health care*. In his book *Just Health*,[10] Daniels extends the right to health to the full range of social determinants of health, arguing that health is something special insofar as it is a condition of possibility for equal opportunity. Daniels articulates more precisely the intuitive articulations of Article 25 of the Universal Declaration of Human Rights between health, access to health care, and social goods ("food, clothing, housing and medical care and necessary social services"). It is challenging to extract Daniels' work from its socio-cultural, political, and institutional context in the United States. However, it is not difficult to understand in what sense the absolute destitution or deprivation of the social determinants of health or lack of access to medical care represents a morally disturbing limitation on the opportunities available to human beings, regardless of any particular cultural context.

A second perspective on the right to health is the capability approach, developed by the economist Amartya Sen, laureate of the 1998 Nobel Prize in Economics and a philosopher in his own right. There are real philosophical tensions between the Rawlsian approach to resources and the capability approach. However, both Norman Daniels, following his theory of distributive justice in health and Amartya Sen, following his capability approach, subscribe to the social determinants of health framework developed by the British social epidemiologist Michael Marmot[11] and significantly contribute to its philosophical foundation. For Sen,[12] the Rawlsian paradigm of formal rights ensuring access to resources is insufficient to guarantee individuals the capacity to convert these resources into effective functioning according to their free choices. In other words, a right to health understood as purely formal access to health care is not enough to guarantee the actual ability to be healthy if the individual lacks the means to feed herself well, live in suitable housing, find transport to reach a health clinic, in all safety, and ultimately exercise meaningful agency. Thus, the capability approach aims to be more encompassing and multidimensional based on what individuals can freely choose to do and to be in their living conditions.

For Sridhar Venkatapuram,[13] the emphasis on access to treatment or quantifiable individual or population health measurements through medical interventions at the national or international level is understandable but masks the real problem. Injustice is at the heart of Venkatapuram's work because if it is true that the socio-political arrangements that determine the more or less unequal entitlements between individuals have a real impact on health inequalities, then we need to think about health justice in societal terms. Our purpose is not to endorse any particular view but to demonstrate that despite the conceptual divergences between Rawls and Sen, Daniels and Venkatapuram, the capability approach to health expresses the same fundamental moral idea at the core of the human right to health: "every human being has a moral entitlement to a capability to be healthy, and to a level that is commensurate with equal human dignity in the contemporary world."[14]

Finally, Henry Shue's basic rights approach best explains the intuitive relationship between health and human security while also allowing us to highlight the intrinsic value of a basic right to health. In Shue's seminal book *Basic Rights. Subsistence, Affluence, and US Foreign Policy*,[15] the author defines three categories of basic rights that underpin all other rights. The basic rights to subsistence, security, and freedom are not defined in terms of the classic dichotomy between negative and positive rights. Shue famously argued that negative rights (protecting the individual from external interference in her private sphere) necessarily imply positive rights (i.e., positive duties and actions incumbent on others or society to ensure an individual's right). According to Shue, the right to health corresponds to a basic right to subsistence, as does the right to food, while the right not to be physically assaulted corresponds to the basic right to security. Shue's philosophical analysis clarifies that the right to enjoy basic health (i.e., access to basic health care) is a condition of subsistence that falls under the right to life. The right to security, in turn, guarantees the protection of physical integrity against any form of external aggression, which includes collective or institutional means to contain arbitrary violence. These three sets of rights to subsistence (right to health, right to food), security (institutional protection against arbitrary violence), and freedom (institutional protection of fundamental political freedoms) are intimately related but conceptually distinct in ensuring the conditions for minimally decent human existence and meaningful agency. To clarify our point, we stress that the minimum enjoyment of the basic rights to subsistence, security, and freedom determines the threshold of a *minimally decent human existence* that is not entirely incapacitated by absolute destitution.

These three philosophical perspectives, however divergent in their theoretical articulation, demonstrate that the right to health rests on an autonomous justification in all views. The right to health represents a fundamental component of a minimally decent human existence that help us to flesh out more concretely the notion of dignity. As such, we argue that the right to health can be translated into the language of fundamental interests, primary social goods, capabilities, or universalisable basic rights.

9.3 The Securitisation of Health in the Name of National Interests

The purpose of this section is to demonstrate that the right to health is unconditional. Although the relationship between health and human security arises naturally in what should be understood as the conditions for a minimally decent human existence, the political language of security can have perverse consequences. As Colin McInnes argues:

> Despite the interest generated in human security in some quarters, and its apparent complementarities with the increased interest in humanitarianism and poverty relief at the turn of the millennium, human security has failed over the last decade to establish itself as the main security narrative. (... ...) Human security is 'slippery by design' (...), a concept that is kept deliberately vague to ensure maximum support from diverse constituencies, but that then makes it ultimately little more than a slogan.[16]

The justification for a human right to health is morally primary, self-sufficient, and conceptually more precise than the notion of human health security. There is no question that good health will produce positive externalities, and there is substantial research to demonstrate the relationship between health, stability, security, and peace.[17] From a strictly prudential point of view, it is understandable why the language of security was mobilised to convince state actors to participate in international cooperation by appealing to their rational interests. The call by WHO Director-General Dr. Tedros for the *Global Health for Peace Initiative* (2023),[18] linking good global health and international peace, undoubtedly aims to converge ethical aspiration and political motivation. However, it is imperative to ground global health policy in the human rights approach, as advocates of "universal health coverage for the global health security architecture"[19] stress. Indeed, as we will demonstrate in the following paragraphs, in the absence of an unconditional and primary defence of the human right to health, the health-security-peace nexus may suggest that health issues are only worthy of consideration when they ensure international political and economic stability in general and the safeguard of national interests in particular.

The securitisation of health refers to the phenomenon whereby health issues are elevated to national security interests.[20] This notion has appeared in the international studies literature since the 9/11 attacks and must be distinguished from human security (which encompasses health in a broader conception of the fundamental interests of every human being). Long before the expression was coined, health risks have preoccupied countries since the Middle Ages and the development of maritime trade and introduced forms of coordination (rather than cooperation) to put in place standard rules of health security in port cities, involving, in particular, the quarantine of suspicious merchant ships. At the turn of the 19th century, cholera, yellow fever, and bubonic plague were the topics of intergovernmental meetings whose agenda was set by the European powers.[21] In the 20th and 21st centuries, global health issues include the risks of bioterrorism, HIV-AIDS, infectious diseases with the potential for regional epidemics (Ebola, yellow fever) or pandemics (influenza, H1N1, MERS, SRAS CoV-2), antimicrobial resistance or the emergence of new human viruses such as zoonoses. Public health imperatives may take precedence over individual freedoms in specific circumstances of health emergencies as stipulated in 1984, the *Siracusa principles on the limitation and derogation provisions in the International Covenant on Civil and Political Rights*. But restrictions on human rights:

> must meet standards of legality, evidence-based necessity, proportionality, and gradualism, (... ...) public health can be used as grounds for limiting certain rights if the state needs to take measures 'aimed at preventing disease or injury or providing care for the sick and injured."

The World Health Organisation (1948) is an intergovernmental structure mandated to determine and implement the International Health Regulations (1969).[22] Member states finance the WHO from contributions based on the GDP and population of each state. The United States and the wealthiest countries are the most significant contributors. Voluntary funding of public and private organisations includes partnerships with the pharmaceutical industry and charities and private actors such as the Bill and Melinda Gates Foundation. In this complex constellation of actors in global health governance, the role of states remains crucial, though weakened by the growing influence of prominent non-state actors in philanthropy, which must be correlated with the undeniable importance of their donations, representing 30% of voluntary donations to WHO. The unequal power of influence is undoubtedly reflected in WHO's public agenda-setting without being subject to public accountability mechanisms. Ted Schrecker[23] claims that the world order has now shifted to a post-Westphalian paradigm to capture salient features of our contemporary globalised era. However, Schrecker argues that these claims overstate that state sovereignty has been substantially eroded. The power of states continues to set the agenda of health issues in the international sphere. The relative strength of countries in the global political and economic arena determines who gets to mobilise resources and to fix priorities. The historical evolution of global health is inseparable from power relations and national interests, which are, by definition, played out on a supra-individual scale. In the words of McInnes, Lee and Youde:

> The determinants and outcomes of global health are not equal, nor is the manner in which issues are constructed and solutions articulated.

The nature of global health is intrinsically political, reflecting power relations which play a significant role in whether various groups can set the political agenda and/or claim resources.[24]

The most disquieting consequence of the contemporary phenomenon of the securitisation of health in the name of national security is the *subordination of basic human rights*. The global order is deeply embedded in a statist conception of the precedence of state sovereignty over fundamental human rights of their nationals or populations outside their borders. The clash between the securitisation of health and the human right to health can be illustrated in at least three ways.

The notion of securitisation of health became more familiar in political discourse after the 9/11 attacks to refer to the threat of bioterrorism and chemical weapons at the heart of the 21st-century national security agenda. However, according to Elbe, who adopts a Foucauldian analysis of biopower, the "medicalization of insecurity"[25] refers to the phenomenon whereby, in addition to the traditional issues of hostility and armed threats from other countries, the identification of health issues and the economic consequences and political instability they entail is added as a source of national insecurity understood in medical terms. The HIV/AIDS crisis in the 1990s is emblematic in this respect, as is the Ebola crisis.[26]

Our first illustration of the securitisation of health at the expense of the human right to health draws from the SARS-Cov-2 pandemic, which shook the world to its core. One of the highlights of the COVID-19 pandemic that needs to be analysed is how countries implement containment measures internationally. In unprecedented global circumstances, the closure of borders for understandable health precautions raises fundamental questions about the double standards of rich and low and middle-income countries and the precariousness of the human rights of individuals caught up in global quarantine. The predatory race by the most affluent countries to procure SARS-Cov-2 vaccines is one of the most disturbing examples of the securitisation of health at odds with international cooperation[27] and global health ethics.[28] In philosophical terms, it is essential to explain how the phenomenon analysed in international studies under the term of health securitisation must be tied to the philosophical notion of moral partiality in favour of co-nationals. Our goal is to demonstrate the conceptual and ethical pitfalls of health nationalism.

In the name of a consequentialist division of labour, one can coherently justify that ensuring the vaccination of one's population is the duty of each responsible government. Some authors argue that a certain degree of moral partiality towards one's co-nationals can be defended in a global health crisis.[29] However, the logic of the securitisation of health disproportionately exacerbates health nationalism, as we have seen during the pandemic.

In July 2021, 75% of the Canadian population had received the first dose of the vaccine, while only 1% of the population received the first dose of the SARS-CoV-2 vaccine in the poorest countries. South Africa and India, which had to deal with the Delta variant and a second tragic wave in the spring of 2021, were the instigators of a request to the World Trade Organization (WTO) in October 2020, supported by nearly a hundred countries, asking for the waver of pharmaceutical patents on vaccines in the context of a global health crisis. The wealthiest countries, including the United Kingdom, Canada, Japan, and the UE, rejected this proposal. Instead, they donated their surplus disorganisedly, despite the efforts of the WHO to set up novel international cooperation mechanisms such as the COVID-19 Tools Accelerator and COVAX, designed to assist vaccines purchase and distribution, and sometimes sending hundreds of thousands of close to expired vaccine doses to countries unable to compete in the open market.

Despite the moral call of the WHO for "vaccine equity" and appeals to the generosity of affluent countries, the rationale behind COVAX does not question the relevance of patents and testifies to a logic of capitalist philanthropy which refuses to change the TRIPS Agreement. Indeed, the logic of economic profits that benefit pharmaceutical giants and the countries that host them runs counter to the claim that COVID-19 vaccines (and vaccines in general) are global public goods, i.e., goods that are non-rivalrous and non-excludable,[30] in the name of human rights to health and principles of global health solidarity.

The second illustration of the securitisation of health is the instrumentalisation of health issues in the context of armed conflict or violent political tensions. The provision of health care by US troops in Afghanistan or Iraq in order to "win hearts and minds" (following Colin Powell's credo that humanitarian aid programmes were a "multiplier force" of US foreign affairs), military offensives against hospitals and health workers in the context of the war in Syria, the use of vaccination campaigns in Pakistan by the CIA to flush out Osama Bin Laden have all contributed to this instrumentalisation of health for national security purposes.[31] From the war in Syria to the attack on the children's hospital in Mariupol, Ukraine, to the US bombing of the MSF hospital in Kunduz, Afghanistan, many other examples tragically illustrate this phenomenon.

Health facilities and personnel represent soft targets, i.e., a target that opposes no defence and is vulnerable to military attack. Regarding empirical analysis, health facilities and personnel are collateral damage arguably more frequent in the context of armed conflict in urban settings. They also become victims of deliberate attacks when no other strategically significant targets remain in the context of complete devastation, as in South Sudan. It is important to consider that religious communities, health clinics, and hospitals are usually the last points of supply for essential goods in survival ecosystems. The MSF (*Médecins Sans Frontières/Doctors Without Borders*) report published in July 2014, *South Sudan Conflict: Violence Against Healthcare* under the international presidency of Dr. Joanne Liu, describes the patients murdered in their beds or lost without trace in the chaos of military attacks. When the last operating INGOs and the International Red Cross become targets of deliberate attacks, hundreds of thousands of people are deprived of primary medical care. The long-term impact is the collapse of the basic structures of health systems for generations to come in these affected countries. In 2016, the Security Council adopted Resolution 2286, co-sponsored by more than 80 Member States.

> The 15-member Council strongly condemned attacks and threats against the wounded and sick, medical personnel and humanitarian personnel exclusively engaged in medical duties, their means of transport and equipment, and hospitals and other medical facilities. It deplored the long-term consequences of such attacks for the civilian populations and health-care systems of the countries concerned. (... ...) The Council demanded that all parties to armed conflict comply fully with their obligations under international law, including international human rights law, as applicable, and international humanitarian law, in particular, their obligations under the Geneva Conventions of 1949 and their Additional Protocols of 1977 and 2005.

Leonard Rubenstein's remarkable book, *Perilous Medicine. The Struggle to Protect Health Care from the Violence of War*[32] provides a comprehensive analysis of case studies and testimonies about the growing violence against health facilities, their staff, and the countless victims. It also presents two conceptions of *jus in bello*, i.e., the normative principles governing military actions in wartime. During the American Civil War, Francis Lieber, a German-American jurist-philosopher, authored *the Code for the Government of Armies in the Field* (1863). *The Lieber Code* undoubtedly echoes a Clausewitzian theory of war and presents a philosophical and systematic defence of the position that all means are justifiable to end a just war as quickly as possible. In many ways, Lieber's philosophical position is reminiscent of General Sherman's credo "War is Hell" and of his strategic justification of the "scorched earth policy" he deployed during the American Civil War (notably to justify the great burning of the city of Atlanta so that it could not be used as a military base for the Confederate States Army, thus causing the exodus and distress of the non-combatant civilian population).

On the other side of the Atlantic, amid the Napoleonic Wars in Italy, the Swiss businessman Henry Dunant witnessed one of the bloodiest battles in the hell of war, the Battle of Solferino (1859). The traumatic experience led him to found the International Red Cross. The principle of humanity was at the heart of the rescue efforts he mobilised with the help of women from neighbouring villages to care for the wounded soldiers regardless of their French, Piedmontese, or Austrian nationality. They only managed to rescue a few hundred soldiers among the 38,000 soldiers lying dead or alive on the battlefield. Since the foundation of the International Red Cross by Henry Dunant, international humanitarian law and the Geneva Conventions condemn attacks on health facilities and personnel, as well as on non-combatant civilian populations in need of care, as violations of *jus in bello*, i.e., as war crimes.[33] From a philosophical perspective, it is crucial to emphasise that these crimes violate fundamental human rights and that the genesis of international humanitarian law is historically embedded in the right to primary health care. Upholding Dunant's legacy, Rubenstein reiterates the need to protect the humanity and dignity of healthcare workers and non-combatant patients. The international community must hold the perpetrators of these immoral abuses accountable for their war crimes. Dr. Joanne Liu forcefully decried in front of the Security Council the repeated violations of Resolution 2286 that are left unpunished and without sanctions.[34]

The securitisation of health serves both the logic of belligerents in conflict and the instrumental reasoning of morally selfish states. The defence of the human right to health without conditionality is imperative. Some may consider our theoretical defence a futile goal. On the contrary, we argue for the necessity of realigning the political discourses in global health and disentangling the human right to health from the language of security. In the absence of any other more robust alternative, all advocates of global health cooperation should endorse the human rights paradigm to counterbalance the securitisation of health in the name of national interests.

9.4 Conclusion

A third and final illustration of the ethical issues raised by the securitisation of health must be presented briefly in conclusion. Refugees, asylum seekers, and irregular migrants driven by political persecution, economic distress, or climate pressures raise severe health issues, not least because the international community leaves behind these populations as they fall into the interstices of no-man's-land between national borders.[35] They are no longer constituents of any country and have no political voice; they depend solely on humanitarian assistance to care for their health needs. However, these migrant populations are perceived as threats to national communities' social and economic instability, which justifies the erection of borders in the name of national security (in some cases, literally barbed wire borders and walls are built as in Hungary and the United States). More recently, Belarus instrumentalised the threat of chaotic illegal migration by leading irregular migrants to the borders of Poland, the point of entry into the European

Union (mostly Iraqi Kurds, likely hundreds, who were thus stranded in a dense forest between the two countries). In the 21st century, "illegal" migration is widely considered a source of national insecurity.[36] The securitisation of health will only exacerbate the perceived threat they pose to the health of national constituents.

Among the selection criteria for new migrants or refugees, the "reasonable public burden on the health system" criterion is often invoked to reject most asylum seekers. This instrumentalisation of health issues in the name of national security has historically been used to justify discriminatory and racist immigration policies – as evidenced by the history of Asian immigration turned away from Angel Island in California and banned by the Chinese Immigration Act of 1923–1947 in Canada.[37]

The Canadian government has now reversed Conservative Prime Minister Harper's suspension of refugee health care by tripling the amount available for refugee care, thereby significantly relaxing the "public charge" criterion. Nevertheless, we argue that the "medicalisation of citizenship," by which we mean the rejection of migrants' request for citizenship on the grounds of health concerns, will become a growing phenomenon if the securitisation of health is not counterbalanced with the recognition of universal human rights. In an era of pandemics, global warming pushing climate refugees to flee,[38] and the rise of xenophobic movements worldwide, the securitisation of health will also determine national admission policies, mainly the exclusion of immigrants and refugees. From a philosophical point of view, we argue that the fundamental right not to be discriminated against based on one's health needs is an essential dimension of the human right to health.

Our contribution is to offer a philosophical reflection on the ethical issues raised by the securitisation of health in the name of national interests that should concern political theorists, international lawyers, humanitarian assistance, and global health scholars and actors. Unless another theoretical and practical alternative proves to be more successful in order to challenge the statist world order, we should endorse and strengthen the human right to health approach in order to promote and implement principles of solidarity and international cooperation in the face of the global health challenges that await us in the 21st century.

Notes

1 World Health Organization (WHO), Constitution of the World Health Organization (1946).
2 Blaxter MB, *Health* (Polity Press 2010).
3 Preamble, WHO Constitution (n 1).
4 Wolff J, *The Human Right to Health* (WW Norton & Company Ltd 2012).
5 United Nations General Assembly, The Universal Declaration of Human Rights (UDHR). (New York: United Nations General Assembly 1948).

6 United Nations Development Programme, Human Development Report 1994: New Dimensions of Human Security (New York 1994).

7 McInnes C and Lee K, Youde J, 'Global health Politics: An Introduction' in McInnes C, Lee K, Youde J (eds.), *The Oxford Handbook of Global Health Politics* (Oxford University Press 2020).

8 Cleghorn E, *Unwell Women. Misdiagnosis and Myth in a Man-Made World* (Dutton 2021); Downs J, *Maladies of Empire. How Colonialism, Slavery, and War Transformed Medicine* (Belknap Press of Harvard University Press 2021); Richardson E, *Epidemic Illusions. On the Coloniality of Global Public Health* (MIT Press 2020).

9 Rawls J, *A Theory of Justice* (Belknap Press of Harvard University Press 1971).

10 Daniels N, *Just Health. Meeting Health Needs Fairly* (Cambridge University Press 2012).

11 Marmot M and Wilkinson RG (co-eds), *Social Determinants of Health* (Oxford University Press 2nd edition 2005).

12 Sen A, *Development as Freedom* (Oxford University Press 1999).

13 Venkatapuram S, *Health Justice. An Argument for the Capabilities Approach* (Polity Press 2011).

14 ibid. 19.

15 Shue H, *Basic Rights. Subsistence, Affluence, and US Foreign Policy* (Princeton University Press, 1980).

16 McInnes C, 'The Many Meanings of Health Security' in Youde J and Rushton S (eds.), *Routledge Handbook of Global Health Security* (Routledge 2015) 13.

17 Davies SE, *Global Politics of Health* (Polity Press 2010).

18 World Health Organization, Global Health for Peace Initiative (2023), https://www.who.int/initiatives/who-health-and-peace-initiative Accessed 30 March 2023.

19 Arush L et al., 'Pandemic Preparedness and Response: Exploring the Role of Universal Health Coverage within the Global Health Security Architecture' [2022] *The Lancet* 10.

20 Elbe S, *Security and Global Health* (Polity Press 2010).

21 Cueto M, 'The History of International Health: Medicine, Politics, and Two Socio-Medical Perspectives, 1851–2000' in McInnes C, Lee K, Youde J (eds.), *The Oxford Handbook of Global Health Politics* (Oxford University Press 2020).

22 Gostin LO, *Global Health Law* (Harvard University Press 2014).

23 Schrecker T, 'The State and Global Health' in McInnes C, Lee K, Youde J (eds.), *The Oxford Handbook of Global Health Politics* (Oxford University Press 2020).

24 C. McInnes and K. Lee, J. Youde, 'Global health Politics: An Introduction' in McInnes C, Lee K, Youde J (eds.), *The Oxford Handbook of Global Health Politics* (Oxford University Press 2020) 8.

25 Elbe S and Voelkner N, 'The Medicalization of Insecurity' in Youde J and Rushton S (eds.), *Routledge Handbook of Global Health Security* (Routledge 2015).

26 Heymann DL et al., 'Global Health Security: The Wider Lessons from the West African Ebola Virus Disease Epidemic' [2015], *The Lancet* 385.

27 Liu J and Chung R, 'Capitalist Philanthropy and Vaccine Imperialism' [2021] *The Hastings Center Bioethics Forum Essay.*

28 Benatar S and Brock G, *Global Health and Global Health Ethics* (Cambridge University Press 2011).

29 Emanuel E et al., 'On the Ethics of Vaccine Nationalism: The Case for Fair Priority for Residents Framework' [2021] *Ethics & International Affairs.*

30 Kaul I, Grunberg I, Stern M (co-eds), *Global Public Goods. International Cooperation in the 21st Century* (Oxford University Press 1999).

31 Chung R, 'The Securitization of Health in the Context of the War on Terror. National Security and Global Health: The Conflict of Imperatives' [2017] *Medicine, Conflict and Survival* 33(1).
32 Rubenstein L, *Perilous Medicine. The Struggle to Protect Health Care from the Violence of War* (Columbia University Press 2021).
33 Allhoff F and Potts K, 'Medical Immunity, International Law and Just War Theory' [2019] *J R Army Med Corps* 165(4).
34 Liu J, International President of MSF Address to the United Nations Security Council, first speech May 3rd 2016, second speech September 28ᵗʰ 2016: https:// www.doctorswithoutborders.org/latest/address-dr-joanne-liu-united-nations- security-council-may-3-2016
35 Parekh S, *No Refuge: Ethics and The Global Refugee Crisis* (Oxford University Press 2020).
36 Guild E, *Security and Migration in the 21st Century* (Polity Press 2009).
37 Lee R and Yung J, *Angel Island. Immigrant Gateway to America* (Oxford University Press 2010).
38 Bell DR, 'Environmental Refugees: What Rights? Which Duties?' [2004] *Res Publica*. Lister M, 'Climate Change Refugees' [2014] *Critical Review of International Social and Political Philosophy* 17(5). Dwyer J., 'Environmental Migrants, Structural Injustice, and Moral Responsibility' [2020] *Bioethics* 34(6).

Bibliography

Allhoff F and Potts K, 'Medical Immunity, International Law and Just War Theory' [2019] Journal of the Royal Army Medical Corps 165(4).
Arush L et al., 'Pandemic Preparedness and Response: Exploring the Role of Universal Health Coverage within the Global Health Security Architecture' [2022] *The Lancet* 10.
Bell DR, 'Environmental Refugees: What Rights? Which Duties?' [2004] *Res Publica*
Benatar S and Brock G, *Global Health and Global Health Ethics* (Cambridge University Press 2011).
Blaxter MB, *Health* (Polity Press 2010).
Chung R, 'The Securitization of Health in the Context of the War on Terror. National Security and Global Health: The Conflict of Imperatives' [2017] *Medicine, Conflict and Survival* 33(1).
Cleghorn E, *Unwell Women. Misdiagnosis and Myth in a Man-Made World* (Dutton 2021).
Cueto M, 'The History of International Health: Medicine, Politics, and Two Socio-Medical Perspectives, 1851–2000' in C. McInnes, K. Lee, and J. Youde (eds.), *The Oxford Handbook of Global Health Politics* (Oxford University Press 2020).
Daniels N, *Just Health. Meeting Health Needs Fairly* (Cambridge University Press 2012).
Davies SE, *Global Politics of Health* (Polity Press 2010).
Downs J, *Maladies of Empire. How Colonialism, Slavery, and War Transformed Medicine* (Belknap Press of Harvard University Press 2021).
Dwyer J., 'Environmental Migrants, Structural Injustice, and Moral Responsibility' [2020] *Bioethics* 34(6).
Elbe S, *Security and Global Health* (Polity Press 2010).
Elbe S and Voelkner N, 'The Medicalization of Insecurity' in J. Youde and S. Rushton (eds.), *Routledge Handbook of Global Health Security* (Routledge 2015).

Emanuel E et al., 'On the Ethics of Vaccine Nationalism: The Case for Fair Priority for Residents Framework' [2021] *Ethics & International Affairs.*

Gostin LO, *Global Health Law* (Harvard University Press 2014).

Guild E, *Security and Migration in the 21st Century* (Polity Press 2009).

Heymann DL et al., 'Global Health Security: The Wider Lessons from the West African Ebola Virus Disease Epidemic' [2015], The Lancet 385.

Kaul I, Grunberg I, and Stern M(co-eds.), *Global Public Goods. International Cooperation in the 21st Century* (Oxford University Press 1999).

Lee R and Yung J, *Angel Island. Immigrant Gateway to America* (Oxford University Press 2010).

Lister M, 'Climate Change Refugees' [2014] *Critical Review of International Social and Political Philosophy* 17(5).

Liu J, International President of MSF Address to the United Nations Security Council, first speech May 3rd 2016, second speech September 28, 2016: https://www.doctorswithoutborders.org/latest/address-dr-joanne-liu-united-nations-security-council-may-3-2016

Liu J and Chung R, 'Capitalist Philanthropy and Vaccine Imperialism' [2021] *The Hastings Center Bioethics Forum Essay.*

Marmot M and Wilkinson RG (co-eds.), *Social Determinants of Health* (Oxford University Press 2nd edition 2005).

McInnes C, 'The Many Meanings of Health Security' in J. Youde and S. Rushton (eds.), *Routledge Handbook of Global Health Security* (Routledge 2015).

McInnes C, Lee K. and Youde J, 'Global health Politics: An Introduction' in C. McInnes, K. Lee and J. Youde (eds.), *The Oxford Handbook of Global Health Politics* (Oxford University Press 2020).

Parekh S, *No Refuge: Ethics and The Global Refugee Crisis* (Oxford University Press 2020).

Rawls J, *A Theory of Justice* (Belknap Press of Harvard University Press 1971).

Richardson E, *Epidemic Illusions. On the Coloniality of Global Public Health* (MIT Press 2020).

Rubenstein L, *Perilous Medicine. The Struggle to Protect Health Care from the Violence of War* (Columbia University Press 2021).

Schrecker T, 'The State and Global Health' in C. McInnes, K. Lee and J. Youde (eds.), *The Oxford Handbook of Global Health Politics* (Oxford University Press 2020).

Sen A, *Development as Freedom* (Oxford University Press 1999).

10

TRANSITIONAL HEALTH JUSTICE

Himani Bhakuni and Lucas Miotto

10.1 Introduction

John Rawls has famously suggested that the need for a concept of justice arises when individuals have competing interests which lead them to lay different claims to the limited available resources.[1] The context of health, particularly healthcare, has always had to reckon with limited resources and competing interests of various stakeholders. But in the past few years, health systems and resources have not only been severely burdened,[2] but also depleted.[3] As a result, both specialised journals and general newspapers have been swarmed with discussions about health justice. Commentators have discussed how to fairly distribute scarce health resources,[4] how to provide just reparations for public health mismanagement,[5] and how to provide fairer working conditions for nurses and midwives.[6] Others have stressed upon the need for starting afresh and rebuilding our health systems to make them both more resilient to health emergencies and less prone to nurturing inequalities.[7]

Discussions about health reform often centre on the ends of reform: the kind of health systems that should be built and the demands of justice that they should be able to satisfy once reformed. However, little has been said about the demands of justice *in* or *during* health reforms. Rebuilding our health systems within a background of material scarcity and inequality will inevitably require the relevant actors to make important choices, choices about how to deal with past failures and the wrongs perpetrated by their respective health systems. These choices, among other things, will require a balance between distributive and reparative demands, blame and forgiveness, truth and efficiency. It is precisely in this context that, what we call, *"transitional health justice"* comes into play.

DOI: 10.4324/9781003399933-15

Transitional health justice (henceforth THJ) can loosely be defined as a set of processes and guiding principles which should be followed by states and communities affected by health emergencies in their attempts to rebuild their (failing) health systems in a just manner. Our idea of THJ derives from transitional justice, a familiar concept to many, but of particular importance to human rights scholars and political theorists. Transitional justice traditionally describes the ways in which countries emerging from periods of conflict and repression address systematic human rights violations and seek certainty about legitimate political authority. For example, an influential characterisation of transitional justice, provided by the United Nations Security Council, describes transitional justice as "the full range of processes and mechanisms associated with a society's attempts to come to terms with a legacy of large-scale past abuses, in order to assure accountability, serve justice and achieve reconciliation".[8] From this characterisation, we can infer that transitional justice finds its place within a specific context: when a given society is riddled with large-scale past wrongs and attempts to transform itself. Hence, "[t]he core problem of transitional justice is how to justly pursue societal transformation".[9]

In this chapter, we intend to set the stage for a larger discussion about the just transformation of our health systems. We argue that an analogous problem of transitional justice exists in health, namely: what constitutes the just transformation of our health systems? We then discuss, and ultimately reject, a sceptical stance towards THJ. After that, we outline some of the key elements of THJ, including some of its demands, practices, and corresponding institutional framework. We conclude by drawing attention to a missing link between THJ and transitional justice more generally: that THJ is often an enabler of transitional justice.

10.2 Health in Transition

THJ is derived from transitional justice, which means that THJ carries some theoretical baggage from its predecessor. For one, just like not every demand of justice is a demand of transitional justice, not every demand of health justice will be a demand of THJ. Thus, to get off the ground, any account of THJ must first show that there is indeed a subset of demands of justice in health-related contexts that closely resemble typical transitional justice demands. This is our task in this section. To do so, it is worth identifying the kind of circumstances that typically give rise to demands of transitional justice. If we can show that similar circumstances are present in health-related contexts, then there will be at least a reason to believe that there are demands of THJ – and thus a genuine problem of THJ.

To identify the circumstances that typically give rise to demands of transitional justice, and to separate them from demands of other kinds of justice, we rely on Colleen Murphy's work.[10] Following David Hume, Murphy sees each kind of justice – e.g., distributive, retributive, corrective, transitional, etc. – as "problem responsive".[11] That is, each kind of justice is a context-sensitive response to problems which are salient to a specific set of circumstances. Thus, to draw the contours of transitional justice, Murphy seeks to find the features that are both typically present and characteristic of the context in which transitional societies find themselves. With the help of empirical literature, Murphy pinpoints four circumstances that typically take place in transitional societies: (i) pervasive structural inequality, (ii) normalised collective and political wrongdoing, (iii) serious existential uncertainty, and (iv) fundamental uncertainty about authority. Murphy calls them the "circumstances of transitional justice", and in such circumstances, "the central issue" that emerges is "what constitutes the just pursuit of societal transformation?".[12]

Given the goal of transitional justice, it is not difficult to reason that in the above circumstances it is the demand of just transformation, rather than a demand of other kinds of justice, that makes itself salient. Take, for example, a core demand of retributive justice: to fittingly punish wrongdoers. It is usually agreed upon that to be fitting, punishment must be administered by an authority to communicate a message of equality between victims and perpetrators.[13] If this is so, then it would be virtually impossible to meet this demand of retributive justice in circumstances of pervasive inequality and fundamental uncertainty of authority. Such a demand would only become salient, and its satisfaction pressing, once some certainty of authority and a minimum degree of equality are achieved. To put it differently, the demand of retributive justice will only become salient once demands of transitional justice – demands of societal transformation – are minimally satisfied.

This is not to say, however, that there is *no* room for retribution, distribution, or correction in transitional contexts. In fact, many think that there cannot be transitional justice without correcting past wrongs or holding perpetrators accountable.[14] The difference is that, in transitional contexts, when retribution, correction, or distribution take place, they do so only if and to the extent that they aid transformation. It is precisely for this reason that it is sometimes appropriate in transitional contexts to abstain from (or to limit) retribution, correction, or distribution. We will return to this point in Section 10.2.5, where we present an argument for the existence of a problem of THJ.

Having adopted Murphy's basic framework, we can now show that the four circumstances of transitional justice find their counterparts in health contexts, principally in health emergencies. We will unoriginally call the health-related circumstances of transitional justice "circumstances of transitional health justice".

10.2.1 The Circumstances of Transitional Health Justice

Before we proceed with the presentation of the circumstances of THJ, three qualifications are in order. The first is that these circumstances do not obtain in communities or states whose health systems have only been momentarily affected by an isolated act of war, armed conflict, or calamity. These transitory calamities do give rise to calls for normalisation, i.e., for the health system (including provision of healthcare) to be back to what it was prior to the calamity. But such calamities do not necessarily trigger calls for *transformation*. In contexts where transformation is called for, returning to where the community or state was in relation to health is morally unacceptable. What we call "circumstances of transitional health justice" are circumstances that involve enduring and systemic wrongs and a deep sense of uncertainty caused or intensified by a health crisis or emergency. When considering states or communities to which the circumstances of THJ apply, we are considering those where a health crisis or emergency has made it evident that transformation is a moral mandate given that the *status quo* is both morally unacceptable and unsustainable in the long run.

We should, however, not see the circumstances of THJ as a set of necessary and jointly sufficient conditions. Each circumstance involves scalar features (e.g., degree of structural inequality) which communities in a transitional health stage typically exhibit to different degrees. Hence, it is likely that there will be some borderline cases of THJ, for example, cases where a community exhibits most of the circumstances to a high degree but exhibits one of the circumstances to a very low or even null degree. The existence of borderline cases, however, should not undermine the value of a THJ framework.[15] In fact, having a theoretical framework that allows us to classify a community as a borderline case may already be valuable. Such a classification may be enough to demonstrate that at least *some* of the demands of THJ may apply, that other forms of justice are *less* salient than in normal circumstances, and that some compromises might be worth making in the name of (partial) transformation.

This brings us to the third qualification; one about the very object of transformation. In a general and unqualified sense, when the circumstances of THJ obtain, a moral demand for the just transformation of health system will emerge. But what must be transformed are not simply material aspects associated with healthcare and the provision of health (e.g., health resources, health personnel, health institutions, rules, etc.) – how we relate to health providers, experts, authorities, institutions, and each other are also, to some extent, the objects of transformation. As we will see next, the circumstances of transitional justice involve circumstances where our social relations are riddled with distrust and uncertainty, which affect the material provision of health as well as health policies.

With these qualifications, we now present the circumstances of THJ.

10.2.2 Pervasive Structural Inequality

Structural inequality suggests a collective failure in recognising or allowing the equal status of either individuals or groups.[16] Such inequality emerges from differences in socioeconomic position, opportunities, or constraints in life which are not essentially dependent on individual choices. In structurally unequal societies, individuals are "differentially limited in the range of opportunities they can feasibly achieve".[17] Up until a few decades ago, inequities in health were described mainly through income inequalities. But this changed with the introduction of the social determinants of health (SDoH), them being various intersecting non-medical factors that impact health.[18] These factors include "conditions in which people are born, grow, work, live, and age"[19] and the policies, agendas, systems, and norms that shape them. The World Health Organisation (WHO) data shows that "[i]n countries at all levels of income, health and illness follow a social gradient: the lower the socioeconomic position, the worse the health".[20]

Health emergencies (like Covid and HIV Aids pandemics) exacerbate existing structural inequalities.[21] Inequality during and after health emergencies can become widespread (for instance, certain groups having a higher infection and morbidity risk due to their living and social conditions), but inequalities soon begin infiltrating institutions that govern health (for instance, institutions privileging people with a certain economic or social background in care and policies). When this happens, not only individuals' basic health needs are put at risk, but inequality also exacerbates social division and affects the ways in which individuals relate to one another. When faced with pervasive systematic unequal health treatment, individuals – especially those from vulnerable groups – are wronged in that they are, as it were, robbed of their capacity to fully trust their health systems and healthcare service providers.[22]

No level of structural inequality is acceptable. However, it is a fact of life that such inequalities are, in non-ideal societies, virtually impossible to eliminate entirely; even good and functioning health systems will exhibit such inequalities to a low degree. Structural inequality is a circumstance of THJ when it is pervasive and unavoidable, to the point of consistently affecting from the most basic, day-to-day, operations (e.g., arranging an appointment with a GP) to the most complex ones (e.g., deciding how to allocate limited space in intensive care units during a crisis). When structural inequality is deeply rooted in a health system, fixing the system is not merely a matter of increasing material resources. A system with health workers that continue to deny members of a minority a simple appointment is still a broken system, one that requires transformation.

10.2.3 Normalised Collective or Individual Wrongdoing

Health emergencies often lead to normalised collective and individual wrongdoing at different levels. Collective wrongdoing includes governments censoring information relevant for management and surveillance of diseases,[23] failure of wealthy states to commit to global health equity,[24] states greenlighting political rallies and mass gatherings during a pandemic,[25] and state policies leading to gross human rights violations either through excessive use of force or inept containment measures.[26] Individual wrongdoing involves, for example, aiding the spread of disease through avoidable actions and behaviour. During health emergencies both collective and individual wrongdoing becomes normalised in the sense that they become so usual and natural that people learn to ignore these wrongdoings and adapt to them. Such normalisation can erode faith in systems that govern public health and create a sense of helplessness. This can only be repaired with a change in the social relations between citizens and their public health systems, which would essentially require a transformation of health systems.

10.2.4 Serious Existential Uncertainty and Fundamental Uncertainty About Authority

Existential uncertainty in the context of a health crisis could be explained in two ways. First, in terms of uncertainty surrounding the probability that health systems will go back to normal, or that things will improve if the current structures and institutions remain in place and function as they normally do. Second, existential uncertainty on a personal level vis-à-vis mental health,[27] including fear and anxiety for one's own longevity and health. Of course, some degree of existential uncertainty is always present, even in moderately just health systems. It is only when this risk becomes serious – that is, when it constitutes a real threat to the day-to-day functioning of health systems – that we can say that it becomes part of the circumstances of THJ.

Regarding fundamental uncertainty about authority, the recent pandemic (alas) provided a good illustration of this circumstance. Not only was the authority of health experts (including epidemiologists, doctors, public health specialists, etc.),[28] called into question by individuals and governments alike, but also the authority of the WHO and of governments in implementing health guidelines. In fact, given the health authority crisis, as it were, some have even argued for *anarchist* solutions to improve our health systems and health inequalities.[29]

10.2.5 From Transitional Justice to Transitional Health Justice

The context of health emergencies displays similar circumstances to those that characteristically give rise to demands of transitional justice. Failing health systems mirror collapsing political systems in conflict-affected states in important ways. Thus, unless there are stronger countervailing reasons against applying the circumstances of transitional justice to the context of health, we can conclude that there is indeed a problem of THJ. But in addition to an argument based on the face-value similarity between the circumstances of transitional justice and the circumstances that obtain in health emergencies, we can also establish that a problem of THJ exists by thinking of how salient the demands of other types of justice are in health emergencies, where health systems fail or are on the brink of failing.

We cannot be exhaustive in this chapter. But to illustrate how this argument goes, let's consider the place of demands of distributive justice in a context where a health system is on the brink of collapse and in need of reform. In such contexts, it is tempting to be swayed by the thought that problems of distributive justice take precedence. After all, the thought goes, a failing health system is likely a system that lacks resources or where resources are poorly allocated – when doctors, nurses, medicines, hospital beds, ventilators, personal protective equipment, and other resources are fairly allocated, a health system is not likely to collapse.

This stance is ultimately mistaken. It is not unlike the thought that the solution to world hunger is cranking up the production and distribution of food. To succeed in doing justice, distributive policies require a minimum degree of institutional normality. There cannot be a just allocation of resources when there is uncertainty around who owes what to whom and who is responsible for managing the relevant resources. Besides, it is unlikely that any allocation of resources will be *regarded* as just in a context of distrust, which is something that can cast a shadow on whether individuals are being respected and treated as moral equals.[30] When the population exhibits distrust in health authorities (or the states), any decision about the distribution of resources will inevitably be met with doubt, criticism, or even resistance. To put the point differently, certainty about who ought to manage the resources and what will be done if resources are mismanaged must be settled before any allocation takes place.

More importantly, in a context of transformation, the just allocation of resources – them being vegetables, vaccines, or ventilators – presupposes a background of norms that ensure not only that each receives their fair share and continues to do so in the long run, but also that the distributions are determined by and conducive to a situation where past wrongs are both absent and repudiated. This means that in health emergencies or other contexts that call for system-level transformation, the main distributive question will not be "what constitutes a just distribution of resources?". Rather, it will be "what constitutes a just distribution *for the purposes of transformation?*". The latter already implies a compromise with full distributive justice; it implies the priority of transformation over distribution. We can say, therefore, that this, and similar questions in similar contexts, belong to the realm of institutional design and transformation. They belong, therefore, to the realm of *transitional* justice. A problem of transitional justice is, therefore, logically prior to questions of distributive justice in the circumstances of health justice. Therefore, we can conclude not only that there is a genuine problem of transitional justice in health, but also that, in the right circumstances, this problem seems to take precedence over other problems of justice that may concern our health systems and institutions.

Having said that, some may still adopt a sceptical attitude towards THJ. In what follows we discuss one form of scepticism towards THJ.

10.3 Why Transitional Health Justice?

Health scholars have been far from oblivious about health justice and health reforms. Yet, THJ has not been part of their concerns. It is, therefore, tempting to think that there might be a good reason for that: maybe health scholars did not speak of a problem of transitional justice in health precisely because – despite what we've said so far – there isn't one. Or, more precisely, there is no *distinct* problem, as problems of transitional justice in health can easily be reduced to familiar problems of health reforms to which health scholars have long applied themselves. To accord THJ a place in health justice discussions – and vindicate the fruitfulness of a THJ framework – we must better understand what motivates this sceptical stance and give reasons to counteract it.

Such sceptical stance is not unheard of. We find a counterpart in the transitional justice literature.[31] According to this sceptical conception, transitional justice demands are not *distinctive* demands of justice; they are instead an aggregate or a compromise between familiar demands of justice that can ultimately be broken down and reduced to more fundamental, and genuine, demands of justice (such as retributive, corrective, and distributive). It follows that, under this conception, we do not need an account of transitional justice (and, similarly, we wouldn't need an account of THJ); all that is needed is an account that allows us to set priorities between the competing demands of justice that emerge in contexts of institutional reform.

A full response to this challenge would require a detailed engagement with the arguments and theories about the distinctiveness of transitional justice, which goes beyond our present purposes. More fundamentally, however, this sceptical challenge *(i.e.,* explaining the distinctiveness of transitional justice) is a challenge we do not need to meet. The reason is that it does not follow from the fact that transitional justice's (and THJ's) demands are not demands of a distinctive kind of justice that we do not need – and would not benefit from – an account of transitional justice (and of THJ).

Even those who see demands of transitional justice as nothing but an aggregate or a compromise between familiar demands of justice (rather than a set of distinct demands) must acknowledge that (i) there are non-trivial questions about which compromises transitional communities are permitted to and ought to make (including which demands of justice must be prioritised); and that (ii) transitional communities may benefit from a set of guiding principles and practices, whether distinct or not, when deciding on which compromises to make in transitional contexts. And if this much is acknowledged, then there is no good reason to object to the usefulness of a theoretical framework dedicated to both explaining the demands of justice that apply to transitional contexts and to laying out a set of guiding principles and practices for transitional communities who ought to satisfy the demands of justice that apply to them. An account of transitional justice is nothing but this framework – and so is an account of THJ.

The sceptical stance thus overlooks the fact that one can be agnostic about the ultimate *nature* of THJ's demands and still propose an account of THJ. To make it clearer, one thing is to ask, "are demands of transitional health justice demands of a distinctive kind of justice?" – another is to ask "what principles and practices does the just transformation of health systems call for?". An answer to the latter – which we take to be the object of an account of THJ – does not depend on an answer to the former.

Now, it may look like we are contradicting ourselves. We have argued in the previous sections that demands of distributive, retributive, corrective, and other types of justice are not salient in the circumstances of THJ. We also explicitly relied on Murphy's circumstances of transitional justice, and it is known that Murphy *does* defend the view that demands of transitional justice are of a distinctive kind. So given what we said before, it seems that we are committed to the view that demands of THJ are distinctive, which contradicts our claim in the present section according to which our account of THJ is agnostic about the distinctiveness issue.

But the contradiction is only seeming. Even though our preferred account is committed to the view according to which demands of THJ are demands of a distinctive kind, it doesn't mean that *every* account of THJ must be so committed. It is, therefore, still possible to hold, for example, that in the circumstances of THJ a particular *bundle* of familiar kinds of demands of justice (corrective, retributive, etc.) typically emerges. And because such bundle of competing demands typically emerges, a problem about which demand to prioritise (and which compromises to make) while aiming at institutional transformation will also emerge. This is precisely the sort of question that those who view transitional justice as compromise focus on.

And because, as we have just shown, this question is still important, there would still be conceptual space for someone to develop a framework to attempt to answer it. In fact, the discussion about THJ may only get richer as alternative views about the nature of transitional justice demands and the institutional frameworks and guiding principles that these views might entail are worked out in detail.

We have so far argued that a problem of THJ exists. The problem, we have suggested, concerns the just transformation of our health systems, as this is the salient question that emerges in the circumstances of THJ. Be this as it may, we have so far been silent on the principles and institutional practices that guide just transformation. In other words, we have not discussed what we call "the structure" of THJ. That is what we will do next.

10.4 The Structure of Transitional Health Justice

THJ does not demand the end of *all* health injustices. Rather, it demands the end of the circumstances of THJ. Ending the circumstances of THJ requires corresponding institutional reforms; reforms which will aid in the rebuilding of social trust in health institutions, abating of existential uncertainty, and tackling the uncertainty regarding the authority of health experts and governments on questions of health. These reforms will also aid in reducing structural health inequalities and in reckoning with the truth of past wrongs. While just transformation will entail some permanent changes in a broad range of institutions, at least some of the principles and institutional arrangements necessary for the implementation of THJ will have a more seasonal character; they will remain in place only insofar as necessary to bring a community above the line of transition. Of course, in practice, this line will never be clear and the decision to suspend or do away with a given transitional principle or practice will rarely be a trivial one, as it will itself be a moral decision.

In the following section, we will outline *some* of the institutional practices and reforms required by THJ. We do not intent to be exhaustive. Our focus will be on reforms that aid to end both the fundamental uncertainty about authority and the normalisation of wrongdoing.

10.4.1 Whose Authority? WHO's Burden?

Governance structures and the degree of decentralisation amongst national, provincial, and municipal structures can often lead to conflicts and confusion related to authority during a health emergency. The governance system of countries (whether unitary or federal) often impacts their health systems' performance during health emergencies. Among the 193 member nations of the United Nations (UN), 25 countries are governed as federal states and

168 are governed as unitary states, while some unitary states display aspects of quasi-federalism.[32] In the early days of the COVID-19 pandemic, for instance, the then President of the United States, which is a federal state, had been considering the idea of imposing a quarantine on parts of Connecticut, New York, and New Jersey. This led to a fierce debate about the powers and authority of the President, the federal government, and responsibility of the states during pandemic response.[33] In the United Kingdom, which is a unitary state with devolved governments, the local governments were fiscally ill-equipped to respond to the critical phase of the Covid crisis[34] and are still struggling to drive recovery of their health systems.[35] There has been a sense that the "central state has more or less disengaged from the layers of governance and public authority that exist at lower levels of the system, including local public health officials, head teachers and local authorities".[36] THJ, first and foremost, demands clarity in the roles and responsibilities of governing authorities. Once the roles of the governing authorities are clearly established, it then looks at rebuilding societal trust in those governing authorities.

A study that included responses from 142 countries found that exposure to a health emergency in individuals aged 18–25 has a "persistent negative effect on confidence in political institutions and leaders".[37] The study also found negative effects on confidence in public health systems.[38] Another study from the United Kingdom showed that government's inability to sustain political trust was "likely to have made the management of public confidence and behaviour increasingly challenging, pointing to the need for strategies to sustain trust levels when handling future crises".[39] Health-governing authorities at the national scale involving federal, state, and municipal governments aided by health experts, public health institutions, and, to some extent, courts are prone to suffer from a lack of trust during and post-emergency. To rebuild such trust, THJ would demand that health institutions that inform government policies are independent, autonomous, and not tied in any form, which would be called a conflict of interest, with the other arms of the state (like the legislative, judiciary, and executive) and private parties. Of course, there would be reasonable checks and balances in place to ensure that such health institution's power is checked often. Such health institutions would be constituted of vetted and respectable health scientists, health economists, community health experts, and other population health professionals.

Some recent studies have shown that courts tended to display a "substantial deference to legislative measures taken by the legislative and executive branches to address COVID-19", but on rare occasions they were able to successfully review government actions and health emergency policies in some jurisdictions.[40] While courts are not strictly health-governing institutions, they provide essential checks on government authority.

Moreover, judicial opinions provide context and guidance for discussions during review of existing health emergency and health system restructuring laws. Courts play an important role as allied health-governing institutions in emergency situations, but their refusal to confront blatantly inept legislative and executive actions accompanied with the high cost and inaccessibility to judicial proceedings can lead to further erosion of trust in legal and political institutions. THJ demands the strengthening of the corpus of health law (including health emergency law) in all jurisdictions to assist the process of just transformation of health systems.

An important point to note here is that in THJ, as opposed to transitional justice, the goal is not "societal transformation". Still, because health is embedded in social relations, for transformation – to be just – it must be sensitive to broader issues. One way to rebuild trust in national-level health-governing authorities would be for health-allied institutions to ensure that the proximal SDoH are, at least, minimally acted upon. Proximate SDoH include lifestyle or behaviour (e.g., fruit, fat, vegetable, alcohol, and tobacco consumption), socioeconomic environment (e.g., wealth), demography (e.g., disabled, or elderly proportion of the total population), and the physical environment (e.g., air pollution).[41] Interestingly, however, despite the goal of THJ not being societal transformation, the fact that health reforms will mobilise health-allied institutions to act upon the social (and even commercial) determinants of health will entail *some* degree of societal transformation. We will come back to this point towards the end of the chapter, where we claim that THJ is an enabler of transitional justice.

Now, if we think of health authority on a global scale, the WHO appears to be close in form and function to such an authority. After years of being reduced to a health emergency bystander, the WHO *suo moto,* and as "an act of executive decision (self-empowerment)"[42], assumed emergency powers after the emergence of the SARS epidemic in 2003. This aided the long-stalled revision process of the International Health Regulations (IHR) and steered the adoption of IHR in 2005 which led to legal normalisation of WHO's emergency powers.[43] The new IHRs gave WHO the legal power to declare a Public Health Emergency of International Concern (PHEIC) based on information acquired through channels other than states' health authorities. Its emergency powers include the competence to issue temporary recommendations on health measures (Article 15 IHR 2005) and requiring states to cooperate with the WHO's monitoring and verification efforts (including deploying operative teams on the ground). Under Articles 10(4) and 11(2) of IHR 2005, the WHO can share and make public the information that it received from state or non-state sources, even if the concerned states or actors decline to collaborate with the organisation. This authorises the WHO to resort to naming and shaming practices concerning non-compliant states.

WHO's emergency powers, along with WHO's authority, have been challenged since it declared H1N1 a PHEIC in 2009, which has since led to constraints on its procedural powers.[44] But more recently, the WHO has been accused of favouring diplomacy over transparency while dealing with powerful states,[45] which is partly due to its reliance on member countries' donations. While the WHO does have emergency powers, they are limited by state sovereignty. Furthermore, it does not have a guaranteed right of access in countries to investigate emerging outbreaks and it cannot ensure compliance with its recommendations. THJ would require the WHO to play a more robust role during emergency and in aiding states during post-emergency rebuilding of health systems (which it does, but to a limited extent, through its Country Readiness Strengthening Department). There are plans to extend WHO's abilities to respond to pandemics and other health crises. As we write this chapter, in early 2023, the WHO has announced that its members states have agreed to draft a convention dedicated to pandemic prevention, preparedness, and response.[46] But it remains to be seen whether such convention will be adequate in eliminating the uncertainty of WHO's authority, strengthening the enforcement of its provisions, and including clear principles and institutional mechanisms for recovery and transformation.[47]

10.4.2 Truth Commissions?

Health emergencies and broken health systems often lead to mass-scale human rights violations that should be acknowledged and possibly re-dressed. In the transitional justice paradigm, this work is done by truth and reconciliation commissions, which are set up to investigate the history of gross violations of human rights in a particular country.[48] It is generally believed that states emerging from conflict or repression need to tackle their recent history of human rights abuses to establish peace and to consolidate new democracies. Most truth commissions combine investigations of human rights abuses with a form of narrative that explains the causes and patterns of wrongdoing in a bid to repair or restore the social fabric damaged by the normalisation of wrongdoing. Truth commissions are not aimed at ret-ribution; they do not punish perpetrators, rather they tend to memorialise the experiences of both victims and perpetrators.

Depending on the type of transitioning society, truth commissions serve several functions, including the promotion of intergroup forgiveness,[49] the re-establishment of procedural justice[50] (by specifying fair procedures in dealing with conflict), the facilitation of respect for human rights, and the recognition of the agency and dignity of the victims by providing a forum for them to narrate their story and (thereby) a public acknowl-edgement of them being wronged.[51] But perhaps the most important purpose of truth commissions is the official acknowledgement of wrong-doing. With public acknowledgement of wrongdoings, truth commissions can cultivate the belief that a period of conflict has come to an end, which in turn can inspire support for the process of reconciliation.[52] Thus, truth commissions can empower victims to become involved in their changing political and social world.[53]

However, critics have doubted the contributions of truth commissions to the transitional justice process.[54] Truth commissions are both products and engineers of political compromises,[55] but they largely exist because society is reluctant to simply forgive and forget. Since truth commissions are not retributive, it is often debated whether victims' dignity and equality can be restored without some form of reparation or criminal prosecution.[56] Critics argue that the kinds of hostility stimulated by the processes of truth commissions only make societal tensions more tangible by opening old wounds and harming people rather than beneficially reconstructing a society in transition.[57]

As evidenced by the recent COVID-19 pandemic, health emergencies often bring with them "a pandemic of human rights abuses".[58] So it could be argued that health systems emerging from crises need to tackle their recent history of human rights abuses to transition into a morally acceptable version of themselves. However, given the nature of health emergencies, the perpetrators of such abuses are difficult to identify. In hindsight, it is sometimes easy to name a few political actors that oversaw certain catastrophic public health measures, but unless their actions demonstrated an element of explicit illegality, there cannot be criminal retribution or civil reparation. Furthermore, during crises, certain viola-tions of civil and political rights are justifiable on grounds of public emergency, and the violations of economic and social rights are not traceable to a single perpetrator. If people are unable to identify the perpetrators of the harms done to them and "unable to forgive what they cannot punish",[59] there is reason to believe that the traditional model of truth commissions would not work for THJ. In fact, traditional truth commissions and reparation mechanisms might hinder health transfor-mations as they might increase societal distrust which is characteristic of transitional health contexts.

Therefore, we posit that instead of traditional truth and reconciliation commissions, THJ would be best served by what we call "best practices commissions". A best practices commission (BPC) would collate information on the successful measures that were adopted within different provinces of a country or by different health systems and make recommendations on the modifications that could be tailored to a country or community which is in a transitional health stage. However, this is not to say that the victims of abuses during health emergencies should be forgotten. Transformation requires that a community is both aware of the present systemic wrongs and inequalities and committed to avoiding these wrongs in the future. Thus, to aid transformation, BPCs must (at least sometimes) also perform a similar investigatory and record-keeping role as traditional truth commissions. They must, for example, investigate and truthfully report on the causes and patterns of failings of previous health systems and human rights abuses during health emergencies. But these reports and investigations should be conducted only to the extent that they advance transformation, therefore, BPCs should focus on *causes* of failings and wrongdoings and not on assigning responsibility. BPCs are, therefore, mostly forward-looking commissions; truth-finding and truth-preservation are treated primarily as means to the development of best health practices and transformation. How exactly BPCs should proceed with their tasks, who should be its members, and what normative framework would bind them are important matters. But these are matters that merit their own discussion and are thus best left for another occasion.

10.5 Conclusion: Enabling Justice

This chapter intended to start a discussion around the value of an account of transitional health justice. Some might argue that the need for a framework of THJ is perhaps more important than we have suggested. After all, health systems are always in transition, as in ever growing and evolving and learning from the past. This is true, if not trivially so. This claim, however, does not capture the kind of transition that we have addressed in this chapter. THJ requires a set of circumstances to obtain, and the demands of THJ only hold true for a health system that shows a serious level of moral and practical collapse. The circumstances of THJ—pervasive structural inequality, normalised individual and collective wrongdoing, serious existential uncertainty, and fundamental uncertainty about authority—typically begin after a chronic public health crisis. But when do these circumstances end *or* when would we say that a health system has transitioned, are questions that require moral assessment or collective deliberation. It could be that a health system, following the structure of THJ, as partly laid out in the chapter, transforms itself enough so that other demands of justice take precedence over transitional questions. It is also possible that a health system might fall back into its transitional state, either because of another health crisis or the misapplication of the transitional health framework.

Now, health and health systems are socially determined; they are embedded in social and political relations. Sometimes, both health crises and the misapplication of the transitional health framework can be ultimately linked to serious political conflict and instability, which are factors that can lead to calls for deeper societal transformation, i.e., for transitional justice (*simpliciter*). It is, therefore, possible that there exist some important relations between THJ and transitional justice.

The relations, it strikes us, go in both directions: from transitional justice to THJ and vice-versa. One such relation we would like to highlight is that THJ can work as an enabler of transitional justice. If transitional justice processes aim at reducing structural inequalities and allowing individuals to develop their capabilities and protecting human rights, they might have to first ensure that the SDoH are minimally acted upon. As pointed out by Erika Blacksher, some forms of political and social participation – "participating as a peer in public life" – are partly constituted by a minimum degree of health.[60] And such forms of public participation exemplify the sort of social relations that traditional transitional justice processes aim at reinstalling. Hence, the lack of health and malfunctioning health systems can pose serious barriers for the success of the broader transformation sought by transitional justice, which suggests that to succeed, transitional justice processes must, at least sometimes, be preceded by or work in tandem with a process of THJ.

Notes

1 Rawls J, *A Theory of Justice (Revised Edition)* (The Belknap Press of Harvard University Press 1999).
2 Ribeiro da Silva SJ and Pena L, 'Collapse of the Public Health System and the Emergence of New Variants during the Second Wave of the COVID-19 Pandemic in Brazil' (2021) 13 One Health 100287; Constantinos Siettos and others, 'A Bulletin from Greece: A Health System under the Pressure of the Second COVID-19 Wave' (2021) 115 Pathogens and Global Health 133; Chang AY and others, 'The Impact of Novel Coronavirus COVID-19 on Noncommunicable Disease Patients and Health Systems: A Review' (2021) 289 Journal of Internal Medicine 450; Williams OD, Yung KC and Grépin KA, 'The Failure of Private Health Services: COVID-19 Induced Crises in Low- and Middle-Income Country (LMIC) Health Systems' (2021) 16 Global Public Health 1320.
3 Barlow P and others, 'COVID-19 and the Collapse of Global Trade: Building an Effective Public Health Response' (2021) 5 The Lancet Planetary Health e102; Khot UN, 'Navigating Healthcare Supply Shortages During the COVID-19 Pandemic' (2020) 13 Circulation: Cardiovascular Quality and Outcomes e006801.
4 Fumagalli R, 'We Should Not Use Randomization Procedures to Allocate Scarce Life-Saving Resources' (2022) 15 Public Health Ethics 87.
5 'Pandemic Reparations and Justice in Global Health Governance | Think Global Health' (*Council on Foreign Relations*) <https://www.thinkglobalhealth.org/article/pandemic-reparations-and-justice-global-health-governance> accessed 22 August 2022.
6 Llop-Gironés A and others, 'Employment and Working Conditions of Nurses: Where and How Health Inequalities Have Increased during the COVID-19 Pandemic?' (2021) 19 Human Resources for Health 112.

7 Fernandes G, Hassan I and Sridhar D, 'Building Resilient Health-Care Supply Chains to Manage Pandemics in Low- and Middle-Income Countries' (2022) 100 Bulletin of the World Health Organization 174; Gebremeskel AT and others, 'Building Resilient Health Systems in Africa beyond the COVID-19 Pandemic Response' (2021) 6 BMJ Global Health e006108; Patel L and others, 'Climate Change and Extreme Heat Events: How Health Systems Should Prepare' 3 NEJM Catalyst CAT.21.0454; Fiske A, McLennan S and Buyx A, 'Ethical Insights from the COVID-19 Pandemic in Germany: Considerations for Building Resilient Healthcare Systems in Europe' (2021) 9 The Lancet Regional Health – Europe <https://www.thelancet.com/journals/lanepe/article/PIIS2666–7762(21)00190-3/fulltext> accessed 24 July 2022; Mustafa S and others, 'COVID-19 Preparedness and Response Plans from 106 Countries: A Review from a Health Systems Resilience Perspective' (2022) 37 Health Policy and Planning 255.

8 'The Rule of Law and Transitional Justice in Conflict and Post-Conflict Societies: Report of Secretary General.' (United Nations Security Council 2004) UN Doc. S/2004/616.

9 Murphy C, *The Conceptual Foundations of Transitional Justice* (Cambridge University Press 2017) <https://www.cambridge.org/core/books/conceptual-foundations-of-transitional-justice/989DAFCD8E1BCCF2716308D0B87AB2CE> accessed 24 July 2022.

10 ibid.

11 ibid 41.

12 ibid 112.

13 Duff RA, *Punishment, Communication, and Community* (Oxford University Press 2001); Murphy (n 9) 93–95.

14 García-Godos J, 'It's About Trust: Transitional Justice and Accountability in the Search for Peace' in Bailliet CM and Larsen KM (eds), *Promoting Peace Through International Law* (Oxford University Press 2015) <https://doi.org/10.1093/acprof:oso/9780198722731.003.0016> accessed 18 March 2023.

15 For a parallel discussion of borderline cases in transitional justice, see Murphy (n 9) 42.

16 Cudd AE, *Analyzing Oppression* (Illustrated edition, Oxford University Press, USA 2006).

17 Murphy (n 9).

18 Marmot M and others, 'Closing the Gap in a Generation: Health Equity through Action on the Social Determinants of Health' (2008) 372 The Lancet 1661.

19 World Health Organisation, 'Health Inequality Monitor' (*WHO Social Determinants of Health: Inequality Monitor*) <https://www.who.int/data/inequality-monitor>.

20 ibid.

21 Finn BM and Kobayashi LC, 'Structural Inequality in the Time of COVID-19: Urbanization, Segregation, and Pandemic Control in Sub-Saharan Africa' (2020) 10 Dialogues in Human Geography 217; Parker R, 'The Global HIV/AIDS Pandemic, Structural Inequalities, and the Politics of International Health' (2002) 92 American Journal of Public Health 343; Fiske A and others, 'The Second Pandemic: Examining Structural Inequality through Reverberations of COVID-19 in Europe' (2022) 292 Social Science & Medicine 114634; Bowleg L, 'We're Not All in This Together: On COVID-19, Intersectionality, and Structural Inequality' (2020) 110 American Journal of Public Health 917.

22 Beller J and others, 'Trust in Healthcare during COVID-19 in Europe: Vulnerable Groups Trust the Least' [2022] Journal of Public Health.

23 Ruan L, Knockel J and Crete-Nishihata M, 'Censored Contagion: How Information on the Coronavirus Is Managed on Chinese Social Media' <https://tspace.library.utoronto.ca/handle/1807/104268> accessed 28 July 2022.

24 Bajaj SS, Maki L and Stanford FC, 'Vaccine Apartheid: Global Cooperation and Equity' (2022) 399 The Lancet 1452.

25 Iacobucci G, 'Covid-19: India Should Stop Mass Gatherings and Consider Postponing Elections, Say Doctors' (2021) 373 BMJ n1102; Domènech-Montoliu S and others, '"Mass Gathering Events and COVID-19 Transmission in Borriana (Spain): A Retrospective Cohort Study"' (2021) 16 PLOS ONE e0256747.

26 Negi C, 'Human Rights Violations of Migrants Workers in India During COVID-19 Pandemic' (Social Science Research Network 2020) SSRN Scholarly Paper 3629773 <https://papers.ssrn.com/abstract=3629773> accessed 28 July 2022; Anand JC and others, 'The Covid-19 Pandemic and Care Homes for Older People in Europe - Deaths, Damage and Violations of Human Rights' (2021) 0 European Journal of Social Work 1; 'From Protection to Repression: State Containment of COVID-19 Pandemic and Human Rights Violations in Nigeria: Victims & Offenders: Vol 0, No 0' <https://www.tandfonline.com/doi/abs/10.1080/15564886.2022.2077494> accessed 28 July 2022.

27 Spitzenstätter D and Schnell T, 'The Existential Dimension of the Pandemic: Death Attitudes, Personal Worldview, and Coronavirus Anxiety' (2022) 46 Death Studies 1031.

28 O'Shea BA and Ueda M, 'Who Is More Likely to Ignore Experts' Advice Related to COVID-19?' (2021) 23 Preventive Medicine Reports 101470.

29 Swann T, '"Anarchist Technologies": Anarchism, Cybernetics and Mutual Aid in Community Responses to the COVID-19 Crisis' [2022] Organization 13505084221090632; Ryan Essex, 'Anarchy and Its Overlooked Role in Health and Healthcare' (2023)] 32 Cambridge Quarterly of Healthcare Ethics 397.

30 Anderson ES, 'What Is the Point of Equality?' (1999) 109 Ethics 287, 314.

31 Posner EA and Vermeule A, 'Transitional Justice as Ordinary Justice' (2004) 117 Harvard Law Review 761; Hull G, 'Justice in Circumstances of Transition: Comments on Colleen Murphy's Theory of Transitional Justice as Justice of a Special Type' (2018) 14 Journal of Global Ethics 147.

32 OECD, *Making Decentralisation Work: A Handbook for Policy-Makers* (Organisation for Economic Co-operation and Development 2019) <https://www.oecd-ilibrary.org/urban-rural-and-regional-development/making-decentralisation-work_g2g9faa7-en> accessed 5 January 2023.

33 Berman E, 'The Roles of the State and Federal Governments in a Pandemic' (2020) 11 Journal of National Security Law and Policy <https://jnslp.com/wp-content/uploads/2020/12/The-Roles-of-the-State-and-Federal-Governments-in-a-Pandemic_2.pdf>.

34 Warner S and others, 'English Devolution and the Covid-19 Pandemic: Governing Dilemmas in the Shadow of the Treasury' (2021) 92 The Political Quarterly 321.

35 Wilkinson E, 'NHS England's Backlog Recovery Plan Is at Serious Risk, Watchdog Warns' (2022) 379 BMJ o2779.

36 Kenny M and Sheldon J, 'How COVID-19 Is Exposing Unresolved Issues about How England Is Governed' (*The British Academy*, 6 July 2020) <https://www.thebritishacademy.ac.uk/blog/how-covid-19-exposing-unresolved-issues-about-how-england-governed/>.

37 Aksoy C, Barry Eichengreen and Saka O, 'The Political Scar of Epidemics | Systemic Risk Centre' (2020) DP 97 LSE Systemic Risks Centre Discussion Papers <https://www.systemicrisk.ac.uk/publications/discussion-papers/political-scar-epidemics> accessed 6 January 2023.

38 ibid.

39 Davies B and others, 'Changes in Political Trust in Britain during the COVID-19 Pandemic in 2020: Integrated Public Opinion Evidence and Implications' (2021) 8 Humanities and Social Sciences Communications 1.

40 Clodfelter CG and others, 'Global Judicial Opinions Regarding Government-Issued COVID-19 Mitigation Measures' (2022) 20 Health Security 97.
41 Arah OA and others, 'Health System Outcomes and Determinants Amenable to Public Health in Industrialized Countries: A Pooled, Cross-Sectional Time Series Analysis' (2005) 5 BMC Public Health 81.
42 Kreuder-Sonnen C, 'WHO Emergency Powers for Global Health Security' in Christian Kreuder-Sonnen (ed), *Emergency Powers of International Organizations: Between Normalization and Containment* (Oxford University Press 2019) <https://doi.org/10.1093/oso/9780198832935.003.0006> accessed 6 January 2023.
43 'International Health Regulations (2005) Third Edition' <https://www.who.int/publications-detail-redirect/9789241580496>.
44 Kreuder-Sonnen (n 42).
45 Maxmen A, 'Why Did the World's Pandemic Warning System Fail When COVID Hit?' (2021) 589 Nature 499.
46 'Pandemic Prevention, Preparedness and Response Accord' <https://www.who.int/news-room/questions-and-answers/item/pandemic-prevention–preparedness-and-response-accord> accessed 25 March 2023.
47 On the role and importance of strengthening enforcement mechanisms in global health, see Weissglass D, 'Justice in Global Health Governance: The Role of Enforcement' in Bhakuni H and Miotto L (eds), *Justice in Global Health: New Perspectives and Current Issues* (Routledge 2023).
48 Hayner PB, 'Fifteen Truth Commissions--1974 to 1994: A Comparative Study' (1994) 16 Human Rights Quarterly 597.
49 Chapman AR, 'Truth Commissions and Intergroup Forgiveness: The Case of the South African Truth and Reconciliation Commission' (2007) 13 Peace and Conflict: Journal of Peace Psychology 51.
50 Nickson R and Braithwaite J, 'Deeper, Broader, Longer Transitional Justice' (2014) 11 European Journal of Criminology 445.
51 Bakiner O, *Truth Commissions: Memory, Power, and Legitimacy* (University of Pennsylvania Press 2015).
52 Murphy C, 'Truth Commissions', *International Encyclopedia of Ethics* (John Wiley & Sons, Ltd 2013) <https://onlinelibrary.wiley.com/doi/abs/10.1002/9781444367072.wbiee446> accessed 25 March 2023.
53 ibid.
54 Robins S, 'Failing Victims? The Limits of Transitional Justice in Addressing the Needs of Victims of Violations' [2017] Human Rights and International Legal Discourse 41.
55 Haldemann F (ed), 'Compromise', *Transitional Justice for Foxes: Conflict, Pluralism and the Politics of Compromise* (Cambridge University Press 2022) <https://www.cambridge.org/core/books/transitional-justice-for-foxes/compromise/8ED1C9D86D3BD6F5A35D68B427945789> accessed 1 March 2023.
56 Robins (n 54).
57 Rotberg RI and Thompson D (eds), *Truth v. Justice: The Morality of Truth Commissions* (Princeton University Press 2000) <https://www.jstor.org/stable/j.ctt7t4sd> accessed 3 March 2023.
58 Guterres A, 'The World Faces a Pandemic of Human Rights Abuses in the Wake of Covid-19' *The Guardian* (22 February 2021) <https://www.theguardian.com/global-development/2021/feb/22/world-faces-pandemic-human-rights-abuses-covid-19-antonio-guterres> accessed 1 March 2023.
59 Arendt H, *The Human Condition* (Second Edition, The University of Chicago Press 1958), 241.

60 Blacksher E, 'Redistribution and Recognition in the Pursuit of Health Justice: An Application of Nancy Fraser's Framework' in Bhakuni H and Miotto L (eds), *Justice in Global Health: New Perspectives and Current Issues* (Routledge 2023).

Bibliography

Aksoy C, Eichengreen B and Saka O, 'The Political Scar of Epidemics | Systemic Risk Centre' [2020] *DP 97 LSE Systemic Risks Centre Discussion Papers* <https://www.systemicrisk.ac.uk/publications/discussion-papers/political-scar-epidemics> accessed 6 January 2023.

Anand JC and others, 'The Covid-19 Pandemic and Care Homes for Older People in Europe – Deaths, Damage and Violations of Human Rights' [2021] 0 *European Journal of Social Work* 1.

Anderson ES, 'What Is the Point of Equality?' [1999] 109 *Ethics* 287.

Arah OA and others, 'Health System Outcomes and Determinants Amenable to Public Health in Industrialized Countries: A Pooled, Cross-Sectional Time Series Analysis' [2005] 5 *BMC Public Health* 81.

Arendt H, *The Human Condition* (Second Edition, The University of Chicago Press 1958).

Bajaj SS, Maki L and Stanford FC, 'Vaccine Apartheid: Global Cooperation and Equity' [2022] 399 *The Lancet* 1452.

Bakiner O, *Truth Commissions: Memory, Power, and Legitimacy* (University of Pennsylvania Press 2015).

Barlow P and others, 'COVID-19 and the Collapse of Global Trade: Building an Effective Public Health Response'[2021] 5 *The Lancet Planetary Health* e102.

Beller J and others, 'Trust in Healthcare during COVID-19 in Europe: Vulnerable Groups Trust the Least' [2022] *Journal of Public Health*

Berman E, 'The Roles of the State and Federal Governments in a Pandemic' [2020] 11 *Journal of National Security Law and Policy* <https://jnslp.com/wp-content/uploads/2020/12/The-Roles-of-the-State-and-Federal-Governments-in-a-Pandemic_2.pdf>

Blacksher, E, 'Redistribution and Recognition in the Pursuit of Health Justice: An Application of Nancy Fraser's Framework' in H. Bhakuni and L. Miotto (eds), *Justice in Global Health: New Perspectives and Current Issues* (Routledge 2023).

Bowleg L, 'We're Not All in This Together: On COVID-19, Intersectionality, and Structural Inequality' [2020] 110 *American Journal of Public Health* 917.

Chang AY and others, 'The Impact of Novel Coronavirus COVID-19 on Noncommunicable Disease Patients and Health Systems: A Review' [2021] 289 *Journal of Internal Medicine* 450.

Chapman AR, 'Truth Commissions and Intergroup Forgiveness: The Case of the South African Truth and Reconciliation Commission' [2007] 13 *Peace and Conflict: Journal of Peace Psychology* 51.

Clodfelter CG and others, 'Global Judicial Opinions Regarding Government-Issued COVID-19 Mitigation Measures' [2022] 20 *Health Security* 97.

Cudd AE, *Analyzing Oppression* (Illustrated edition, Oxford University Press, USA 2006).

David Williams O, Yung KC and Grépin KA, 'The Failure of Private Health Services: COVID-19 Induced Crises in Low- and Middle-Income Country (LMIC) Health Systems' [2021] 16 *Global Public Health* 1320.

Davies B and others, 'Changes in Political Trust in Britain during the COVID-19 Pandemic in 2020: Integrated Public Opinion Evidence and Implications' [2021] 8 *Humanities and Social Sciences Communications* 1.

Domènech-Montoliu S and others, 'Mass Gathering Events and COVID-19 Transmission in Borriana (Spain): A Retrospective Cohort Study' [2021] 16 *PLoS One* e0256747.

Duff RA, *Punishment, Communication, and Community* (Oxford University Press 2001).

Essex R, 'Anarchy and Its Overlooked Role in Health and Healthcare' [2023] *Cambridge Quarterly of Healthcare Ethics* 32 397–405

Fernandes G, Hassan I and Sridhar D, 'Building Resilient Health-Care Supply Chains to Manage Pandemics in Low- and Middle-Income Countries' [2022] 100 *Bulletin of the World Health Organization* 174.

Finn BM and Kobayashi LC, 'Structural Inequality in the Time of COVID-19: Urbanization, Segregation, and Pandemic Control in Sub-Saharan Africa' [2020] 10 *Dialogues in Human Geography* 217.

Fiske A and others, 'The Second Pandemic: Examining Structural Inequality through Reverberations of COVID-19 in Europe' [2022] 292 *Social Science & Medicine* 114634.

Fiske A, McLennan S and Buyx A, 'Ethical Insights from the COVID-19 Pandemic in Germany: Considerations for Building Resilient Healthcare Systems in Europe' [2021] 9 *The Lancet Regional Health – Europe* <https://www.thelancet.com/journals/lanepe/article/PIIS2666–7762(21)00190-3/fulltext> accessed 24 July 2022.

'From Protection to Repression: State Containment of COVID-19 Pandemic and Human Rights Violations in Nigeria: Victims & Offenders: Vol 0, No 0' <https://www.tandfonline.com/doi/abs/10.1080/15564886.2022.2077494> accessed 28 July 2022.

Fumagalli R, 'We Should Not Use Randomization Procedures to Allocate Scarce Life-Saving Resources' [2022] 15 *Public Health Ethics* 87.

García-Godos J, 'It's About Trust: Transitional Justice and Accountability in the Search for Peace' in C. M. Bailliet and K. M. Larsen (eds), *Promoting Peace Through International Law* (Oxford University Press 2015) <10.1093/acprof:oso/9780198722731.003.0016> accessed 18 March 2023.

Gebremeskel AT and others, 'Building Resilient Health Systems in Africa beyond the COVID-19 Pandemic Response' [2021] 6 *BMJ Global Health* e006108.

Guterres A, 'The World Faces a Pandemic of Human Rights Abuses in the Wake of Covid-19' *The Guardian* (22 February 2021) <https://www.theguardian.com/global-development/2021/feb/22/world-faces-pandemic-human-rights-abuses-covid-19-antonio-guterres> accessed 25 March 2023.

Haldemann F (ed), 'Compromise', *Transitional Justice for Foxes: Conflict, Pluralism and the Politics of Compromise* (Cambridge University Press 2022) <https://www.cambridge.org/core/books/transitional-justice-for-foxes/compromise/8ED1C9D86D3BD6F5A35D68B427945789> accessed 25 March 2023.

Hayner PB, 'Fifteen Truth Commissions--1974 to 1994: A Comparative Study' [1994] 16 *Human Rights Quarterly* 597.

Hull G, 'Justice in Circumstances of Transition: Comments on Colleen Murphy's Theory of Transitional Justice as Justice of a Special Type' [2018] 14 *Journal of Global Ethics* 147.

Iacobucci G, 'Covid-19: India Should Stop Mass Gatherings and Consider Postponing Elections, Say Doctors' (2021) 373 *BMJ* n1102.

'International Health Regulations (2005) Third Edition' <https://www.who.int/publications-detail-redirect/9789241580496>

Kenny M and Sheldon J, 'How COVID-19 Is Exposing Unresolved Issues about How England Is Governed' (The British Academy, 6 July 2020) <https://www.thebritishacademy.ac.uk/blog/how-covid-19-exposing-unresolved-issues-about-how-england-governed/>

Khot UN, 'Navigating Healthcare Supply Shortages During the COVID-19 Pandemic' [2020] 13 *Circulation: Cardiovascular Quality and Outcomes* e006801.

Kreuder-Sonnen C, 'WHO Emergency Powers for Global Health Security' in C. Kreuder-Sonnen (ed.), *Emergency Powers of International Organizations: Between Normalization and Containment* (Oxford University Press 2019) <10.1093/oso/9780198832935.003.0006> accessed 6 January 2023.

Llop-Gironés A and others, 'Employment and Working Conditions of Nurses: Where and How Health Inequalities Have Increased during the COVID-19 Pandemic?' [2021] 19 *Human Resources for Health* 112.

Marmot M and others, 'Closing the Gap in a Generation: Health Equity through Action on the Social Determinants of Health' [2008] 372 *The Lancet* 1661.

Maxmen A, 'Why Did the World's Pandemic Warning System Fail When COVID Hit?' [2021] 589 *Nature* 499.

Murphy C, 'Truth Commissions', *International Encyclopedia of Ethics* (John Wiley & Sons, Ltd 2013) <https://onlinelibrary.wiley.com/doi/abs/10.1002/9781444367072.wbiee446> accessed 25 March 2023.

Murphy C, *The Conceptual Foundations of Transitional Justice* (Cambridge University Press 2017) <https://www.cambridge.org/core/books/conceptual-foundations-of-transitional-justice/989DAFCD8E1BCCF2716308D0B87AB2CE> accessed 24 July 2022.

Mustafa S and others, 'COVID-19 Preparedness and Response Plans from 106 Countries: A Review from a Health Systems Resilience Perspective' [2022] 37 *Health Policy and Planning* 255.

Negi Advocate C, 'Human Rights Violations of Migrants Workers in India During COVID-19 Pandemic' (Social Science Research Network 2020) SSRN Scholarly Paper 3629773 <https://papers.ssrn.com/abstract=3629773> accessed 28 July 2022.

Nickson R and Braithwaite J, 'Deeper, Broader, Longer Transitional Justice' [2014] 11 *European Journal of Criminology* 445.

OECD, *Making Decentralisation Work: A Handbook for Policy-Makers* (Organisation for Economic Co-operation and Development 2019) <https://www.oecd-ilibrary.org/urban-rural-and-regional-development/making-decentralisation-work_g2g9faa7-en> accessed 5 January 2023.

O'Shea BA and Ueda M, 'Who Is More Likely to Ignore Experts' Advice Related to COVID-19?' (2021) 23 *Preventive Medicine Reports* 101470.

'Pandemic Prevention, Preparedness and Response Accord' <https://www.who.int/news-room/questions-and-answers/item/pandemic-prevention–preparedness-and-response-accord> accessed 25 March 2023.

'Pandemic Reparations and Justice in Global Health Governance | Think Global Health' (*Council on Foreign Relations*) <https://www.thinkglobalhealth.org/article/pandemic-reparations-and-justice-global-health-governance> accessed 22 August 2022.

Parker R, 'The Global HIV/AIDS Pandemic, Structural Inequalities, and the Politics of International Health' [2002] 92 *American Journal of Public Health* 343.

Patel L and others, 'Climate Change and Extreme Heat Events: How Health Systems Should Prepare' 3 *NEJM Catalyst CAT*. 21.0454.

Posner EA and Vermeule A, 'Transitional Justice as Ordinary Justice' [2004] 117 *Harvard Law Review* 761.

Rawls J, *A Theory of Justice (Revised Edition)* (The Belknap Press of Harvard University Press 1999).

Robins S, 'Failing Victims? The Limits of Transitional Justice in Addressing the Needs of Victims of Violations' [2017] *Human Rights and International Legal Discourse* 41.

Rotberg RI and Thompson D (eds), *Truth v. Justice: The Morality of Truth Commissions* (Princeton University Press 2000) <https://www.jstor.org/stable/j.ctt7t4sd> accessed 25 March 2023.

Ruan L, Knockel J and Crete-Nishihata M, 'Censored Contagion: How Information on the Coronavirus Is Managed on Chinese Social Media' <https://tspace.library.utoronto.ca/handle/1807/104268> accessed 28 July 2022.

Siettos C and others, 'A Bulletin from Greece: A Health System under the Pressure of the Second COVID-19 Wave' [2021] 115 *Pathogens and Global Health* 133.

Silva SJR da and Pena L, 'Collapse of the Public Health System and the Emergence of New Variants during the Second Wave of the COVID-19 Pandemic in Brazil' [2021] 13 *One Health* 100287.

Spitzenstätter D and Schnell T, 'The Existential Dimension of the Pandemic: Death Attitudes, Personal Worldview, and Coronavirus Anxiety' [2022] 46 *Death Studies* 1031.

Swann T, '"Anarchist Technologies": Anarchism, Cybernetics and Mutual Aid in Community Responses to the COVID-19 Crisis' [2022] *Organization* 13505084221090632

'The Rule of Law and Transitional Justice in Conflict and Post-Conflict Societies: Report of Secretary General.' (United Nations Security Council 2004) UN Doc. S/2004/616

Warner S and others, 'English Devolution and the Covid-19 Pandemic: Governing Dilemmas in the Shadow of the Treasury' [2021] 92 *The Political Quarterly* 321.

Weissglass D, 'Justice in Global Health Governance: The Role of Enforcement' in H. Bhakuni and L. Miotto (eds), *Justice in Global Health: New Perspectives and Current Issues* (Routledge 2023).

Wilkinson E, 'NHS England's Backlog Recovery Plan Is at Serious Risk, Watchdog Warns' [2022] 379 *BMJ* o2779.

World Health Organisation, 'Health Inequality Monitor' (*WHO Social Determinants of Health: Inequality Monitor*) <https://www.who.int/data/inequality-monitor>

PART V

Global Health Justice

New Frames, New Approaches

11

REDISTRIBUTION AND RECOGNITION IN THE PURSUIT OF HEALTH JUSTICE

An Application of Nancy Fraser's Framework

Erika Blacksher

11.1 Introduction

As long as there have been empiric studies of population health, they have raised questions of responsibility and justice. In the middle of the 19th century, when pioneering studies established that adverse social conditions led to poor health and early death, judgements varied widely regarding who was to blame and what, if any, responsibility society had to fix poor living and working conditions.[1] Similarly, at the turn of the 21st century, a "rediscovery of the social determinants of health" has produced thousands of empiric studies of health inequalities and debate about whether and why we should judge some to be unjust.[2]

To answer such questions, philosophers and ethicists have drawn on and adapted prominent theories of justice, such as Rawls's distributive theory of justice, capability approaches, and luck egalitarianism.[3] One account of justice that has received scant attention is that by philosopher Nancy Fraser. Fraser's writings on justice have evolved over time, often in dialogue with recognition theorists, especially Alex Honneth.[4] Her account aims to overcome what she takes to be recognition theory's neglect of distributive injustices (deprivations in the "economic order", e.g., education, income, wealth, healthcare, and housing) and distributive theory's neglect of recognitional injustices (deficiencies in the "cultural order", e.g., racism, sexism, heterosexism, colonialism, nativism, and other "isms"). Unlike approaches that ignore one or the other or attempt to subsume one into the other, Fraser argues that any viable theory of justice today must address both and treat them as distinct and irreducible forms of social stratification and subordination that interact and overlap in real people's lives. These forms of

DOI: 10.4324/9781003399933-17

domination and subordination matter, she argues, because they impede people's opportunity to participate as peers in public life, the positive goal of justice. She calls this "participatory parity".[5]

My aim in this chapter is to test the potential utility of Fraser's framework for questions of health justice. The scope of a book chapter precludes advancing a definitive interpretation of it for such purposes. To my knowledge, Fraser has never extended her theory to questions of health and health inequalities. Nor have I yet found such uses in the literature, other than my own.[6] However, to the extent that Fraser's account tilts toward relational justice—given its overarching concern with equal social relations—analyses of the implications of relational egalitarianism for debates about health justice may apply here as well.[7] I will also occasionally note the ways in which Fraser's model of justice compares to alternative approaches, but will do so selectively, looking often to capability approaches or those that draw upon them because, in my view, they offer the strongest statements to date on why human health and social inequalities in health may matter to justice.

I examine the utility of Fraser's framework for considerations of health (in)justice by two criteria. The first concerns the conceptual resources it provides to identify, interrogate, and assess injustices and, when need be, adjudicate among them. To that end in Section 11.2, I describe Fraser's approach to theorising about justice and outline the two main planks of her framework: a bifocal formulation of injustice and positive goal of justice, participatory parity. Together they clarify the moral status of socioeconomic and cultural subordination as injustices and create normative scaffolding for assessing a deeper and wider terrain of health inequalities generated by "intersectional" health studies, by which I mean those that examine a health indicator by multiple axes of difference simultaneously. I also briefly note the ways in which these concepts can provide ethical guidance for health equity research, action, and policy.

The second criterion concerns the framework's real-world fit with contemporary population inquiry. To that end in Section 11.3, I map key elements of Fraser's framework and theory onto debates about the appropriate purpose and models of population health science. I argue that Fraser's critical, sociological, and egalitarian social theory makes it purpose built for a 21st-century population health inquiry that seeks to overcome ahistorical, individualistic models of health, and to document and explain the social forces that produce and distribute health at the population level. While some consider this second criterion to be the ultimate test of theories of justice (do they track with real-world social struggles and egalitarian movements?), others argue that normative theory should be judged by the criteria it supplies to critically assess these movements and distinguish among legitimate and illegitimate claims of injustice.[8] Fraser's framework has something to offer on both scores.

In the conclusion, I summarise the strengths of Fraser's framework of justice, including its potential to meet several criteria that have been proposed by Sridhar Venkatapuram in this volume as key criteria of a global health justice theory. I also note a potentially serious limitation of Fraser's account, namely, whether it has the conceptual resources to address the needs of people who are not yet adults, that is, children whose capabilities for health and other important capabilities, are undergoing formation and development. Given the profound impact of early life development on health over the life course and the devastating effects of poverty, malnutrition, war, abuse and neglect, and other forms of trauma on children around the globe, a theory of global health justice must address the needs of its future citizens.

11.2 Fraser's Normative Framework

Fraser takes a "critical" stance in theorising about justice. Critical theory seeks to provide an empirically accurate picture of society's struggles, foregrounding the "social conditions, social changes, and social actors that we ought to be attending to" so they can be evaluated and transformed.[9] Its vantage point is that of non-ideal theory, in contrast to ideal theory. Ideal theory brackets real-world struggles, hierarchies, and harms in order to articulate "principles meant to govern the operation of just institutions, embedded within the background of a just social structure".[10] Perhaps the most prominent contemporary example of ideal theory is Rawls' theory of justice, whose idealising assumption that all persons are normal functioning adults had to be relaxed in order to serve as a basis for considerations of health justice.[11] Ideal theory has been criticised for ignoring relations of structural domination, exploitation, coercion, and oppression that have historically and presently systematically shape people's life chances, much to the detriment of minoritised groups, women, and those who are poor.[12]

Ideal theory neglects precisely the power relations and people that occupy Fraser's framework of justice. Her bifocal formulation of injustice delineates two processes of social subordination. One is distributive in nature ("maldistribution") and the other is recognitional in nature ("misrecognition"). Maldistribution refers to processes rooted in the socioeconomic order that create class-like groups, some of which are subject to socioeconomic exploitation, deprivation, marginalisation, and exclusion. Misrecognition refers to processes rooted in the sociocultural order that involve patterns of representation, interpretation, and communication that subject some to discrimination, stigmatisation, marginalisation, and exclusion on the basis of ascribed characteristics such as race, ethnicity, gender, sexual orientation, religion, language, social class, etc.

Fraser argues that maldistribution's and misrecognition's separate tap roots require a theory of justice that treats them as distinct harms, even as they intersect and interpenetrate people's lives to varied degrees. She argues that recognition theories either ignore harms of maldistribution or, in their attempts to incorporate or subsume them, suppress or distort the phenomena in question. Distributive theories, she asserts, commit the error in reverse, eliding harms of misrecognition.[13]

Fraser shows how maldistribution and misrecognition always intersect and interact in the real world, using the four major sociological categories of social stratification—class, race, gender, and sexual orientation—to make her case. Race, she explains, functions both as an organising principle of the economy, creating racially specific forms of maldistribution, and as an organising principle of the cultural order, creating racially specific forms of status subordination. To the first point, people of colour are over-represented in low-wage work and in the ranks of the unemployed and impoverished. To the second, everything coded as non-white is racialised and stigmatised, subjecting minoritised people to daily harassment, discrimination, stereotypes, criminalisation, incarceration, and violence.[14]

Gender, too, can be dually parsed. Gender is used to structure a division between paid and unpaid labour (e.g., reproductive/care labour), and a division within paid labour—e.g., lower paid "pink collar" work.[15] Gender also operates in the sociocultural order by devaluing all things "feminine", subjecting women to trivialisation, stereotypes, harassment, domestic violence, rape, and murder.[16]

These are not exceptions. Even class and sexual orientation, which may seem solely the product of the economic order or cultural order, respectively, involve both maldistribution and misrecognition. For example, class-like groups whose primary struggle is economic impoverishment may seem to suffer only from the economic structure of a capitalist society, a harm remediable by redistribution. Yet, class-like groups that are not subject to racisms based on skin colour are subject to other forms of misrecognition based on culture, e.g., ugly tropes and stereotypes that demean them ('white trash,' 'rednecks,' and 'degenerate families') and their ways (e.g., 'culture of poverty').[17] The primary cause of injustice here is the economy, Fraser argues, but with traces of misrecognition.

Sexual orientation, too, entails both. The primary cause of injustice for LGBTQ people, Fraser argues, is misrecognition, reflected in the slurs, shaming, threats, and violence to which they are subject. But there are also serious economic and employment risks associated with making one's status known and liabilities associated, for example, with taxes and inheritance laws, where same-sex marriage is not legally protected.

The need for a two-dimensional account of justice becomes still "more pressing as soon as one ceases considering axes of subordination singly and begins considering them together. After all gender, race, sexuality, and class are not neatly cordoned off from one another. Rather all these axes of subordination intersect one another in ways that affect everyone's interests and identities. No one is a member of only one such collectivity. And individuals who are subordinated along one axis of social division may well be dominant along another".[18] Fraser's framework is in this way "intersectional." It is structured to account for a multiplicity of power relations and thus has the capacity to identify, interrogate, and address an array of socially salient differences that shape social positions, life chances, and social struggles.[19]

The second plank of her framework is the standard of justice, participatory parity. Participatory parity is the criterion for establishing the requirements of justice and judging claims of injustice. Participatory parity requires that social and economic arrangements "permit all (adult) members of society to interact with one another as peers".[20] Fraser argues that this standard must be construed as structural and sociological, rooted in the social systems and patterns that govern collective life, not in the psychology of individuals. This matters because claims of injustice can then be judged by whether economic arrangements and institutionalised patterns of cultural value prevent some from participating on a par with others in social life, not by whether an individual claims to feel impoverished or demeaned. For example, claims of maldistribution made by individuals whose expensive tastes fuel a feeling of economic insufficiency, despite being materially comfortable enough to achieve participatory parity, would not have a legitimate basis for claiming injustice. Similarly, claims of misrecognition made by white racists who feel their self-worth is compromised by a social order that values people of all races equally have no legitimate claim of injustice.

Justice is secured, and legitimate claims of maldistribution and misrecognition are remedied, by two conditions. The objective condition requires that people have the socioeconomic resources they need to promote "independence" and "voice". Such conditions preclude "institutionalized deprivation, exploitation, and gross disparities in wealth, income, and leisure time".[21] The intersubjective condition requires that institutionalised patterns of interpretation and communication express moral respect for all, creating conditions that support the equal opportunity of all to achieve self-respect and social esteem. It thereby precludes social relations distorted by racism, sexism, heterosexism, colonialism, ableism, classism, ageism, and other systemic power relations that demean and devalue some social identities.

This basic outline of Fraser's normative framework is incomplete but sufficient to explore what utility it may have for considerations of health justice. To my knowledge, Fraser has never said anything about the potential relevance of her notion of justice to health or the disproportionate incidence of preventable morbidity and premature death among minoritised and otherwise marginalised and exploited groups.

11.2.1 Why and How Health Matters to Justice

One of the first questions a theory of health justice has to answer is why health is relevant to justice. What about health and its lack, as reflected in health inequalities, suggests a problem of justice? How might achieving some level of health or not falling below a certain level of health be important to being able to participate as a peer in social life? Fraser has not provided much elaboration of what participatory parity entails. Like other relational egalitarians, she has focused more on what she opposes than what she proposes.[22] But, as already described, she has identified objective and intersubjective conditions that must be met to secure justice and those conditions could be further specified in ways that support different interpretations of why health matters to participatory parity.

The interpretive work could head in a few directions. One approach is to argue that health is instrumentally valuable to participatory parity. That is, all people need some level of physical and mental health to participate as peers in public life. People cannot be so debilitated by poor health or disability that they are unable to participate as equals, or at all, in public life. They cannot be so overwhelmed by chronic worry over their health or whether they can access the care needed to treat disease that they cannot participate in public life. More would need to be said about the meaning of health and the level needed to achieve participatory parity, but Fraser's objective and intersubjective criteria could be built out to protect human health at whatever level was posited. For example, the objective condition could detail the necessary social resources, e.g., healthful nutrition, quality education, living wages, safe housing and streets, and timely healthcare services. The intersubjective condition could likewise detail the social relations necessary for healthy human development (e.g., attachment and care in early life), intrapersonal and interpersonal respect, and social trust. On this interpretation, health is valued not in itself but for what it enables, much like Norman Daniels's argument for why health is a "special good" in his adapted Rawlsian approach to health justice.[23] People need, he argues, some degree of mental and physical health over the course of their lives to have fair equality of opportunity to pursue their life projects. On this interpretation, then, health is instrumentally valuable to participatory parity.

Another approach is to argue that health is intrinsically valuable to participatory parity, namely, that having some threshold level of health is a constitutive element of what it means to participate as a peer in public life. Participatory parity would have to undergo further specification to describe what it looks like to engage as a peer in social life and how health features as an element of it. For example, participatory might entail being able to navigate the world without impediments based on one's health status, which would have implications for the objective and intersubjective conditions of participatory parity (e.g., wheelchairs and curb cuts, gender-affirming healthcare, service animals, and corresponding regulation thereof). Or it might involve being able to achieve functionings widely deemed valuable, like bearing a child that survives beyond infancy or living a normal lifespan. Such an argument might find further footing in the view that health in late modernity has come to be seen as an achievement, something people should be "supported to work at to enhance their quality of life".[24] On this interpretation, then, health is intrinsically valuable as a constitutive element of participatory parity.

This approach arguably moves toward a thick description of participatory parity, which might raise questions about whether it violates Fraser's commitments to a deontological account of justice, one that can avoid arguments over what constitutes a good life. But her account has already been taken to task along such lines.[25] Any interpretation of her account for purposes of health justice would have to address the matter.

One might find neither approach satisfactory or convincing, yet still view the study of health and health inequalities imperative to the pursuit of participatory parity. Because the objective and intersubjective conditions that secure justice also correspond neatly to the social resources (e.g., income, employment, education, housing, healthcare) and social relations (e.g., racism, sexism, heterosexism, nativism, colonialism) that drive health outcomes, population-level inequalities in morbidity and mortality may signal deprivations and deficiencies in the economic and/or sociocultural orders, and thus failures of participatory parity. On this interpretation, the measurement of population health functions as an empiric test of whether the conditions of justice are present.

Capability theorists sometimes do something similar. "Capabilities" refer to people's genuine opportunities to be and do things they have reason to value, which are intrinsic goods justice should protect and promote. Because this sort of human freedom can be difficult to measure directly, people's actual "functionings" may be measured to gauge whether people have genuine freedom to pursue their ends. Studies of famine, poverty, health, school attendance, literacy, and other basic 'beings and doings' can provide clues to which capabilities are substantive and real.[26] Some capability theorists build a capability for health directly into justice, as with Martha Nussbaum's inclusion of capabilities for life and for bodily health within her list of central human capabilities and Sridhar Venkatapuram's specification of health as a capability.[27] But Amartya Sen purposefully provides no such list or elaboration specific to health. Sen prefers to leave the question of what capabilities matter most to the deliberative decision making of communities and localities. Yet, over his decades of writings across many disciplines, he seems to always include measures of health (e.g., 'being free of preventable morbidity') as examples of important capabilities or as deficiencies in capabilities (e.g., premature death).

For current purposes, it is enough to have established that an argument could be made as to why and how health might matter to participatory parity and that those arguments are not unlike those made in other theories used to address questions of health justice.

11.2.2 Determinations of Health Injustice

A second important question is whether Fraser's framework—once retrofitted to include health as special to justice—can provide guidance in determining which health inequalities constitute health inequities. That question is important in the base case, as there are many health inequalities. But it becomes imperative against the backdrop of intersectional health studies that examine health indicators by multiple axes of social stratification simultaneously (e.g., by race, class, and gender). Mapping health in this way can unmask health shortfalls that are papered over by studies of health indicators that use only one analytic category (e.g., race only, or class only), reveal the depth of poor health and early death in groups disadvantaged along multiple axes (e.g., poor, Black, transgender persons), and map a broad and complex landscape of health inequalities.

Two inter-related aspects of Fraser's framework are useful to thinking about health (in)justice "intersectionally". First, health inequalities rooted in either maldistribution or misrecognition or some combination are candidate cases of injustice. Socioeconomic and sociocultural harms interpenetrate actual people's lives to different degrees, depending on their social position and identity. But in theory, these harms have independent moral standing and equal moral status. Were they expressed as action-guiding norms or principles (e.g., put negatively, do no distributive harm and do no recognitional harm), we might say they have *prima facie* standing. Prima facie principles are obligatory, other things being equal.[28]

This formulation matters to the study of health justice precisely because it foregrounds class alongside other forms of social subordination and domination. In doing so, Fraser's framework could help correct a tendency in intersectional analyses and contemporary social justice discourse to neglect or suppress class as a difference that makes a difference in people's life chances.[29] As Patricia Hill Collins notes, even when class is mentioned, "it remains underutilised as an analytic category to explain complex social inequalities".[30] Foregrounding harms in the economic order is especially important in political contexts such as the United States where class has been a suppressed system of power relations since the nation's founding.[31] That suppression is reflected in the history of public health and the struggle to make data collection by measures of socioeconomic status routine and robust, a task still incomplete.[32]

This neglect is especially problematic for considerations of health justice, because socioeconomic status (e.g., education and income) is a potent predictor of health and longevity. Any framework of justice built for questions of health justice cannot ignore maldistribution in the economic order.

Second, Fraser's framework pivots determinations of health justice from "single axis" to "matrix" investigations.[33] Although Fraser's framework is two dimensional, the categories of maldistribution and misrecognition can be further disaggregated into multiple dimensions. Misrecognitions may take several health-harming forms—racism to be sure, but also colonialism, sexism, heterosexism, nativism, ableism, ageism, classism, etc. Maldistributions, too, may be refined into subcategories that have well-documented health-harming effects, such as disproportionate exposures to early life adversity among poor children of all races, birth cohort effects associated with serious economic upheavals (e.g., the Great Recession), geographic localities that lack resources and amenities (e.g., some urban and rural areas), and so on.

The investigation of any health inequality as a potential injustice would need to be informed by additional considerations, including the theory's tolerance for inequality. Theories of justice are typically guided not only by an account of the good or right but also by standards of allocation. Those standards range from utilitarianism's maximisation principle, which is neutral with regard to the good's distribution; to strict equality, which tolerates no inequality; to some form of prioritarian principle, which prioritises the least advantaged.[34] Fraser does not address such matters directly. However, one can interpret Fraser's basic commitments to mean that she would reject utilitarian's distributive neutrality as unacceptable, given its disregard for socially disadvantaged groups, and possibly would accept some degree of inequality, namely, that which does not undermine participatory parity. Fraser's commitments are arguably prioritarian.

Here, too, there are choices about the kind of prioritarianism that would support Fraser's account of justice. There are prioritarian principles, such as John Rawls's "difference" principle, that aim to improve the situation of the worst off, but which also tolerates considerable inequality.[35] There are "sufficiency" principles that aim to establish some basic minimum or threshold level of the good in question, such as that articled by Madison Powers and Ruth Faden.[36] The scope of this chapter precludes working out this facet of Fraser's account in detail. What can be said is that questions about which health inequalities constitute health inequities would need to be informed not only by their causal story—whether they are traceable to maldistribution and misrecognition—but also by whether the health shortfalls threaten or compromise participatory parity.

Consider the case of U.S. inequalities in infant mortality. U.S. infant mortality data show that college-educated mothers, regardless of race, generally have much better outcomes than women without a high school diploma (i.e., women who have not completed 12 years of primary education). Data also show that black college-educated women have much higher rates of infant mortality than their college-educated white counterparts. Studies show that high infant mortality rates among women with little formal education can be traced to hardships of poverty.[37] Numerous studies also show that high infant mortality rates among college-educated Black women are likely attributable to lifelong exposure to racisms—interpersonal, cultural, structural.[38] Because Fraser specifies maldistribution and misrecognition as distinct harms with independent moral standing, attention to infant mortality rates traceable to racism and to socioeconomic deprivations, regardless of race, both raise concerns of justice. Thus, on their face, the high rates of infant mortality in college-educated black women and poor women of all races who have lacked the opportunity for formal education are unjust.

Such a judgement would need to be further supported by a determination that these rates of infant mortality violate an account of participatory parity that incorporated health in some way, work I do not do here. But several considerations seem relevant. The first is the gravity of infant mortality. Infant mortality refers to the death of a baby before its first birthday, an event that is experienced as a tragedy by parents, who may consider childbearing integral to their identity and culture. Second, infant mortality is considered a good gauge of population health and societal well-being broadly, because of its association with social and economic conditions, racial discrimination and civil rights, and access to healthcare and public health practices.[39] Third, the U.S. infant mortality rate is more than twice that of nations with the lowest rates; roughly five U.S. infants per 1,000 live births die before their first birthday compared to two infants per 1,000 live births in Japan and Finland.[40] Infant mortality rates are, as already noted, even higher among racially minoritised and socioeconomically marginalised women. Fourth, rates vary by state residence, possibly a function of divergent state policy contexts that reflect varying degrees of social protections, such as the generosity of unemployment insurance, sickness benefits, and pension programs.[41] This degree of uncertainty, variability, and tragedy in human reproduction in the 21st century, when much lower rates are achievable, arguably violates a health-sensitive standard of participatory parity.

Consider a second especially tough case. Multiple studies demonstrate worsening mortality trends in white people who have a high school diploma or less. Those trends include an absolute decline in life expectancy documented in white women and men who lack high school diplomas and rising midlife mortality in white people with a high school degree or less.[42] These trends are attributable in part but not exclusively to what have been called "deaths of despair" associated with the opioid epidemic, suicide, and alcohol poisoning.[43] The causal story is multifaceted and remains subject to study and debate, but prominent among causal explanations is the role of sustained socioeconomic deprivation set in motion by decades of globalisation, automation, and the attendant loss of steady living wages, guaranteed benefits (e.g., healthcare and pensions), and social connections and support (e.g., marriage). On the face of it, such maldistributions are serious matters of justice in Fraser's account.

However, there are possible explanations for these trends. Some research, for example, attributes high rates of opioid deaths to racism within healthcare systems that facilitate white patients' access to highly addictive opioids, while denying appropriate pain management to people of colour.[44] Another study suggests that white despair itself is rooted in a (mis)perception that their social status is in decline relative to people of colour.[45] Other arguments suggest that racist beliefs animate working class white people's resistance to government programs (e.g., universal healthcare). All three of these alternative explanations suggest that various forms of racisms may be causally implicated in these white mortality trends. If racisms are involved–in Fraser's terms, if misrecongition is involved–how should these inequalities be assessed ethically? Do they constitute an injustice? I know of only one systematic ethical analysis that has taken up the question.[46]

What guidance might Fraser's account provide on the question? The causal story matters considerably to Fraser's account of justice because of the moral status of maldistribution and misrecognition as injustices. Yet, the upstream causal story for such complex trends is likely to involve many forms of subordination and oppression and there are likely multiple stories. It might be important, for example, to distinguish the absolute decline in life expectancy in white people who lack a high school degree, who may come from intergenerational poverty and so know only poverty, from rising midlife mortality in white working-class people, who have experienced a *decline* in their economic and social status. The effects of socioeconomic hardship may differ between those who are inured to poverty and have lower expectations for their lives and those to whom hardship is new and experienced as a status loss and an affront to their expectations.[47] It might also be important to examine why deaths of despair began to ensnare communities of colour around 2013.[48] Are they too falling victim to deteriorating socioeconomic conditions and forms of despair?

If we accept that deteriorating socioeconomic conditions have contributed to these phenomena, we still might ask, *why* they have been deteriorating. But the further upstream we look for ultimate explanations, the more we might disagree. Some will see the ills of structural racism at work.[49] Others will see capitalist ideologies and policies that protect the economic rights of the elite class.[50] Importantly, Fraser's intersectional framework makes space for *both explanations, their intersection with each other and with other systems of power*—e.g., colonialism, imperialism, patriarchy and sexism, heterosexism, nativism, etc. Fraser's justice rejects reductionist tendencies to explain all social struggles in terms of one single metanarrative, e.g., a capitalist-class order, *or* a racialised social order, *or* a patriarchal order, etc. The perspicacity of Fraser's account is precisely its insight that manifold power relations are driving social inequalities.

With regard to the 'tough case' under consideration, Fraser's approach would not allow the serious maldistribution at work in these mortality trends to be ignored. Any determination of injustice would also need to be judged by whether these mortality trends violate a health-sensitive standard of participatory parity, for which the following considerations are relevant. People are dying in their prime working years, including in their younger years, often by suicide. People are also dying prematurely of chronic diseases, which are presaged by many years of poor health, chronic pain, mental distress, and fear, all accompanied by major disruptions in life plans and projects that people care about. Add to this a healthcare system, on which sick people heavily rely, that is excessively expensive and fails to deliver timely quality care to low-income people. These sorts of facts suggest that current arrangements do not support all persons to participate as peers in public life.

11.2.3 Priority Setting Among Health Inequities

The fact that intersectional health inequalities will unmask a broader more complex landscape of social locations and formations of inequality that may all be judged unjust raises a related question. What criteria or process should guide prioritising some inequities for collective action and resources when not all can be? The account of justice that has addressed this question most directly is advanced by Powers and Faden. Although they do not refer to intersectionality *per se*, their notion of justice is centrally concerned with the "interacting" and "cascading" effects of social determinants that form "densely woven, systematic patterns of disadvantage" that jeopardise "essential dimensions of well-being".[51] Intersectional analyses also focus on social groups and identities marginalised by multiple social hierarchies.[52] Powers and Faden argue that the most urgent inequalities to address are those that entail "overlapping social determinants with profound and pervasive effects on a cluster of well-being dimensions".[53] Worrisome, too, but less so are three other categories of health inequalities, in ranked order: (1) "one social determinant with profound and pervasive effects on one dimension of well-being", (2) "overlapping social determinants with profound and pervasive effects on one dimension of well-being", and (3) "one social determinant with profound and pervasive effects on a cluster of dimensions of well-being".[54] Each category (i.e., 1,2,3) grows in urgency as a problem of social justice.

There are two potential problems with this approach to normative assessments of intersectional health inequalities. First, rarely will health inequalities involve only one social determinant. Take our "tough case" of worsening white mortality trends. The men in this case are advantaged by their skin colour and gender but disadvantaged by their class position, thus their decline in life expectancy might seem to qualify as Powers and Faden's third kind of health inequality—one social determinant with profound and pervasive effects on a cluster of dimensions of well-being. But on closer inspection one finds other social determinants at work: in this era, their lack of a high school diploma suggests these white men likely grew up in poor, chaotic, and abusive or neglectful families, which have lifelong impacts on health.[55] Early life adversity is an often-overlooked social determinant of health.[56]

The premature deaths of white women who lack high school diplomas also involve multiple social determinants. Like their male counterparts, the lack of a high school diploma is likely traceable to early life adversity, which then translates into sustained socioeconomic stressors throughout adulthood (unsteady work, low wages, and poverty). Unlike their male counterparts, these women also labour under the burden of "gendered, unwaged care work care" that is assigned to women in a sexist society.[57] If this is correct, then the absolute decline in life expectancy documented in these two groups arguably fits in Powers and Faden's most urgent category of health inequalities—overlapping social determinants with profound and pervasive effects on a cluster of dimensions of well-being dimensions. I would argue that many cases of health inequalities, if closely examined, can be shown to implicate a cluster of social determinants and have profound and pervasive effects on a cluster of well-being dimensions (rather than one dimension of well-being). This would place many health inequalities in Powers and Faden's "most urgent" category.

A second potential problem with Powers and Faden's approach is that it seems to support an "additive" interpretation of intersectionality in which layers of disadvantage "add up" in a straightforward linear way. Intersectional theorists view this interpretation as a mistake. The relevant intersections do not just add up; they create something altogether new.[58] If each "ingredient" of difference (e.g., location in an economic hierarchy) changes as it intersects with another difference (e.g., location in a racial hierarchy) and changes again as it intersects with another difference (e.g., location in a gender hierarchy), and so on, then intersectionality is not simple arithmetic. Many new, complex, and unique formations of inequality are forged. The task of determining which among them warrants collective action is unlikely to be amenable to an algorithm that can be easily applied. What is likely required is a fair democratic process. Fraser suggests just that. Tough cases will require democratic processes of public deliberation "in which conflicting judgments are sifted and rival interpretations are weighed".[59] The "tough case" used in this chapter bears this out (Wilson 2018; Lee and Hicken 2018; Wray 2018; Zaidi and Sederstrom 2018).[60]

11.2.4 Ethical Guidance for Health Equity Research, Action, and Policy

Fraser's framework can also be mined for ethical guidance for health equity research, action, and policy. As I have written on these topics elsewhere, I quickly summarise the main points here. First, I have extended Fraser's standard of participatory parity to develop the idea of "participatory parity in health" (Blacksher 2012).[61] In this application, I argue that minoritised and otherwise marginalised social groups and communities should have meaningful opportunities to inform the development, content, and implementation of health-relevant research and policy. Because they shoulder a disproportionate burden of preventable disease and premature mortality and are likely to be often targeted by health research, policies, and programs, these communities can more accurately identify and articulate the challenges to health as well as opportunities for remedies that resonate with their beliefs, values, and lifeways. Engagement that identifies their priorities and that continues throughout the research process through to implementation may also avoid harms of misrecognition. Fraser explains that misrecognition can occur by either amplifying difference in ways that depict groups as aberrant or deviant or by denying difference via expectations of assimilation. In the first instance, misrecognition places groups and communities on the margins or outside of our shared humanity; in the second, distinctive and important life experiences, traditions, and histories are ignored. Sustained and meaningful engagement with communities may be the best guide to respectful research and action. This sort of participatory engagement is particularly important in light of the complex formations of health and social inequality identified by intersectional health studies.[62] The acuity of lived experience may be essential to making research both effective and respectful.

Second, I have argued that stigmatisation is an ethically unacceptable tool of public health.[63] Although some have argued that an anti-stigma ethic has overtaken public health, ethical debates over the use of stigmatization to prevent disease and promote health are active.[64] One need only examine anti-tobacco or anti-obesity efforts to see that the use of stigmatisation is alive and well in public health. Although the meaning and implications of stigmatisation vary, key elements overlap with Fraser's notion of misrecognition. The point of stigma is to mark some people as different and deviant, to denormalise them or their behaviour, or exclude them from public life.[65] This process denies shared humanity to those targeted and can only be exercised in the context of power relations that Fraser's account of justice seeks to end.

More could be said about how these conceptual resources apply to questions of health justice and other conceptual resources that I have not mentioned could be brought to bear, such as Fraser's formulation of "affirmative" and "transformative" approaches to remedying injustice. But this treatment is sufficient to establish that the framework could be very useful to considerations of health justice, with some adaptation.

11.3 21st-Century Population Health Inquiry and Fraser's Critical Social Theory

The second criterion for judging the adequacy of justice frameworks is the degree to which they track with real world social movements. Fraser's framework appears purpose-built for a 21st-century population health inquiry that seeks to document, explain, and end the social relations and social conditions that produce stark health inequalities. That close fit relates to both the framework's purpose and content.

11.3.1 Purpose

Contemporary population health inquiry and Fraser's account of justice share emancipatory aspirations. They seek not only to describe and explain processes of social ordering but to denounce some as unjust. Indeed, for some population health researchers, the study of health inequalities *is and should be* a form of moral critique.

That view has long been subject to debate within public health. Pioneering studies from the 17th and 18th centuries documented associations between poverty, morbidity, and mortality, and more refined such studies dominated public health practices during the first half of the 19th century.[66] Despite this history, contemporary interest in the social determinants of health and health inequalities represents a paradigm shift within the epidemiological sciences, because the intervening decades saw the rise of modern epidemiology's "risk factor" approach. Its focus on biological and behavioural risk factors, measurable at the individual level within a small window of time, abstracts the study of disease away from the social and economic conditions, and the social and political choices, that jeopardise human health. A "rediscovery of the social determinants of health" at the turn of the 21st century, however, is fully underway.[67] Referred to variously as social epidemiology, eco-epidemiology, or population health, this ascendant paradigm seeks to explain what a risk factor approach alone cannot—persistent and significant social inequalities in health. Proponents of this approach aim not to exclude biology and behaviour from inquiry but rather to develop frameworks with the theoretical and methodological power to contextualise them within broader social and political structures and systems.

But within population health, there is also debate about how and why to measure health inequalities.[68] That debate turns on whether to measure health inequalities across individuals in a population or across social groups that are differentiated by some proxy of social (dis)advantage, such as socioeconomic status, race, ethnicity, gender, and such. In 1999, Murray noted that in "much of the published literature, health inequalities are taken to be synonymous with social group differences in health".[69] One year later, the World Health Organization's 2000 report's recommendation to measure health across individuals without any form of social group categorisation or differentiation provoked an outcry. Critics argued that such an approach "removes equity and human rights considerations from the routine measurement and reporting of health disparities".[70] What gets removed more specifically are the social structures that systematically set health inequalities in motion, which persistently and significantly burden people who are already socially disadvantaged, thus depriving them of an essential component of well-being: good health.[71] What also gets erased, critics implied, is the capacity to document, explain, and build an evidence base to remedy health inequalities that are unjust.

11.3.2 Content

Whether these egalitarian ends have won the day in population health inquiry is unclear, but they are reflected in the workaday machinery and models of population health studies. The use of social group categories (e.g., education, income, occupation, race/ethnicity, gender, and sexual orientation) to measure and report health inequalities is ubiquitous and the list of relevant social categories continues to grow. Conceptual models of the "social determinants" of health number in the dozens and routinely include an array of social group variables alongside other salient features of social, material, and environmental conditions. Definitions of social determinants foreground categories of social resources and social relations, such as that advanced by Jones and colleagues, who explain that an economic class structure and a range of "isms" based on interpretations of how one looks create "systems of power" that determine the range of social contexts and situate populations within them.[72] A seminal textbook of social epidemiology frontloads chapters on socioeconomic position; discrimination based on race, ethnicity, gender, sexual orientation, disability, immigrant status, age, and social class; income inequality; and working conditions.[73] Class and race are treated as "fundamental causes" of health inequalities.[74]

These examples, among many others that could be given, all reflect population health inquiry's overarching aim to situate health inequalities within broader sociological and historical contexts and power relations that systematically shape who stays healthy and who gets sick. Those contexts and power relations are precisely the social systems that comprise Fraser's bifocal formulation of injustice. This is the first of three ways in which the content of Fraser's framework fits that of contemporary population health studies.

The second is the intersectionality of Fraser's framework, described in Section 11.2, which aligns with an 'intersectional turn' underway in the study of health inequalities.[75] Population health researchers increasingly are documenting health inequalities by multiple analytic categories simultaneously to capture the complexity of social locations and multiplicity of social processes that compromise human health.[76] Some such studies are "intra-categorical", meaning they may document health inequalities for a demographic group disadvantaged along several axes, such as studies that examine LGBTQ black women or transgender Latinx men. Others are "inter-categorical", meaning they document health inequalities across a wider array of social groups and locations (e.g., race, class, and gender) that may involve a mix of advantage (e.g., whiteness) and disadvantage (e.g., poverty).[77]

The case for studying health by race and class simultaneously is especially strong, as they are both potent predictors of health and longevity and they interact. Studying them together can uncover social locations and formations of inequality that may be hidden otherwise. For example, studies that sort populations by only a proxy of class, such as education or income, mask the added effects of racism and other forms of stigmatisation and marginalisation to which people of colour are subject.[78] Studies that examine health only by race mask the effects of socioeconomic deprivation and discrimination that affect all people, including white people who are poor.[79]

U.S. inequalities in infant mortality and life expectancy, again, are illustrative. The life expectancy of those with the most education (16+ years) is more than a decade longer than those with the least education (less than 12 years).[80] Infant mortality exhibits a similar pattern. Mothers who lack a high school diploma are twice as likely to lose an infant before its first birthday as women with a college degree.[81] But for both health outcomes, the "health dividend" paid to those with higher levels of education pays less to African Americans than to white people.[82] College-educated African American men and women have life expectancies roughly 4 years shy of their white college-educated counterparts.[83] College-educated African American women are roughly 2.5 times more likely to lose an infant before its first birthday than are college-educated white women.[84] One sees a similar pattern in other widely used measures of health, such as self-rated health. Regardless of race, health status is best for people living well above the poverty level and worst for those living at or below the poverty level. But within each income group, racial disparities generally prevail, with white people typically faring better than their African American counterparts.[85]

The third alignment between population health studies and Fraser's bifocal formulation of injustice is a shared focus on macro-social causes of harm, two in particular. Maldistribution and misrecognition are well-established drivers of health inequalities. The effects of socioeconomic deprivation—such as early life adversity, poor quality schools, low educational attainment, low paying and/or high-risk jobs, lack of healthcare, resource-poor and unsafe neighbourhoods, and the chronic chaos and stress of it all—get under the skin no matter its colour. Harms rooted in the economic order help explain why white people who are poor have health outcomes more similar to black people who are poor than to that of their college-educated white counterparts.[86] The health outcomes of black and brown people at each level of education/income are, however, typically worse, reflecting the additional assaults of structural, institutional, cultural, and interpersonal racism. The health effects of other "isms," such as heterosexism and structural sexism, are also being studied.

Fraser's dual formulation may hold explanatory power for other long-studied cases and causes of health inequalities. Take the "Hispanic paradox". Upon arrival to the United States, Hispanic/Latinx people generally have better health and longer lives than white people, despite their overall lower socioeconomic status. But with longer residence, the health of Hispanic people declines. While the causal story is not fully understood, social processes of racialisation, discrimination, and stigmatisation may be implicated.[87]

Another example is the "income inequality hypothesis", which posits that the magnitude of income inequality in a political community (e.g., a nation, state, and province) impacts the health of its residents.[88] While experts debate its effect in many political contexts, a clearly established relationship between income inequality and increased mortality has been documented in the United States.[89] What remains open to debate is whether income inequality itself is the cause or rather the social relations that tolerate, or even encourage, significant income inequality. The evidence from the United States suggests that race/racism may be a key factor in the degree of income inequality and associated excess mortality that is tolerated.

Notice that in each of these examples, neither racism nor poverty on its own can tell the whole story. One needs to take seriously both sources of harm *and* investigate how they intersect and combine in particular subgroups to the detriment of health and longevity.

Fraser has also suggested that her bifocal formulation of justice may need to be extended to include a third form of social ordering, specifically, governance structures and political decision making.[90] Political decision making and governance systems have come under increasing study in population health inquiry. The "political determinants of health" refer to systems of governance, political institutions, and decision-making procedures that impact whose interests are represented, subsequent policymaking by elected representatives, and the consequent health effects for those who are un- or underrepresented.[91] Political determinants are likely to be particularly salient in countries with non-democratic systems of governance, where democratic systems of governance are under threat, or as seen in the United States, where governance systems enable extreme polarisation. Increasingly in the United States, one's health and longevity prospects have come to depend on the state within which one lives due to its federalist government structure.[92] Mounting evidence shows that divergent state policies—enabled by shifts in power from the federal government to state governments over the last four decades—are implicated in state-level variations in COVID-19 mortality, life expectancy, infant mortality, and working-age mortality.[93]

11.4 Concluding Remarks

This chapter has examined the potential utility of Nancy Fraser's critical social theory as a framework for global health justice. Although more interpretive spadework would need to be done to advance a Fraser-based account of health justice, this chapter has gone some distance in establishing its value to that end. Fraser's critical, sociological, and egalitarian social theory provides a fitting framework for a population health inquiry that seeks to document, elucidate, and transform the social forces that drive health inequities. Its perspicuous description of global social movements and their struggles map directly onto the definitions, explanatory theories and frameworks, and aspirations of population health and health equity movements. In this regard, a Fraser-based account of health justice meets the criterion of "intertheoretic coherence", one of several proposed by Sridhar Venkatapuram for a global health justice.[94] This criterion refers to the need for a global health justice to be able to accommodate the disciplines (e.g., social epidemiology, demography, sociology, etc.) and fields that document and explain health inequalities.

Fraser's framework also provides conceptual and normative resources that can guide questions of health justice and the conduct of health equity research, action, and policy. The framework's bifocal formulation of injustice and the norm of participatory parity provide some normative scaffolding for the assessment of health inequalities, including in complex cases wherein health outcomes are examined simultaneously by multiple axes of social difference. Because such studies reveal social locations and complex formations of inequality, they are likely to identify multiple health injustices and thus to raise tough questions about which merit prioritisation for collective concern and resources. Tough cases may be resolvable only by deliberative processes. This is not a fatal flaw for theories of justice, as they often have to specify some sort of "fair process" to set priorities and allocate resources in the real world.[95] With more conceptual development for applications in population health, these resources could provide practical actionable guidance in the real world and thus meet the criterion of "relevance" that Venkatapuram proposes a theory of global health justice must meet.[96]

Fraser's standard of participatory parity and concept of misrecognition also have direct relevance to health equity research and action. As I have elsewhere interpreted the first two concepts, they supply ethical guardrails for research and interventions that target minoritised and socioeconomically marginalised groups and communities, by creating space for their voices, views, and values and as messengers of healthy living.[97] While more would need to be said about these concepts as ethical guideposts for health equity action and policy, I believe that work would show that Fraser's account meets another criterion that Venkatapuram proposes a theory of global health justice should meet, namely, that it can inform health policy.[98]

For all of its promise as a framework of health justice, Fraser's account has at least one potential serious limitation. It is not immediately clear how the theory can attend to the early developmental needs of humans who are not yet adults. The positive goal of justice is that all *adults* have the opportunity to participate as peers in public life. The origins of health begin early in human development and are compromised by exposure to malnutrition, chronic trauma and stress, poverty, and abuse and neglect. Social gradients in health—the stepwise relationship between social position and health that holds for all 14 major causes of death—are foreshadowed in social gradients in children's developmental health.[99] The social gradient in developmental health, as with the social gradient in population health generally, shows a stepwise relationship between the degree of disadvantage of a child's family and that child's health and healthy development.

It is not uncommon for theories of justice and health justice to be critiqued as unable to meet the needs of persons who are not yet competent adults. But that does not mean they do not need to. Rawls's theory of justice has long struggled with the question of whether and how the family should be treated as a basic institution that shapes people's life chances.[100] Capability approaches are perhaps best at addressing the needs of children and here I note one reason why. Capabilities protect and promote not only what Sen calls "agency freedom" but also their "well-being freedom". The former refers to one's freedom to achieve valuable ends through one's choices and actions. The latter refers to one's freedom to achieve the constituents of wellbeing, regardless of whether individuals choose or act to protect their well-being. When a swamp is drained, the people living in its midst are better protected against malaria. When water is fluoridated, people drinking and brushing their teeth with that water are better protected against dental caries. People need not drain the swamp or place fluoride in the water, or even vote in order to incur benefits to their health and well-being. Capabilities in this way are protective of those who cannot yet make, or may never be able to make, informed decisions. This feature of capability approaches is sometimes overlooked yet arguably it is a signal feature of the approach and contributes to its wide application around the globe.

Children would certainly be healthier in a world governed by Fraser's idea of justice. Freedom from socioeconomic deprivations and economic exploitation would protect them and those caring for them. So too would freedom from demeaning treatment on the basis of how they and their caregivers look, love, pray, speak, and so on. But children need additional protections that are not obvious ingredients in the objective and inter-subjective conditions that Fraser's account specifies. Children need attachment and love, and they need to be free from abuse and neglect. I do not resolve this challenge to Fraser's account of justice but note only that a global health justice needs to be able to reach its youngest residents. Like much else in this chapter, that analysis awaits future treatment.

Notes

1 Krieger N, and Birn AE, 'A Vision of Social Justice as the Foundation of Public Health: Commemorating 150 Years of the Spirit of 1848.' (1998) 88 American Journal of Public Health 1603; Birn A, 'Making It Politic(al): Closing the Gap in a Generation: Health Equity Through Action on the Social Determinants of Health' (2009) 4 Social Medicine 166.
2 Mechanic D, 'Book Review Essay: Rediscovering The Social Determinants Of Health' (2000) 19 Health Affairs 269.
3 Powers M, and Faden R, *Social Justice: The Moral Foundations of Public Health and Health Policy* (Oxford University Press 2006); Daniels N, *Just Health: Meeting Health Needs Fairly* (Cambridge University Press 2008) <https://www.cambridge.org/core/books/just-health/
1322AC95E8FEA51A978F200200A103A4>; Segall S, *Health, Luck, and Justice* (Princeton University Press 2010) <https://press.princeton.edu/books/hardcover/9780691140537/health-luck-and-justice>; Sridhar Venkatapuram, *Health Justice* (Polity Press 2011).
4 Fraser F, and Honneth A, *Redistribution or Recognition? A Political-Philosophical Exchange* (Verso 2003).
5 ibid 36–37.
6 Blacksher E, 'Redistribution and Recognition: Pursuing Social Justice in Public Health' (2012) 21 Cambridge quarterly of healthcare ethics: CQ: the International Journal of Healthcare Ethics Committees 320; Blacksher E, 'Public Health and Social Justice: An Argument Against Stigma as a Tool of Health Promotion and Disease Prevention' in B Link, J Dovidio and B Major (eds), *The Oxford Handbook of Stigma, Discrimination and Health* (Oxford University Press 2018) <https://search.library.uq.edu.au/primo-explore/fulldisplay/61UQ_ALMA21202529940003131/61UQ>.
7 Voigt K, and Wester G, 'Relational Equality and Health' (2015) 31 Social Philosophy and Policy 204; Zhuang X, 'World Citizenship and Global Health' in Bhakuni H and Miotto L (eds), *Justice in Global Health: New Perspectives and Current Issues* (Routledge 2023).
8 Voigt K, 'Relational Egalitarianism' [2020] Oxford Research Encyclopedia of Politics.

9 Zurn C, 'Arguing Over Participatory Parity: On Fraser's Conception of Social Justice' (2003) 47 Philosophy Today <https://www.academia.edu/737276/Arguing_Over_Participatory_Parity_On_Fraser_s_Conception_of_Social_Justice>.

10 Powers and Faden (n 3) 30.

11 Daniels (n 3).

12 Mills CW, '"Ideal Theory" as Ideology' (2005) 20 Hypatia 165.

13 Ingrid Robeyns argues that Fraser fails to engage with Sen's capability approach and questions whether her critique to it. See Robeyns I. 'Is Nancy Fraser's Critique of Theories of Distributive Justice Justified?' (2003) 10 Constellations.

14 Fraser and Honneth (n 4) 22–23.

15 ibid 20.

16 ibid 21.

17 ibid 23–24; Wray M, *Not Quite White: White Trash and the Boundaries of Whiteness* (Duke University Press 2006).

18 Fraser and Honneth (n 4) 25–26.

19 Collins PH, 'Intersectionality's Definitional Dilemmas' (2015) 41 Annual Review of Sociology 1.

20 Fraser and Honneth (n 4) 36.

21 ibid.

22 Voigt (n 8).

23 Daniels (n 3).

24 Cockerham WC, 'Health Lifestyle Theory and the Convergence of Agency and Structure' (2005) 46 Journal of Health and Social Behavior 51.

25 Zurn (n 9).

26 Sen A, 'Missing Women.' (1992) 304 British Medical Journal 587; Sen A, *Inequality Reexamined* (Russell Sage Foundation Books at Harvard University Press 1992); Alkire S, *Valuing Freedoms: Sen's Capabilities Approach and Poverty Reduction* (Oxford University Press 2002) <https://doi.org/10.1093/0199245797.001.0001.002.002>.

27 Nussbaum MC, *Women and Human Development: The Capabilities Approach* (Cambridge University Press 2000) <https://www.cambridge.org/core/books/women-and-human-development/58D8D2FBFC1C9E902D648200C4B7009E>; Venkatapuram (n 3).

28 Beauchamp TL, and Childress JF, *Principles of Biomedical Ethics* (Seventh, Oxford University Press 2009) <//global.oup.com/ushe/product/principles-of-biomedical-ethics-9780190640873>.

29 Coole D, 'Is Class a Difference That Makes a Difference?' [1996] Radical Philosophy <https://www.radicalphilosophy.com/article/is-class-a-difference-that-makes-a-difference>; Collins (n 18).

30 Collins (n 19) 13.

31 Isenberg N, *White Trash: The 400-Year Untold History of Class in America* (Viking Press 2016) <https://history.wisc.edu/publications/white-trash-the-400-year-untold-history-of-class-in-america/>.

32 Krieger N, and Fee E, 'Measuring Social Inequalities in Health in the United States: A Historical Review, 1900–1950' (1996) 26 International Journal of Health Services: Planning, Administration, Evaluation 391.

33 May VM, *Pursuing Intersectionality, Unsettling Dominant Imaginaries* (Routledge, Taylor & Francis Group 2015).

34 Marchand S, Wikler D, and Landesman B, 'Class, Health and Justice' (1998) 76 The Milbank Quarterly 449; Parfit D, 'Equality and Priority' (1997) 10 Ratio 202.

35 Rawls J, *A Theory of Justice* (Belknap Press 1971).

36 Powers and Faden (n 3).
37 Braveman PA and others, 'The Role of Socioeconomic Factors in Black-White Disparities in Preterm Birth' (2015) 105 American Journal of Public Health 694.
38 Colen CG and others, 'Maternal Upward Socioeconomic Mobility and Black–White Disparities in Infant Birthweight' (2006) 96 American Journal of Public Health 2032; Braveman and others (n 37).
39 MacDorman MF, and Mathews TJ, 'The Challenge of Infant Mortality: Have We Reached a Plateau?' (2009) 124 Public Health Reports 670.
40 Kindig D, 'Using Uncommon Data to Promote Common Ground for Reducing Infant Mortality' (2020) 98 The Milbank Quarterly 18.
41 Beckfield J and Bambra C, 'Shorter Lives in Stingier States: Social Policy Shortcomings Help Explain the US Mortality Disadvantage' (2016) 171 Social Science & Medicine (1982) 30.
42 Harris KM, Becker T, and Majmundar MK (eds), *High and Rising Mortality Rates Among Working-Age Adults* (National Academies Press (US) 2021) <http://www.ncbi.nlm.nih.gov/books/NBK568187/>.
43 Case A, and Deaton A, *Deaths of Despair and the Future of Capitalism* (Princeton University Press 2020) <https://press.princeton.edu/books/hardcover/9780691190785/deaths-of-despair-and-the-future-of-capitalism>.
44 Pletcher MJ, and others, 'Trends in Opioid Prescribing by Race/Ethnicity for Patients Seeking Care in US Emergency Departments' (2008) 299 JAMA 70.
45 Siddiqi A, and others, 'Growing Sense of Social Status Threat and Concomitant Deaths of Despair among Whites' (2019) 9 SSM - population health 100449.
46 Blacksher E, 'Public Health and Social Justice: An Argument Against Stigma as a Tool of Health Promotion and Disease Prevention' (n 6).
47 Neff D, 'The Satisfied Poor: Evidence from South India' (2009) BWPI Working Paper 72 Science & Social Medicine <https://www.academia.edu/70157100/The_Satisfied_Poor_Evidence_from_South_India>; Blacksher E, 'On Being Poor and Feeling Poor: Low Socioeconomic Status and the Moral Self' (2002) 23 Theoretical Medicine and Bioethics 455.
48 Case A, and Deaton A, 'The Great Divide: Education, Despair, and Death' (2022) 14 Annual Review of Economics 1.
49 McGhee H, *The Sum of Us: What Racism Costs Everyone and How We Can Prosper Together* (Random House Publishing Group 2021).
50 MacLean N, *Democracy in Chains: The Deep History of the Radical Right's Stealth Plan for America* (Penguin Random House 2017) <https://history.wisc.edu/publications/democracy-in-chains-the-deep-history-of-the-radical-rights-stealth-plan-for-america/>.
51 Powers and Faden (n 3) 69–71.
52 Bowleg L, 'The Problem With the Phrase Women and Minorities: Intersectionality—an Important Theoretical Framework for Public Health' (2012) 102 American Journal of Public Health 1267.
53 Powers and Faden (n 3) 65.
54 ibid.
55 Blacksher, 'Public Health and Social Justice: An Argument Against Stigma as a Tool of Health Promotion and Disease Prevention' (n 6).
56 Hertzman C, 'The Case for Child Development as a Determinant of Health' (1998) 89 Canadian Journal of Public Health.
57 Macintosh J, and Nelson RH, 'Social Reproductive Labor, Gender, and Health Justice' (2018) 18 The American Journal of Bioethics: AJOB 26.
58 Bowleg (n 52).
59 Fraser and Honneth (n 4) 43.

60 Wilson Y, 'Shrinking Poor White Life Spans and the Requirements of Justice' (2018) 18 The American Journal of Bioethics: AJOB 19; Lee H, and Hicken MT, 'Racism and the Health of White Americans' (2018) 18 The American journal of bioethics: AJOB 21; Wray M, 'A Crisis of Identity, a Crisis of Place' (2018) 18 American Journal of Bioethics 23; Zaidi D, and Sederstrom N, 'The Racist Underbelly of Health Disparities in America' (2018) 18 The American Journal of Bioethics: AJOB 25.

61 Blacksher, 'Redistribution and Recognition: Pursuing Social Justice in Public Health' (n 6).

62 Hankivsky O, and Christoffersen A, 'Intersectionality and the Determinants of Health: A Canadian Perspective' (2008) 18 Critical Public Health 271.

63 Blacksher, 'On Being Poor and Feeling Poor' (n 47).

64 Bayer R, 'Stigma and the Ethics of Public Health: Not Can We but Should We' (2008) 67 Social Science & Medicine (1982) 463; Burris S, 'Stigma, Ethics and Policy: A Commentary on Bayer's "Stigma and the Ethics of Public Health: Not Can We but Should We"' (2008) 67 Social Science & Medicine (1982) 473.

65 Link BG, and Phelan JC, 'Conceptualizing Stigma' (2001) 27 Annual Review of Sociology 363.

66 Susser M, and Susser E, 'Choosing a Future for Epidemiology: I. Eras and Paradigms' (1996) 86 American Journal of Public Health 668; McMichael AJ, 'Prisoners of the Proximate: Loosening the Constraints on Epidemiology in an Age of Change' (1999) 149 American Journal of Epidemiology 887.

67 Mechanic (n 2).

68 Murray CJ, Gakidou EE, and Frenk J, 'Health Inequalities and Social Group Differences: What Should We Measure?' (1999) 77 Bulletin of the World Health Organization 537.

69 ibid 537.

70 Braveman PA, Starfield B, and Geiger HJ, 'World Health Report 2000: How It Removes Equity from the Agenda for Public Health Monitoring and Policy' (2001) 323 BMJ: British Medical Journal 678, 678.

71 Braveman PA, and Gruskin S, 'Defining Equity in Health' (2003) 57 Journal of Epidemiology and Community Health 254.

72 Jones CP, and others, 'Addressing the Social Determinants of Children's Health: A Cliff Analogy' (2009) 20 Journal of Health Care for the Poor and Underserved 1, 8.

73 Berkman LF, and Kawachi I, 'Social Cohesion, Social Capital, and Health', Social Epidemiology (1st edn, Oxford University Press 2000).

74 Link BG, and Phelan JC, 'Social Conditions As Fundamental Causes of Disease' [1995] Journal of Health and Social Behavior 80; Jo C Phelan and Bruce G Link, 'Is Racism a Fundamental Cause of Inequalities in Health?' (2015) 41 Annual Review of Sociology 311.

75 Schulz AJ, and Mullings L, Gender, Race, Class, and Health: Intersectional Approaches (1st ed, Jossey-Bass 2006) <http://catdir.loc.gov/catdir/toc/ecip061/2005028724.html>; Bowleg (n 52); Bauer GR, 'Incorporating Intersectionality Theory into Population Health Research Methodology: Challenges and the Potential to Advance Health Equity' (2014) 110 Social Science & Medicine (1982) 10.

76 Krieger N, 'The Making of Public Health Data: Paradigms, Politics, and Policy' (1992) 13 Journal of Public Health Policy 412; Schulz and Mullings (n 75); Bowleg (n 52).

77 Bauer GR, and Scheim AI, 'Methods for Analytic Intercategorical Intersectionality in Quantitative Research: Discrimination as a Mediator of Health Inequalities' (2019) 226 Social Science & Medicine (1982) 236.

78 Kawachi I, Daniels N and Robinson DE, 'Health Disparities By Race And Class: Why Both Matter' (2005) 24 Health Affairs 343; Williams DR, and Collins C, 'U.S. Socioeconomic and Racial Differences in Health: Patterns and Explanations' (1995) 21 Annual Review of Sociology 349.

79 Isaacs SL and Schroeder SA, 'Class — The Ignored Determinant of the Nation's Health' (2004) 351 New England Journal of Medicine 1137.

80 Sasson I, 'Trends in Life Expectancy and Lifespan Variation by Educational Attainment: United States, 1990–2010' (2016) 53 Demography 269; Olshansky SJ and others, 'Differences in Life Expectancy Due to Race and Educational Differences Are Widening, and Many May Not Catch Up' (2012) 31 Health Affairs (Project Hope) 1803.

81 Braveman PA, Egerter SA, and Mockenhaupt RE, 'Broadening the Focus: The Need to Address the Social Determinants of Health' (2011) 40 American Journal of Preventive Medicine S4.

82 Montez JK and others, 'Trends in the Educational Gradient of U.S. Adult Mortality from 1986 to 2006 by Race, Gender, and Age Group' (2011) 33 Research on Aging 145.

83 Olshansky and others (n 80); Sasson (n 80).

84 Kindig DA, 'Using Uncommon Data to Promote Common Ground for Reducing Infant Mortality' (2019) 98 The Milbank Quarterly <https://www.milbank.org/quarterly/articles/using-uncommon-data-to-promote-common-ground-for-reducing-infant-mortality/>.

85 Braveman, Egerter and Mockenhaupt (n 81).

86 Kawachi, Daniels and Robinson (n 78).

87 Abraído-Lanza AF, Echeverría SE, and Flórez KR, 'Latino Immigrants, Acculturation, and Health: Promising New Directions in Research' (2016) 37 Annual Review of Public Health 219.

88 Kawachi I, Kennedy BP and Wilkinson RC (eds), *The Society and Population Health Reader: Income Inequality and Health*, vol 1 (The New Press 1999) <https://thenewpress.com/books/society-population-health-reader-volume-i>.

89 Marmot M, *The Status Syndrome: How Social Standing Affects Our Health and Longevity* (Macmillan 2004) <https://us.macmillan.com/books/9780805078541/thestatussyndrome>.

90 Fraser and Honneth (n 4) 67–68.

91 Navarro V, and Shi L, 'The Political Context of Social Inequalities and Health' (2001) 52 Social Science & Medicine (1982) 481; Dawes DE, *The Political Determinants of Health* (Johns Hopkins University Press 2020) <https://www.press.jhu.edu/books/title/12075/political-determinants-health>.

92 Woolf SH, 'The Growing Influence of State Governments on Population Health in the United States' (2022) 327 JAMA 1331.

93 Montez JK and others, 'US State Policies, Politics, and Life Expectancy' (2020) 98 The Milbank Quarterly 668; Woolf (n 92); Beckfield and Bambra (n 41); Montez JK and others, 'U.S. State Policy Contexts and Mortality of Working-Age Adults' (2022) 17 PloS One e0275466; Montez JK, 'Policy Polarization and Death in the United States' (2020) 92 Temple law review 889.

94 Venkatapuram S, 'What do we want from a theory of global health justice?' in Bhakuni H and Miotto L, *Justice in Global Health: New Perspectives and Current Issues* (Routledge 2023).

95 Daniels (n 3).

96 Venkatapuram (n 94).

97 Blacksher, 'Redistribution and Recognition: Pursuing Social Justice in Public Health' (n 6).

98 Venkatapuram (n 94).

99 Mechanic (n 2); Hertzman C and Boyce T, 'How Experience Gets under the Skin to Create Gradients in Developmental Health' (2010) 31 Annual Review of Public Health 329.
100 Nussbaum MC, *Sex and Social Justice* (Oxford University Press 1999) <https://global.oup.com/academic/product/sex-and-social-justice-9780195110326?cc=us&lang=en&>.

Bibliography

Abraído-Lanza AF, Echeverría SE and Flórez KR, 'Latino Immigrants, Acculturation, and Health: Promising New Directions in Research' [2016] 37 *Annual Review of Public Health* 219.

Alkire S, *Valuing Freedoms: Sen's Capabilities Approach and Poverty Reduction* (Oxford University Press 2002) <10.1093/0199245797.001.0001.002.002>

Bauer GR, 'Incorporating Intersectionality Theory into Population Health Research Methodology: Challenges and the Potential to Advance Health Equity' [2014] 110 *Social Science & Medicine (1982)* 10.

Bauer GR and Scheim AI, 'Methods for Analytic Intercategorical Intersectionality in Quantitative Research: Discrimination as a Mediator of Health Inequalities' [2019] 226 *Social Science & Medicine (1982)* 236.

Bayer R, 'Stigma and the Ethics of Public Health: Not Can We but Should We' [2008] 67 *Social Science & Medicine (1982)* 463.

Beauchamp TL and Childress JF, *Principles of Biomedical Ethics* (Seventh, Oxford University Press 2009) <//global.oup.com/ushe/product/principles-of-biomedical-ethics-9780190640873>

Beckfield J and Bambra C, 'Shorter Lives in Stingier States: Social Policy Shortcomings Help Explain the US Mortality Disadvantage' [2016] 171 *Social Science & Medicine (1982)* 30.

Berkman LF and Kawachi I, 'Social Cohesion, Social Capital, and Health', *Social Epidemiology* (1st edn, Oxford University Press 2000).

Birn A, 'Making It Politic(al): Closing the Gap in a Generation: Health Equity Through Action on the Social Determinants of Health' [2009] 4 *Social Medicine* 166.

Blacksher E, 'On Being Poor and Feeling Poor: Low Socioeconomic Status and the Moral Self' [2002] 23 *Theoretical Medicine and Bioethics* 455.

Blacksher E, 'Redistribution and Recognition: Pursuing Social Justice in Public Health' [2012] 21 *Cambridge Quarterly Of Healthcare Ethics: CQ: The International Journal of Healthcare Ethics Committees* 1.

Blacksher E, 'Public Health and Social Justice: An Argument Against Stigma as a Tool of Health Promotion and Disease Prevention' in B. Link, J. Dovidio and B. Major (eds), *The Oxford Handbook of Stigma, Discrimination and Health* (Oxford University Press 2018) <https://search.library.uq.edu.au/primo-explore/fulldisplay/61UQ_ALMA21202529940003131/61UQ> accessed 24 March 2023

Bowleg L, 'The Problem With the Phrase Women and Minorities: Intersectionality—an Important Theoretical Framework for Public Health' [2012] 102 *American Journal of Public Health* 1267.

Braveman P and Gruskin S, 'Defining Equity in Health' [2003] 57 *Journal of Epidemiology and Community Health* 254.

Braveman P, Starfield B and Geiger HJ, 'World Health Report 2000: How It Removes Equity from the Agenda for Public Health Monitoring and Policy' [2001] 323 *BMJ: British Medical Journal* 678.

Braveman PA and others, 'The Role of Socioeconomic Factors in Black-White Disparities in Preterm Birth' [2015] 105 *American Journal of Public Health* 694.

Braveman PA, Egerter SA and Mockenhaupt RE, 'Broadening the Focus: The Need to Address the Social Determinants of Health' (2011) 40 *American Journal of Preventive Medicine* S4.

Burris S, 'Stigma, Ethics and Policy: A Commentary on Bayer's "Stigma and the Ethics of Public Health: Not Can We but Should We"' [2008] 67 *Social Science & Medicine (1982)* 473.

Case A and Deaton A, *Deaths of Despair and the Future of Capitalism* (Princeton University Press 2020) <https://press.princeton.edu/books/hardcover/9780691190785/deaths-of-despair-and-the-future-of-capitalism>

Case A and Deaton A, 'The Great Divide: Education, Despair, and Death' [2022] 14 *Annual Review of Economics* 1.

Cockerham WC, 'Health Lifestyle Theory and the Convergence of Agency and Structure' [2005] 46 *Journal of Health and Social Behavior* 51.

Colen CG and others, 'Maternal Upward Socioeconomic Mobility and Black–White Disparities in Infant Birthweight' [2006] 96 *American Journal of Public Health* 2032.

Collins PH, 'Intersectionality's Definitional Dilemmas' (2015) 41 *Annual Review of Sociology* 1.

Coole D, 'Is Class a Difference That Makes a Difference?' [1996] Radical Philosophy <https://www.radicalphilosophy.com/article/is-class-a-difference-that-makes-a-difference> accessed 24 March 2023

Daniels N, *Just Health: Meeting Health Needs Fairly* (Cambridge University Press 2008) <https://www.cambridge.org/core/books/just-health/1322AC95E8FEA51A978F200200A103A4>

Dawes DE, *The Political Determinants of Health* (Johns Hopkins University Press 2020) <https://www.press.jhu.edu/books/title/12075/political-determinants-health>

Fraser N and Honneth A, *Redistribution or Recognition? A Political-Philosophical Exchange* (Verso 2003).

Hankivsky O and Christoffersen A, 'Intersectionality and the Determinants of Health: A Canadian Perspective' [2008] 18 *Critical Public Health* 271.

Harris KM, Becker T and Majmundar MK (eds), *High and Rising Mortality Rates Among Working-Age Adults* (National Academies Press (US) 2021) <http://www.ncbi.nlm.nih.gov/books/NBK568187/>

Hertzman C, 'The Case for Child Development as a Determinant of Health' [1998] 89 *Canadian Journal of Public Health = Revue Canadienne De Sante Publique* S14.

Hertzman C and Boyce T, 'How Experience Gets under the Skin to Create Gradients in Developmental Health' [2010] 31 *Annual Review of Public Health* 329.

Isaacs SL and Schroeder SA, 'Class—The Ignored Determinant of the Nation's Health' [2004] 351 *New England Journal of Medicine* 1137.

Isenberg N, *White Trash: The 400-Year Untold History of Class in America* (Viking Press 2016) <https://history.wisc.edu/publications/white-trash-the-400-year-untold-history-of-class-in-america/>

Jones CP and others, 'Addressing the Social Determinants of Children's Health: A Cliff Analogy' [2009] 20 *Journal of Health Care for the Poor and Underserved* 1.

Kawachi I, Daniels N and Robinson DE, 'Health Disparities By Race And Class: Why Both Matter' [2005] 24 *Health Affairs* 343.

Kawachi I, Kennedy BP and Wilkinson RC (eds), *The Society and Population Health Reader: Income Inequality and Health*, vol 1 (The New Press 1999) <https://thenewpress.com/books/society-population-health-reader-volume-i>

Kindig D, 'Using Uncommon Data to Promote Common Ground for Reducing Infant Mortality' [2020] 98 *The Milbank Quarterly* 18.

Kindig DA, 'Using Uncommon Data to Promote Common Ground for Reducing Infant Mortality' [2019] 98 *The Milbank Quarterly* <https://www.milbank.org/quarterly/articles/using-uncommon-data-to-promote-common-ground-for-reducing-infant-mortality/> accessed 24 March 2023

Krieger N, 'The Making of Public Health Data: Paradigms, Politics, and Policy' [1992] 13 *Journal of Public Health Policy* 412.

Krieger N and Birn AE, 'A Vision of Social Justice as the Foundation of Public Health: Commemorating 150 Years of the Spirit of 1848' [1998] 88 *American Journal of Public Health* 1603.

Krieger N and Fee E, 'Measuring Social Inequalities in Health in the United States: A Historical Review, 1900-1950' [1996] 26 *International Journal of Health Services: Planning, Administration, Evaluation* 391.

Lee H and Hicken MT, 'Racism and the Health of White Americans' [2018] 18 *The American Journal of Bioethics: AJOB* 21.

Link BG and Phelan J, 'Social Conditions As Fundamental Causes of Disease' [1995] *Journal of Health and Social Behavior* 80.

Link BG and Phelan JC, 'Conceptualizing Stigma' [2001] 27 *Annual Review of Sociology* 363.

MacDorman MF and Mathews TJ, 'The Challenge of Infant Mortality: Have We Reached a Plateau?' [2009] 124 *Public Health Reports* 670.

Macintosh J and Nelson RH, 'Social Reproductive Labor, Gender, and Health Justice' [2018] 18 *The American Journal of Bioethics: AJOB* 26.

MacLean N, *Democracy in Chains: The Deep History of the Radical Right's Stealth Plan for America* (Penguin Random House 2017) <https://history.wisc.edu/publications/democracy-in-chains-the-deep-history-of-the-radical-rights-stealth-plan-for-america/>

Marchand S, Wikler D and Landesman B, 'Class, Health and Justice' [1998] 76 *The Milbank Quarterly* 449.

Marmot M, *The Status Syndrome: How Social Standing Affects Our Health and Longevity* (Macmillan 2004) <https://us.macmillan.com/books/9780805078541/thestatussyndrome>

May VM, *Pursuing Intersectionality, Unsettling Dominant Imaginaries* (Routledge, Taylor & Francis Group 2015).

McGhee H, *The Sum of Us: What Racism Costs Everyone and How We Can Prosper Together* (Random House Publishing Group 2021).

McMichael AJ, 'Prisoners of the Proximate: Loosening the Constraints on Epidemiology in an Age of Change' [1999] 149 *American Journal of Epidemiology* 887.

Mechanic D, 'Book Review Essay: Rediscovering The Social Determinants Of Health' [2000] 19 *Health Affairs* 269.

Mills CW, '"Ideal Theory" as Ideology' [2005] 20 *Hypatia* 165.

Montez JK, 'Policy Polarization and Death in the United States' [2020] 92 *Temple Law Review* 889.

Montez JK, 'Trends in the Educational Gradient of U.S. Adult Mortality from 1986 to 2006 by Race, Gender, and Age Group' [2011] 33 *Research on Aging* 145.

Montez JK, 'US State Policies, Politics, and Life Expectancy' [2020] 98 *The Milbank Quarterly* 668.

Montez JK, 'U.S. State Policy Contexts and Mortality of Working-Age Adults' [2022] 17 *PLoS One* e0275466.

Murray CJ, Gakidou EE and Frenk J, 'Health Inequalities and Social Group Differences: What Should We Measure?' [1999] 77 *Bulletin of the World Health Organization* 537.

Navarro V and Shi L, 'The Political Context of Social Inequalities and Health' [2001] 52 *Social Science & Medicine (1982)* 481.

Neff D, 'The Satisfied Poor: Evidence from South India' [2009] *BWPI Working Paper* 72 *Science & Social Medicine* <https://www.academia.edu/70157100/The_Satisfied_Poor_Evidence_from_South_India> accessed 24 March 2023

Nussbaum MC, *Sex and Social Justice* (Oxford University Press 1999) <https://global.oup.com/academic/product/sex-and-social-justice-9780195110326?cc=us&lang=en&>

Nussbaum MC, *Women and Human Development: The Capabilities Approach* (Cambridge University Press 2000) <https://www.cambridge.org/core/books/women-and-human-development/58D8D2FBFC1C9E902D648200C4B7009E>

Olshansky SJ and others, 'Differences in Life Expectancy Due to Race and Educational Differences Are Widening, and Many May Not Catch Up' [2012] 31 *Health Affairs (Project Hope)* 1803.

Parfit D, 'Equality and Priority' [1997] 10 *Ratio* 202.

Phelan JC and Link BG, 'Is Racism a Fundamental Cause of Inequalities in Health?' (2015) 41 *Annual Review of Sociology* 311.

Pletcher MJ and others, 'Trends in Opioid Prescribing by Race/Ethnicity for Patients Seeking Care in US Emergency Departments' [2008] 299 *JAMA* 70.

Powers M and Faden R, *Social Justice: The Moral Foundations of Public Health and Health Policy* (Oxford University Press 2006).

Rawls J, *A Theory of Justice* (Belknap Press 1971).

Sasson I, 'Trends in Life Expectancy and Lifespan Variation by Educational Attainment: United States, 1990–2010' [2016] 53 *Demography* 269.

Schulz AJ and Mullings L, *Gender, Race, Class, and Health: Intersectional Approaches* (1st ed, Jossey-Bass 2006) <http://catdir.loc.gov/catdir/toc/ecip061/2005028724.html>

Segall S, *Health, Luck, and Justice* (Princeton University Press 2010) <https://press.princeton.edu/books/hardcover/9780691140537/health-luck-and-justice>

Sen A, *Inequality Reexamined* (Russell Sage Foundation Books at Harvard University Press 1992).

Sen A, 'Missing Women' [1992] 304 *British Medical Journal* 587.

Siddiqi A and others, 'Growing Sense of Social Status Threat and Concomitant Deaths of Despair among Whites' [2019] 9 *SSM – Population Health* 100449.

Susser M and Susser E, 'Choosing a Future for Epidemiology: I. Eras and Paradigms' [1996] 86 *American Journal of Public Health* 668.

Venkatapuram S, *Health Justice* (Polity Press 2011).

Venkatapuram S, 'What do we want from a theory of global health justice?' in Bhakuni H and Miotto L, *Justice in Global Health: New Perspectives and Current Issues* (Routledge 2023).

Voigt K, 'Relational Egalitarianism' [2020] *Oxford Research Encyclopedia of Politics* <https://> accessed 24 March 2023

Voigt K and Wester G, 'Relational Equality and Health' (2015) 31 *Social Philosophy and Policy* 204.

Williams DR and Collins C, 'U.S. Socioeconomic and Racial Differences in Health: Patterns and Explanations' [1995] 21 *Annual Review of Sociology* 349.

Wilson Y, 'Shrinking Poor White Life Spans and the Requirements of Justice' [2018] 18 *The American Journal of Bioethics: AJOB* 19.

Woolf SH, 'The Growing Influence of State Governments on Population Health in the United States' [2022] 327 *JAMA* 1331.

Wray M, *Not Quite White: White Trash and the Boundaries of Whiteness* (Duke University Press 2006).

Wray M, 'A Crisis of Identity, a Crisis of Place' [2018] 18 *American Journal of Bioethics* 23.

Zaidi D and Sederstrom N, 'The Racist Underbelly of Health Disparities in America' [2018] 18 *The American Journal of Bioethics: AJOB* 25.

Zhuang X, 'World Citizenship and Global Health' in H. Bhakuni and M. Miotto (eds), *Justice in Global Health: New Perspectives and Current Issues* (Routledge 2023).

Zurn C, 'Arguing Over Participatory Parity: On Fraser's Conception of Social Justice' [2003] 47 *Philosophy Today* <https://www.academia.edu/737276/Arguing_Over_Participatory_Parity_On_Fraser_s_Conception_of_Social_Justice> accessed 24 March 2023

12

BEYOND EGALITARIANISM

A Confucian Approach to Global Health Justice

Man-to Tang

12.1 Introduction

Drawing on the contemporary debate and the pre-Qin texts in Confucianism, this chapter presents an overview of a Confucian approach to justice that can be applied to global health issues. Starting with a brief explanation of the debate on whether Confucian justice adopts the principle of egalitarianism, this article continues by arguing that Confucians reject the principle of egalitarianism, even though it may sometimes agree with egalitarian considerations. The fundamental principle of Confucian justice is sufficiency for all. This article then argues in defence of the principle of sufficiency and discusses the essence of Confucian justice in the pre-Qin period. The essence of Confucian justice lies in its emphasis on harmonious human relations. It is also based on cardinal virtues such as benevolence (*ren*仁), justice (*yi* 義), and rites (*li* 禮). Ultimately, Confucians would propose that to achieve justice in global health is to create a world where sufficient material conditions are provided to everyone for a flourishing life, while the allocation of resources is fair. It is mistaken, according to this version of Confucianism, simply to require institutions to be the sole bearers of responsibility for global health justice; rather, because all stakeholders belong together to the world; they share the responsibility for providing basic medical care and fair resource distribution.

12.2 Confucian Justice With or Without Egalitarianism

In this section, I reformulate a recent debate on Confucian justice. Many Confucian scholars like Joseph Chan and Ruiping Fan argue that Confucianism advocates a non-egalitarian account of justice, whereas Chun Hin Tsoi

DOI: 10.4324/9781003399933-18

counterargues that Confucianism appreciates the principle of egalitarianism in his account of Confucian justice.

Tsoi asserts that Confucian justice consists of three principles: egalitarianism, prioritarianism, and sufficientarianism. According to Tsoi, "egalitarianism stresses the equality, prioritarianism stresses the priority of benefits to the less advantaged, and sufficientarianism stresses that everyone has enough".[1] At first glance, the three ideas are mutually exclusive. If we support the priority of benefits to the less advantaged, it is impossible to treat everyone equally. Facing this tension, Tsoi adds the adequacy thesis. The adequacy thesis suggests that "a society that has achieved *full sufficiency* is *morally acceptable*".[2] It means that sufficientarianism is fundamental, while egalitarianism and prioritarianism are supplementary. Kings who work to ensure that people have enough are moral enough, and yet, kings who work for equality or priority are even better.

Tsoi is correct in his assertion about the fundamentality of sufficientarianism. When resources are limited, people are constantly under temptation and struggle. In years of famine, for example, people must choose between their own lives and the lives of others. In such extreme situations, even benevolent people would not typically be keen on sacrificing themselves to save others – and it would even be difficult to demand, as a matter of morality, that the common people do so. Lack of sufficiency thus leads to suffering, death, and situations where individuals prioritise their biological needs; situations where moral conduct and knowledge cannot be cultivated. Insufficientarianism should be of inherent disvalue to all people.

However, despite arguing for the fundamentality of sufficientarianism, Tsoi also admits that sufficientarianism is not necessarily at odds with egalitarianism (and prioritarianism). According to his interpretation of Confucian doctrine, Confucians can be considered egalitarians of opportunity in relation to resources: in a background of material scarcity, the deserved benefit should strictly correspond to an individual's level of contribution, regardless of other arbitrary personal factors. To support this view, Tsoi relies on the classic works of *Mengzi* and suggests that Mengzi himself hinted at the value of equality. He claims that, for Mengzi, "[t]here is no *prima facie* reason for the ruler to have more than what is necessary, to possess much more than the people. Furthermore, the ruler should enjoy and suffer together with the people".[3] Thus, it follows from this interpretation, that the ruler and the people have equal social and economic status; none of them is superior to the other. Neither the ruler nor the people should receive much more than others. Resources should thus be distributed equally. Hence, Confucianism may support egalitarianism with regard to distributions. Or, more broadly, Confucianism can embrace sufficientarianism, egalitarianism, and prioritarianism as distributive ideals.

This account may meet with much criticism. Even though some Confucian passages can be related to sufficientarianism, egalitarianism, and prioritarianism, it is doubtful if all three values can serve as guidelines for interpreting distributive justice in Confucianism. The theoretical framework of distributive ideals introduced by Tsoi may cause difficulty in the Confucian idea of distributive justice that did not belong to Confucianism initially.[4] Some scholars such as Joseph Chan and Ruiping Fan have also made this point and argued that Confucianism, when properly understood, is incompatible with some of the core values shared by egalitarianism and, therefore, that egalitarianism cannot be a principle of Confucian justice.

To advance this argument, we should make a distinction between the principle of egalitarianism and egalitarian consideration. Egalitarianism advocates equal social and economic status of the ruler and the people, whereas egalitarian consideration means taking equality into consideration. The former assumes egalitarianism as a principle applicable in all circumstances, whereas the latter considers egalitarianism as an acceptable value in some issues. So, Confucianism being incompatible with egalitarianism – as scholars like Chan, Fan, and I have argued – does not entail that Confucianism negates or is incompatible with egalitarian consideration. Confucianism agrees that the ruler should enjoy and suffer together with the people, but, *pace* Tsoi, Confucianism does not imply that the ruler and the people have equal social and economic status. For example, the Confucian principle of benevolence (*ren* 仁), with its internal requirement of "love with distinction", does not emphasise egalitarianism in social and economic status. According to this principle, the social hierarchy should be maintained to harmonise human relations.[5]

Moreover, it is important to highlight the context in which the claim that the ruler should enjoy and suffer together with the people appears. This claim appears when Mengzi criticises the ruler's policy of hoarding in years of famine. However, Mengzi had no objection to the policy of hoarding in good years, which suggests that economic and social inequality is morally permissible if sufficient material conditions are provided to all members. Egalitarian consideration is only occasionally applicable in some extreme situations where resources are insufficient to main basic human needs, so it cannot be regarded as a principle in Confucian justice.

Other commentators share the same view and further explicate an essential difference between the principle of equality in egalitarianism and egalitarian consideration in Confucianism. Chan, for example, has argued that the principle of equality in egalitarianism is grounded on human rights and civil liberties. These rights and liberties are justified by the fundamental idea that people have sovereign rights over their bodies and actions. Thus, social justice is premised on the self-ownership right or the right to equal respect and concern. However, as per Chan, Confucianism justifies the idea of justice in relation to the contribution to a good life. According to Confucianism, sufficient resources should be provided for everyone to live an ethical life while allowing economic inequality to arise from merit and contribution.[6] Even though Confucianism has implicit ideas of rights and liberties, rights and liberties must be exercised with a balanced consideration of individual interest in leading an ethical life with moderate personal autonomy. Confucianism does not take sovereign rights for granted. Sovereign rights are essential only if they can promote the well-being of individuals and their relatives.

So far, we have encountered objections to the view espoused by Tsoi and other commentators that Confucian justice is compatible with the principle of egalitarianism. But despite this misapprehension, Tsoi still makes a substantial contribution in highlighting sufficiency as one of the principles of Confucian justice. On this point, Chan also asserts that,

> The fundamental principle of social justice for early Confucians is sufficiency for all, which is neither a libertarian nor an egalitarian conception of justice. Social justice aims to enable every member of a community to have sufficient resources to live a good life.[7]

There seems, therefore, to be some agreement amongst Confucian scholars that sufficiency is the fundamental principle of Confucian justice. Sufficiency implies that each person should have basic needs that are sufficient for their well-being and also their life. Without basic needs, one cannot have a flourishing life. In this regard, a virtuous person (*junzi* 君子) does not require – and is not entitled to hoard – more than they need. Chan draws textual evidence from the *Analects*,

> I have heard that a virtuous person helps the distressed but does not add to the wealth of the rich.[8]

吾聞之也，君子周急不繼富。

When a virtuous person deliberates on distributing resources, they must conclude that they should help the poor rather than the rich. A virtuous person does not apply the principle of egalitarianism to achieve substantive equality in all circumstances, but they distribute according to the principle of sufficiency. A virtuous person must understand other people's background, and more importantly, distinguish between those members of society who are in need and those who are not. It is based on this information that a virtuous person offers help. If people were rich enough, no help would be provided; whereas if people were too poor, "sufficient" help would be given. One should not take more than one needs out of consideration of the needs of others. We have seen that once the level of material sufficiency has been attained, Confucians do not object to economic inequalities that arise from personal factors such as merit and contribution, which are primarily based on the possession of abilities (moral character and intelligence).

To sum up, Confucian scholars disagree about the extent to which Confucianism is committed to egalitarianism. But despite disagreeing on this point, scholars at both ends of the spectrum share the same view about the fundamentality of sufficientarianism. I have illustrated this with the views of Chan and Tsoi, the former clearly stating that "Confucian justice is not of an egalitarian but a sufficientarian view" while also acknowledging that "justice as sufficiency for all (...) is only part of the larger Confucian conception of the social ideal".[9] Though it may be argued that a principle of egalitarianism still has an important role to play in Confucian justice, I still doubt in what sense, the principle of egalitarianism can be seen as a "principle" of justice in Confucianism when Confucians have always resisted to take it seriously, and when its application is reserved to exceptional circumstances. However, to make this point more convincing, it is necessary to evaluate how Confucian justice is explicated in ancient Classical Confucianism, particularly in the works of Kongzi, Mengzi, and Xunzi. This is what I will do in the next section.

12.3 A Review of Justice in Pre-Qin Confucianism

The foregoing analysis of Confucian justice is correct as far as it goes, yet it is incomplete. A comprehensive illustration of Confucian justice must reflect upon its essence. Bongrae Seok makes some substantial contributions in describing the essence of Confucian justice,

> Confucian justice is not based on the moral or legal rights of autonomous individuals but the communal life of human beings (...) the essence of Confucian justice lies in its emphasis on the well-balanced interest for one's well-being and that of others and, ultimately, on the harmonious human relations. These ideas, properly extended and applied to the global front, could make today's conflicted world safe, united, and peaceful.[10]

Confucianism emphasises a harmonious society in which human relations within communal human life rather than the moral or legal rights of autonomous individuals are preserved. This is not to say that Confucianism neglects the moral or legal rights of autonomous individuals. Their view is, instead, that harmonious human relations within communal human life outweigh moral or legal rights of autonomous individuals. Some questions, however, remain puzzling: for Confucians, what kinds of laws or standards should a society have in order to manifest the idea of justice? Is Confucian justice constituted by members of society? Is it based on social convention? How can Confucian justice help preserve a stable and harmonious society? In this section, let me review Confucian justice by deep diving into the pre-Qin Confucian texts.

In the *Analects*, Confucius considers harmony as a criterion for the superior person. He states that "the superior person harmonises (*he* 和) and does not merely agree (*tong* 同)".[11] Other than harmony, justice is another criterion for the moral person. He also asserts that "the superior person admires justice (*yi* 義) above all".[12] The superior person must be a just person, but a just person does not simply equalise the moral or legal rights of autonomous individuals. He must harmonise human relations within a community and harmonising human relations is never identical to equal-ising the moral or legal rights of autonomous individuals. *Yi* literally means righteousness, justice, or appropriateness, and it refers to the call of duty in a community. It primarily means having a sense of what is appropriate in a given context;[13] it is the measure of fairness and impartiality. Fairness and impartiality, however, are never identical to equality. Mengzi explicates the distinction in his critique of Mohism. He argues against the Mohist doctrine of universal love. Mohists propose a society based on universal love in which everyone loves all equally. But Mengzi criticises such doctrine because it distorts the principle of justice in the sense that loving all equally ignores the relevant context and social conventions which make different expressions of love appropriate.[14] For example, there are different ways to express our love to our parents and colleagues. We may kiss and hug our parents without asking for explicit consent, but it would be inappropriate, and even rude, to greet our colleagues with the same level of affection without their consent. This is because physical touch can have different meanings and levels of appropriateness depending on the context and relationship. Loving all equally without considering the relevant context and social conventions disrespects others' boundaries and consent. As a result, harmonising requires partiality rather than equality. We should treat others based on the sense of appropriateness in a given circumstance rather than based on a context-insensitive principle of equality.

Thanks to Mengzi's critique of Mohism, we find that harmony in human relations requires consideration of context. The sense of appropriateness is neither simply motivated to some degree to abide by our moral judgements nor merely involves subjecting ourselves to any fact that our sense of appro-priateness is so constituted. But rather, while our sense of appropriateness is primarily and necessarily motivated by our compassion, it is secondarily and contingently amended by conventions. This is why Mengzi argues for the intertwining of cardinal virtues such as *ren*, *yi*, and *li*.[15] Here we can find a direct connection between harmony and *li* (rites). Kongzi asserts that "the function of *li* is to harmonise, and harmony is the [most] precious".[16]

Xunzi shares the same view by claiming that "following rites is to harmonize and regulate".[17] Scholars such as Chenyang Li and Ruiping Fan confirm that the observance of rites constitutes harmonious human relations in Confucian social and political philosophy. "A major function of *li* (rites, rituals of propriety) is precisely to harmonize people of various kinds".[18] "It is the skills of participating in the Confucian *li* that contributes to a harmonious society".[19] These ritual practices integrate various human interests into a possibly harmonious system where individuals are taught and trained virtues which allow them to interact appropriately and cooperatively.

Rites provide formal rules for human relationships. However, if formal rules for human relationships are not practiced sincerely, rituals become a mere formality and can eventually cause disorder within a community.[20] For Confucians, moral conduct is directly motivated by moral principles. Before that, people follow their parents' or teachers' demands to observe the rituals, then in the process of such practices, gradually coming to understand that this is precisely the way of following the requirements of the moral principles and subsequently being motivated by the principles.[21] *Li* is a necessary but insufficient condition for harmonious human relations. Mengzi explains this point by giving an example of a village paragon (*xiangyuan* 鄉愿). A village paragon is a thief of virtue who has no sense of appropriateness. They simply follow traditional ritual practices without critical reflection. This deeply misleads people. Mengzi resents the village paragon because they might be confused with the virtuous.

What distinguishes the virtuous from the village paragon is *ren*. The notion of *ren* literally means compassion, benevolence, and kindness, and it refers to the motivation and desire of caring for oneself and for others. Shun explains that "*ren* 仁 (humanity, benevolence), as a Confucian ethical ideal, has to do with one's concern for the well-being of others".[22] *Ren* is a necessary condition for harmonious human relations. For the village paragon and a hypocrite can blindly follow the conventional sense of appropriateness and insincerely practice ritual rules. Only the virtuous, with compassion, can critically examine the sense of appropriateness in a given context, thereby sincerely practicing suitable ritual rules. Benevolence motivates one's wholehearted concern for the well-being of others. *Ren*, however, is an insufficient condition for harmonious human relations because one is ignorant of proper expressions of benevolence without ritual practices and the sense of appropriateness. In *Liji, The Doctrine of the Mean*, the Confucian notion of *ren* was further distinguished into two levels. The first is loving relatives, and the second is honouring the worthy.[23] On this point, Confucian thinkers state that,

> Benevolence is the characteristic element of humanity, and the great exercise of it is in loving relatives. Justice is the accordance of actions with

what is right, and the great exercise of it is in honoring the worthy. The decreasing measures of love due to relatives, and the steps in honor due to the worthy, produces by the principle of propriety.[24]

仁者人也，親親為大；義者宜也，尊賢為大。親親之殺，尊賢之等，禮所生也。

This passage asserts the connections between benevolence (ren), justice (yi), and rites (li). Benevolence is the fundamental motivation for loving relatives, whereas justice is the grounding principle for honouring the worthy. The principle of ritual propriety offers expressive guidance for loving relatives and honouring the worthy. Despite the requirement to love both our nearest relatives and strangers, it is natural and practically neces- sary that love should start with our nearest. So according to this interpre- tation, when there is not enough food to save both our nearest relatives and strangers, we must save our nearest relatives.[25]

An essential lesson of Confucianism is that one should love all with differ- entiation and relativity of importance. Based on our finitude, Confucianism always requires that there ought to be a clear and definite order, distinction, and differentiation in the application of love.[26] In the pre-Qin context, Mengzi was aware of the seriousness of injustice and, to that effect, stated that "nowadays, the means laid down for the people are sufficient neither for the care of parents nor for the support of wife and children. In good years life is always hard, while in bad years, there is no way of escaping death".[27] Although benevolence requires loving all humans, this requirement is not that one should love all humans equally or similarly. Expanding our love to everyone in the world is ethically ideal, but Confucianism puts more weight on practical feasibility.

As an ethical ideal, everyone in the world should be capable of having a stable livelihood. But Confucianism also acknowledges the existence of practical constraints, particularly, in years of famine. As we've seen before, Mengzi contrasts people's livelihood in good years and in years of famine.[28] In good years, people have enough to serve their fathers and mothers, as well as to nurture their wives and children. But that is not the case in years of famine. To provide the means to escape death in years of famine, an enlightened ruler must tax people's livelihood. But the taxation should be done according to "the assistant method" – a method focused on community service – rather than according to "the equality method", which boils down to taxing according to proportionate contribution.[29] The equality method lacks the sense of appropriateness because it takes a constant amount of taxation in both good years and years of famine. If the constant amount is guaranteed in years of famine, then people are unable to care for their parents and must go into debt to make up for their quota. In this way, Mengzi argues against an extremely unequal distribution of material goods responsible for killing many people from hunger while maintaining the privileges and luxurious standard of living of the few. This is why when Mengzi evaluates different forms of ruling, he appreciates monarchy the most, then the hegemony, and tyranny the least. In the first two ways of governance, he claims, enlightened rulers (including both sage-kings and hegemons) issue a "do not hoard grain" order.[30]

Confucianism's practical feasibility can be explained in three ways. First, we should prioritise giving the minimum to those close to us. Once this is satisfied, we should move on and give it to others. It is natural for us to take the nearest into the most serious consideration. Without violating our human nature, we can sincerely motivate ourselves to give. Second, Confucianism considers the minimum amount in a given context and sets an extremely feasible bottom line. Unlike common egalitarian doctrines that try to guarantee a decent minimum for everyone from a top-down approach, Confucianism pursues the amount of the minimum from a bottom-up approach. It begins with the bottom line that it must be unjust to allow death as a result of starvation, and it gives room for further discussion of just regulation. Third, to avoid death due to starvation, the virtuous should always care for the well-being of others, including the nearest and the strangers. Especially in years of famine, an enlightened ruler should establish different regulations to ensure people's livelihood. This would include, as a minimal, a rejection of any proposal of hoarding material goods in such circumstances.

To promote a Confucian ethical ideal, Mengzi suggests expanding our love to not only the nearest but also strangers. He suggests using oneself as a standard to discover other people's needs and thus regulate one's conduct depending on what one finds. The way of expansion of our love emphasises an inference by analogy (*tui* 推). Confucian inference by analogy is a methodological procedure that firstly considers one's concern for oneself and then expands this concern to his relatives, neighbours, friends, and finally to people in the world. In Mengzi's words

> When we know how to enlarge and bring these four sprouts to fulfillment within us, it will be like a fire beginning to burn or a spring finding an outlet. If one is able to bring them to fulfillment, they will be sufficient to enable him to protect 'all within the four seas'; if one is not, they will be insufficient even to enable him to serve his parents (*Mengzi* 2A6).

凡有四端於我者，知皆擴而充之矣，若火之始然，泉之始達。苟能充
之，足以保四海；苟不充之，不足以事父母。

The four sprouts, which include benevolence and justice, are innate to us. Since they are sprouts, one must develop and bring them to fulfilment. Mengzi makes an analogy. Benevolence and justice are like a fire beginning to burn and a spring finding an outlet. Without "flourishing" the fire and spring, the fire will burn out rapidly and the spring will cease to flow easily. Analogically speaking, if one fails to develop and bring four sprouts to fulfilment, one will not be able to take care of his parents. If he cannot show his concern for his relatives, it is also impossible for him to care for the well-being of strangers worldwide. The development of benevolence can motivate one to become a virtuous person who wholeheartedly and sincerely acts according to justice. Another similar passage points out that

> The ode says he set an example for his wife; it extended to his brothers and from there to the state's family.[31]

> 《詩》云：『刑于寡妻，至于兄弟，以御于家邦。』言舉斯心加諸彼而已。故推恩足以保四海，不推恩無以保妻子。

This ode simply speaks of taking kindness and extending it to others. Thus, if one extends his kindness, it will be enough to protect all within the four seas, whereas if one fails to extend it, he will have no way to protect his wife and children. One should extend kindness from relatives to strangers. The way of expansion arouses our sense of responsibility for protecting all people in the world, including relatives and strangers. Such an expansion is based on inference by analogy that one extends one's primary concerns for oneself to others. Mengzi does not demand one to bear an obligation to care for the well-being of others, but rather, he encourages one to love others as one's relatives or even oneself.

12.4 A Confucian Approach to Global Health Justice

The Confucian account of global health justice is a two-level account. On the one hand, Confucian justice requires all individuals who have medical resources to offer help to the needy. It demands the complete exercise of complete virtue in relation to others, not only in matters that concern oneself. The demand is based on human nature, that love starts with our nearest relatives who are in need, then strangers. On the other hand, Confucian justice requires rulers (the State) to regulate people's livelihood by preventing hoarding and shortages. The control measure is carried out in years of emergency and should be removed when the emergency has been resolved. It is based on the method of assistance rather than the method of contribution. This approach has two advantages. First, it is practical and realistic. Taking the early COVID-19 pandemic in Hong Kong Special Administrative

Region of China (HKSAR) as an example, the role of community and social mobilisation took a decisive role in fighting against the pandemic, as the HKSAR government responded slowly and inefficiently in sustaining health services and reducing the risk of spread. Regardless of governmental policies, a community-based mobilisation of mutual assistance was implemented. The most salient case in demonstrating Confucian justice is the sharing and distribution of community-based personal protective equipment (PPE), particularly surgical masks and hand sanitisers. The supply of surgical masks was limited for several reasons, *e.g.*, the temporary suspension of trans- porting material goods during the Lunar New Year Holiday, and the export bans implemented by other countries. Facing these obstacles, people in Hong Kong (HK) first provided information and PPE to their dearest rela- tives then shared with strangers, and eventually, circulated information and extra PPE within a community-based network formed by these self-help models.[32] The community-based network has promoted the protection of the public, especially that of disadvantaged groups and high-risk workers. The fast and transparent circulation of information has enabled citizens to overcome the collective challenges in the early COVID-19 pandemic.[33] It is not surprising for people of HK, who have roots in Confucian culture and an emphasis on filial love, to take these actions, although none explicitly stated that the sharing and distribution were based on Confucian justice. Interestingly enough, the community-based network formed by self-help models was helpful. Still, many people in HK expected the government to control hoarding and to regulate PPE in drugstores.

I believe that the Confucian approach to global health justice can match up with important cultural elements, and perhaps with the ethical intuitions, of many Chinese and East Asians. Therefore, couching certain health prac- tices in Confucian terms may prove beneficial – at least in these regions. Overall, by applying Confucian justice to global health issues, we can find three basic principles:

1 Sufficiency: Each person should have basic medical care that is sufficient for their well-being and life;
2 Fairness: The allocation of medical resources should follow a graded love or love with distinction approach (more resources will be given to the nearest and dearest who are in need, and fewer resources will be offered to strangers); and
3 Responsibility: The individuals and governments must ensure that care is "properly drawn" and the distribution of resources according to the well-field system is fair and just.

The first and third principles clarify the responsibility-bearers in global health issues. Political institutions such as the government are indeed responsible for promoting justice in the global world. However, according to Confucianism, this is insufficient because everyone has both a claim to material sufficiency and also an obligation to work to provide that sufficiency for all.[34] Confucianism endorses the idea of "human flourishing". It obligates the government to distribute medical resources in a fair and just way. However, it also motivates people to promote justice in global health. Erin Cline elaborates that Confucianism "specifically concerns the ability to take a wider view and exercise good judgment out of a sense of accountability to other members of society".[35] It is improper if one person, including the rich and the powerful, causes others to suffer in order to become wealthy and avoid poverty. If one person eliminates poverty properly, this is something worth celebrating. Cline also believes that justice involves a lack of greed and a sense of fairness. Even though this sense of justice does not concern fairness in the sense of a disposition to adhere to the law or in regard to distribution and retribution, it certainly concerns a sense of fairness that is likely to shape one's views about the kinds of laws or standards that a society should have, as well as one's willingness to adhere to them. The amalgamation of both individual and institutional obligation with compassionate motivation is essential for promoting a world where all people can be healthy. Besides, the first principle sets the minimal action guidance for responsibility-bearers. Everyone should have basic medical care that is sufficient for their well-being and life. In an ideal situation, we should have medical care and allocate medical resources to everyone. In an extreme situation where medical resources are limited, we should still have medical care for everyone, but the second principle justifies our natural tendency to prioritise our dearest relatives over strangers in allocating medical resources. So, the second principle applies only after sufficiency is satisfied. Sufficiency is undeniably a core principle of Confucian justice. Of course, classical texts like the *Analects* mention fairness and fair distribution – many passages concern the source of our attitudes and responsibilities towards other members of society, specifically with respect to questions of fairness. But commentators such as Cline clarify that fair distribution in the *Analects* concerns the kinds of laws or standards that a society should have.[36] Justice is also undeniably one of the many important capacities that cultivated persons exemplify in the *Analects*, so that cultivated persons appreciate the institutions that help preserve a stable and harmonious society. But the main focus of Confucianism remains sufficient distribution.

Crucial to the application of Confucian justice to global health issues is the emphasis on responsibilities of individuals – rather than institutions – to promote health justice. Rather than laws or rights, benevolence binds the patient, family members, and physicians together in the family based and harmony-oriented model. All stakeholders are invited to "regard critical medical decisions as located in families, structured by ritual practices and guided by Confucian virtue in order to achieve a harmonious agreement for the health care of patients".[37] Such an approach to global health justice goes for an agent-focused account.

The agent-focused account can be divided into two levels. The first level argues for the charity of the common people. People should "assist one another in their protection and defence, and sustain one another through illness and distress, the hundred surnames will live together in affection and harmony".[38] Those who assist others will be appreciated, but those who fail to assist others will not be blamed. If people assist one another in their protection and defence and sustain one another through illness and distress, they will eventually want to live together in affection and harmony. Living together in affection and harmony motivates sustaining one another through illness and distress. A harmonious society is not a society without distinctions. People treat others according to some well-established social dimension, *e.g.*, the relationship between relatives and strangers and between the worthy and the unworthy. The appropriate treatment for each social dimension may relate to different factors, for example, the degree of proximity or social hierarchy. And these factors reveal different virtues; for example, loving relatives reveal benevolence while honouring the worthy reveals righteousness. The proper response in accordance with the distinctions follows the rules of propriety. The second level argues for the obligations of the rulers. An enlightened ruler should implement regulations to avoid hoarding in years of famine. A sage-king ruler such as King Wen (文王) will know how to nourish people. For example, King Wen "regulated fields and dwellings, taught people about planting and animal husbandry, and guided the women and children in caring for the old".[39] Under the rule of King Wen, people could avoid death due to starvation or suffering due to freezing. It is not only a charity but also an obligation for rulers to give the minimum to the needy. If rulers fail to give the minimum to the needy, they are blamed as tyrannical or fatuous rulers.

This is different from the institution-focused account. For example, in Gillian Brock's recent account of global health justice, she argues against the dichotomy between cosmopolitanism and statism, as well as the distinction between the state-level institution and the international (global)-level institution. State-level institutions are highly significant in promoting human beings' prospects for flourishing lives and constitute an important site of cooperation that ought to aspire to fairness.[40] In most cases, it is challenging for citizens to achieve global justice without state-level institutions that can ensure fair distribution at the international level. Her account remains focused on the responsibilities of institutions responsible for sustaining the ongoing health vulnerabilities.[41] By contrast, the Confucian approach develops a sense of justice based on the gradual expansion of complete virtue.

The corresponding responsibility-bearers are all individual stakeholders and not solely institutions. The principles of justice, benevolence, and rites provide a moral foundation for everyone to promote and protect their health as well as the health of others.

In this way, Confucian justice can avoid paternalistic concerns typically associated with institution-focused accounts. Institution-focused accounts of global health justice are defined by opposition to inequality and thus demand an equitable distribution of material goods and medical resources.[42] Such a demand justifies paternalistic interventions that override individual autonomy. To clarify the term paternalistic intervention, Gerald Dworkin defined it as "interference with a person's liberty of action justified by reason referring exclusively to the welfare (...) of the person being coerced".[43] When an institution presumptively believes that certain policies or actions are just, then it is justified in seeking to override others' decisions. It provides authoritative support for an institution restricting individual autonomy to protect and promote global health. But people may criticise that people may put more weight on pursuing goals other than health. Unlike institution-focused accounts, the Confucian account leaves much room for individual autonomy. On empirical grounds, the sharing of PPE in the community-based network shows that the greatest degree of individual autonomy also enjoys the best health, even better than institutional interventions. The community-based network has recently expanded to mainland China and some surrounding regions. Based on such experiences, a prominent and prevalent stance in global health can be explained through Confucian justice, a stance signified by appending "graded love" or "love with distinction" to justice. This position holds that individuals should provide medical care to others, and such care can begin with the dearest because of human finitude and nature.

12.5 Conclusion

This chapter outlined some of the core tenets of a Confucian-inspired idea of justice in global health. Confucian justice can contribute to global health through the reconsideration of non-egalitarian principles of medical care and allocation, as well as the explication of the motivational foundation of being a virtuous person within a harmonious society. Such a non-egalitarian tendency marks the difference between Confucian justice and modern Western justice theory. The virtue consanguinism and family oriented favouritism of traditional Confucianism support the conception of non-equality which is, at first sight, antithetical to modern liberal and western justice theories that insist on seeing equality as the core principle of justice.[44] The non-egalitarian idea of fairness not only differs from modern Western theories of justice theory, but also represents a challenge to it. Whether these challenges can be overcome is up for debate. But the uniqueness of Confucian justice outlined in this chapter provides an alternative way to approach global health issues, one that may help shed light on the place of equality, priority, and sufficiency in our theories of global health justice.

Notes

1 Tsoi CH, 'Distributive Justice in Pre-Qin Confucianism: Equality, Priority, and Sufficiency' in R. A. Carleo III, Y. Huang (eds.), *Confucian Political Philosophy* (Springer 2021) 140.
2 Ibid. 156, emphasis in original.
3 Ibid. 159.
4 Ibid 140. Tsoi argues that sufficientarianism is compatible with egalitarianism and prioritarianism in Confucian political philosophy. He admits that there is a fine but significant difference between egalitarianism and prioritarianism. However, he also claims that he does "not intend to imply that the three values (equality, priority, and sufficiency) are mutually exclusive," and "if the three values can be embraced separately, then they may have different weightings and trump each other in different situations". Ibid 52. It is worth noting that discussing whether the potential conflict between egalitarianism and prioritarianism can be solved in Confucianism is not Tsoi's focus.
5 Fan RP, 'Social Justice: Rawlsian or Confucian?' in Mou Bo (ed.), *Comparative Approaches to Chinese Philosophy* (Routledge 2003) 180.
6 Chan J, *Confucian Perfectionism: A Political Philosophy for Modern Times* (Princeton University Press 2015) 22.
7 Ibid. 162.
8 Kongzi, *Analects: With Selections from Traditional Commentaries* (Edward Slingerland tr, Hackett Publishing 2003) 53, with my modification.
9 Chan J, *Confucian Perfectionism: A Political Philosophy for Modern Times* (Princeton University Press 2015) 22.
10 Seok BG, 'Justice and Religion: Confucianism', *Encyclopedia of Global Justice* (2011) 595.
11 Kongzi, *Analects: With Selections from Traditional Commentaries* (Edward Slingerland tr, Hackett Publishing 2003) 149.
12 Ibid. 210.
13 Yu offers some comparisons between Confucianism and Aristotle. According to his analysis, Confucian notion of *yi* corresponds to Aristotelian notion of phronesis. Yu JY, 'Virtue: Confucius and Aristotle' *Philosophy East and West* (1998) 323, 344 note 24. However, he also argues that "the lack of an Aristotelian notion of practical wisdom turns out to be the weakness in Confucius' thinking" in the same article. Ibid 331. While Aristotle suggests an attitude that is not one of blind compliance with tradition, Confucius insists on the continuity and authenticity of the tradition. I believe Confucius also agrees that one should not act in blind compliance with tradition. One of the clearest examples is his critique of the village paragon who blindly and insincerely follows traditions. Confucius describes them as "the thief of virtue". Therefore, both Confucius and Aristotle argue for the attitude that one should not blindly comply with tradition even though tradition has a significant role. Hence, to a large extent, the Confucian notion of *yi* corresponds to Aristotelian notion of phronesis.

14 Mengzi, *Mencius* (Philip J. Ivanhoe tr, Columbia University Press 2009) 150.
15 Ibid. 35 & 123–124.
16 Kongzi, *Analects: With Selections from Traditional Commentaries* (Edward Slingerland tr, Hackett Publishing 2003) 5.
17 Xunzi, *Xunzi: The Complete Text* (Eric Hutton tr, Princeton University Press 2014) 11.
18 Li CY, 'The Philosophy of Harmony in Classical Confucianism' *Philosophy Compass* (2008) 423, 427.
19 Fan RP, *Reconstructionist Confucian: Rethinking Morality After the West* (Springer 2010) 177.
20 Ritual formalism emphasises ritual and propriety over the situation and the sincerity of a ritual performer.
21 Fan RP, 'Confucian Ritualization: How and Why?' in D. Solomon, R. P. Fan, and P. C Lo (eds), *Ritual and the Moral Life: Reclaiming the Tradition* (Springer 2012) 155. Aristotle has famously claimed that human beings are primarily family oriented. He states that "a human is a social being and his nature is to live in the company of others.". Aristotle, *Nicomachean Ethics* (Roger Crisp tr. Cambridge University Press 2000) 177. And more importantly, the community is clearly by nature prior to the family, and the individual since the whole is of necessity prior to the part. The part-whole logic shows that all men must live in a community as a whole, while a member of a community can be regarded as a part of the whole. Men are primarily social beings in their practical life. Only in their theoretical reflection men are separated into individuals. All men, by nature, have inevitable social ties. Our first social tie is with our family. Unsurprisingly, men typically love their families more than strangers. When men distribute their resources, they tend to care for one's interests and those of the nearest and dearest. Berry Tholen correctly addresses that "special concern for one's interests and those that are most near and dear may threaten the cohesion and support necessary for achieving the good life under the common good, but it is also a necessary part of it". Tholen B, 'Political Responsibility as a Virtue: Nussbaum, MacIntyre, and Ricoeur on the Fragility of Politics' (2018) *Alternatives* 22, 29.
22 Shun KL, 'Early Confucian Moral Psychology' in V. Shen (ed.). *Dao Companion to Classical Confucian Philosophy* (Springer 2014) 267.
23 In contrast, benevolence refers to humane love, which is different from charity, the love of God. The essential difference between Confucian benevolence and charity is whether they love with or without distinctions. Confucian benevolence is love with distinctions through practical reason, stemming from the love of dear ones, a universal and natural spiritual fact of human beings. In contrast, charity is love without distinctions through unconditional passion, coming from the all-embracing grace of God, which is the nature of the omnipotent God. Although some contemporary discussion uses terms such as "love," "compassion," "empathy," and "benevolence" interchangeably, these terms often carry specific connotations. Empathy and compassion are linked to being benevolent or showing loving-kindness to one's fellow human beings. Benevolence is deeply rooted in innate human feelings of compassion and empathy. Barton KC, and Ho LC, 'Cultivating Sprouts of Benevolence: A Foundational Principle for Civic and Multicultural Education Curriculum' (2020) *Multicultural Education Review* 157, 157.
24 Legge J, *The Chinese Classics* (Hong Kong University Press 1960) 405–406.
25 It is noteworthy to mention that relatives (*qin* 親) should not be understood as those who are blood related to us. Mengzi discusses the doctrine of loving relatives (*qin qin* 親親) in two passages. In *Gaozi II* while explaining his idea of graded love or love with distinction, Mengzi uses "relatives" to refer to those who

are blood related. Mengzi, *Mencius* (Philip J. Ivanhoe tr, Columbia University Press 2009) 134. However, in *Jin Xin I*, the notion of relative is extended to the nearest in society, including brothers, spouses and friends. Ibid 147.

26 Fan RP, 'Confucian Ritualization: How and Why?' in D. Solomon, R. P. Fan, and P. C. Lo (eds), *Ritual and the Moral Life: Reclaiming the Tradition* (Springer 2012) 53.

27 Mengzi, *Mencius* (Philip J. Ivanhoe tr, Columbia University Press 2009) 35 & 123–124.

28 Ibid. 11–12.

29 Ibid. 54.

30 Ibid. 139.

31 Mengzi, *Mencius* (Philip J. Ivanhoe tr, Columbia University Press 2009) 9.

32 Wan KM, et al, 'Fighting COVID-19 in Hong Kong: The Effects of Community and Social Mobilization' (2020) *World Development* 1; Wong WC, et al, 'The Resilience of Social Service Providers and Families of Children with Autism or Development Delays during the Covid-19 Pandemic—A Community Case Study in Hong Kong' (2021) *Frontiers in Psychiatry* 1.

33 Ibid.

34 Chan J, 'Is There a Confucian Perspective on Social Justice?' in T. Shogiman and C. J. Nederman (eds.). *Western Political Thought in Dialogue with Asia* (Roman and Littlefield 2008) 178–261.

35 Cline EM, 'Two Senses of Justice: Confucianism, Rawls, and Comparative Political Philosophy' (2007) *Philosophy Compass* 361, 369.

36 Ibid. 371.

37 Chen XY and Fan RP, 'The Family and Harmonious Medical Decision Making: Cherishing an Appropriate Confucian Moral Balance' (2010) *Journal of Medicine and Philosophy* 573, 574.

38 Mengzi, *Mencius* (Philip J. Ivanhoe tr, Columbia University Press 2009) 54.

39 Ibid. 148.

40 Brock G, 'Global Justice, Cosmopolitan Duties and Duties to Compatriots: the Case of Healthcare' (2015) *Public Health Ethics* 110, 113.

41 Ibid. 117.

42 Buchanan DR, 'Autonomy, Paternalism, and Justice: Ethical Priorities in Public Health' (2008) *American Journal of Public Health* 15, 16.

43 Dworkin G, 'Defining Paternalism' in Thomas Schramme (ed.), *New Perspectives on Paternalism and Health Care* (Springer 2015).

44 Murphy T, and Weber R, 'Ideas of Justice and Reconstructions of Confucian Justice' (2016) *Asian Philosophy* 99, 111.

Bibliography

Aristotle, *Nicomachean Ethics* (Roger Crisp tr. Cambridge University Press 2000).

Barton K C and Li C Ho, 'Cultivating Sprouts of Benevolence: A Foundational Principle for Civic and Multicultural Education Curriculum' [2020] *Multicultural Education Review* 157.

Brock G, 'Global Justice, Cosmopolitan Duties and Duties to Compatriots: the Case of Healthcare' [2015] *Public Health Ethics* 110.

Buchanan D R, 'Autonomy, Paternalism, and Justice: Ethical Priorities in Public Health' [2008] *American Journal of Public Health* 200815.

Chan J, 'Is There a Confucian Perspective on Social Justice?' in T. Shogiman and C. J. Nederman (eds.), *Western Political Thought in Dialogue with Asia* (Roman and Littlefield 2008).

Chan J, *Confucian Perfectionism: A Political Philosophy for Modern Times* (1st edn, Princeton University Press 2015).

Chen XY and Fan RP, 'The Family and Harmonious Medical Decision Making: Cherishing an Appropriate Confucian Moral Balance' [2010] Journal of Medicine and Philosophy 573.

Cline E. M., 'Two Senses of Justice: Confucianism, Rawls, and Comparative Political Philosophy' [2007] Philosophy Compass 361.

Dworkin G, 'Defining Paternalism' in T. Schramme (ed.), *New Perspectives on Paternalism and Health Care* (Springer, New York 2015).

Fan RP, 'Confucian Ritualization: How and Why?' in D. Solomon, R. Fan, and Ping-cheung Lo (eds), *Ritual and the Moral Life: Reclaiming the Tradition* (Springer 2012).

Fan RP, 'Social Justice: Rawlsian or Confucian?' in M. Bo (ed.), *Comparative Approaches to Chinese Philosophy* (Routledge 2003).

Fan RP, *Reconstructionist Confucian: Rethinking Morality After the West* (1st edn, Springer 2010).

Kongzi, *Analects: With Selections from Traditional Commentaries* (E. Slingerland tr, Hackett Publishing 2003).

Legge J, *The Chinese Classics* (1st edn, Hong Kong University Press 1960).

Li CY, 'The Philosophy of Harmony in Classical Confucianism' [2008] *Philosophy Compass* 423.

Mengzi M (Philip J. Ivanhoe tr, Columbia University Press 2009).

Murphy T and Weber R, 'Ideas of Justice and Reconstructions of Confucian Justice' [2016] *Asian Philosophy* 99.

Seok B, 'Justice and Religion: Confucianism', *Encyclopedia of Global Justice* [2011].

Shun KL, 'Early Confucian Moral Psychology' in V. Shen (ed.), *Dao Companion to Classical Confucian Philosophy* (Springer 2014).

Tholen B, 'Political Responsibility as a Virtue: Nussbaum, MacIntyre, and Ricoeur on the Fragility of Politics' [2018] *Alternatives* 22.

Tsoi CH, 'Distributive Justice in Pre-Qin Confucianism: Equality, Priority, and Sufficiency' in Robert A. Carleo III, Y. Huang (eds), *Confucian Political Philosophy* (Springer 2021).

Wan KM and others, 'Fighting COVID-19 in Hong Kong: The Effects of Community and Social Mobilization' [2020] *World Development* 1.

Wong WC and others, 'The Resilience of Social Service Providers and Families of Children with Autism or Development Delays during the Covid-19 Pandemic—A Community Case Study in Hong Kong' [2021] *Frontiers in Psychiatry* 1.

Xunzi, *Xunzi: The Complete Text* (Eric Hutton tr, Princeton University Press 2014).

Yu JY, 'Virtue: Confucius and Aristotle' (1998) *Philosophy East and West* 323.

13

WHAT DO WE WANT FROM A THEORY OF GLOBAL HEALTH JUSTICE?

Sridhar Venkatapuram

13.1 Introduction

This chapter presents a rough sketch of my nascent thinking regarding a theory or approach to global health justice. It has three parts. The first is an introduction and background to the topic of global justice, and a brief overview of the state of the global health justice literature. In the second part, I present some criteria for what we want from a theory of global health justice or, perhaps, a theory of global justice that appropriately centres on health. Then, in the third part, I conclude with a discussion for what a human capabilities-centred theory of global health justice would or could look like. Indeed, I recognise that against the norm or standard practice in political philosophy academic literature where a line of argument is clearly presented and defended, presenting a rough sketch looks incomplete. However, the present discussion is purposefully and consciously tentative because the real-world institutions seeking to improve global health as well as the broader global governance architecture (or world order) are under great stress and undergoing great transformations. For a few months early in the Covid-19 pandemic, there was doubt if many global institutions or the global order would survive. The Covid-19 pandemic, like HIV/AIDS in the 1990s, is also profoundly challenging and transforming social, economic, and political institutions within and across countries. To carry on with pre-pandemic thinking and projects, conceptual vocabulary, and methodologies as if nothing has substantively changed would run the great risk that the effort is born stillborn, irrelevant to real-world concerns. It would also be disrespectful to tens of millions of people who have died and suffered, are still suffering, and will predictably suffer in the future as a result of our

DOI: 10.4324/9781003399933-19

human actions and neglect since Covid-19 appeared in late 2019 and began to spread. But even before Covid-19, there were dramatic global transformations happening that required a reassessment of global justice and global health justice philosophy such as the growth of authoritarian governments across the world; increasing number of billionaires who can influence governments, international agendas, and laws; growth of technology companies and the impact of their products; climate heating, and so forth.

A second and equally important reason for this present discussion on a theory of global health justice being tentative is that various events and social movements have come together over the past three years in such a way that some of us, at the least, are now able to openly name and question the epistemic domination by certain cultures, institutions, social groups and individuals, countries, and so forth. Such domination was clearly visible, for those who were willing to see, in the global justice literature that developed after 2000. It would not be unfair to describe the central question being addressed in that literature as being, "What do we owe those poor and suffering people over there in those far-away places"?[1] An approach or theory of global health justice, and potentially global justice, has to do much better than assume the subjective position of being one of the well-off societies or individuals in the world, or erasing the history of how the "we" became wealthy while "they" become poor and stay poor. Indeed, "doing better" philosophy than those who tried before is the standard for which we should aim. Aiming for the one final and true approach to global health justice would be repeating the errors and epistemic hubris that pervades European Enlightenment philosophy and its modern progenitors. The great advantage of philosophers now is that, if we choose to do so, we can take ideas from anywhere in the world, build on them, and offer them up for truly global scrutiny. If the ideas survive such global public scrutiny, that process will itself be a form of moral justification.

13.2 Global Justice with Health or Global Health Justice: The Background

Let me begin by explaining that I chose the title "What do we want from a theory of global health justice?" not only because it reflects the topic of this book and the preparatory workshops, but also because it raises the following question: is a theory of global health justice the same as a theory of global justice with adequate consideration of health? Or, is it global health practice and theory as it is now or should be with justice being more explicit in it? These definitional issues are not the focus here, but it is worth noting that conversations would be different and go in different directions if we had global health scholars asking, "What should we do when health involves justice?" versus global justice philosophers discussing what global justice philosophy with health would look like. I believe that both kinds of conversations should be seen as one and the same. What I'm going to try to do here is to show how we can bring these conversations together based on the criteria we want a theory of global health justice to satisfy.

Perhaps to put it another way, recall John Rawls's original 1971 publication of a Theory of Justice.[2] He gives significant importance to and space discussing economics and economic theory. Before Rawls's publication, some economists did seriously consider justice. And some philosophers thought seriously about economic issues and theories. But Rawls developed his theory of social justice with some criteria in mind, and these criteria motivated bringing together, integrating, and further evolving previously siloed discussions in economics as well as philosophy. Such serious consideration and integration are reflected in Rawls's understanding of what causes countries to be wealthy or poor, how incentives work, how innovation happens, and the role of income and wealth. I would ask that, like Rawls and other philosophers think about economics, we think about global health. Twenty or more years ago, asking political philosophers to give serious consideration to public and global health like they do economics would have been received with confusion or laughter. If your understanding of public and global health is that they are concerned about sanitation, clean water, and so forth, then, such matters don't really match up to the grand ideas and great thinkers of political philosophy and economics. I tell you this from experience of having tried to do this.

There is likely to be much less resistance at present in asserting that health needs to be a more central consideration of social and global justice theories. Every person on the planet is now aware of what kind of grand impact a public/global health issue can have on our lives, and what kind of grand response it requires. In bringing together the grand ideas of social and global justice with the concerns of global health, this present discussion is simply stating that we need to first identify the criteria or desideratum of theory or approach to global health justice. I sometimes say approach because it may be that a complete theory of global justice may not be possible or justifiable.[3] The lack of consideration of what we want from a theory or the standards according to which we should assess global health justice would produce some bad things – lots of poor reasoning could be labelled as being theories or approaches to global health justice, perpetuate the blind spots in justice theorising, continue to erase or ignore some of the most glaring health injustices, and so forth.

As many will be aware, Anglo-American global justice scholarship really took off around 1999 or 2000. Ostensibly, as the story is told, the birth of this area of scholarship was because of John Rawls's publication of *The Laws of Peoples* (LOP), which made the concept of global justice a popular and accessible topic.[4] Up until Rawls's LOP publication, there were disparate discussions and very few publications that explicitly used the word "global justice". Those familiar with the literature post-2000 would hopefully agree with me that global justice philosophy essentially was – in the early 2000s – a debate between "statists" and cosmopolitans. While the initial problem of global justice may have been frequently identified as being the preventable deaths and low life expectancy of those poor people in faraway places, the underlying philosophical issue that was of interest to academic philosophers was whether and what kinds of demands of justice there are across societies/national borders. Does justice demand that my country or I do something about those people's preventable deaths and suffering? Statists argued that the concept of justice does not exist outside of our own social and political boundaries based on some basic ideas regarding the social contract and circumstances of justice. There are various kinds of statists, most notably David Miller,[5] but also John Rawls. Moreover, as it is well known, Rawls thought it is best to begin by imagining the world as having only one society. He asserted that it is best to get the theory of social justice right in our own society first, and then reason about justice in a world with many other societies. The consequences of this step-wise reasoning – first domestic then global – about justice are many, and the evaluation of this reasoning is beyond the scope of the present discussion. However, one consequence is that outside of a Rawlsian just society the scope of justice is fairly minimal.

Cosmopolitans can be represented along a spectrum. On one end of the spectrum, you have what I am going to call the "extreme cosmopolitans" such as Peter Singer. Singer, the standard bearer of utilitarian philosophers, basically argues that international borders don't mean much ethically.[6] What really matters is whatever your choice of thing that you value – your health, life expectancy, life, or whatever that might be. Justice requires maximising the outcome or thing that is valuable, which usually relates to positive wellbeing. But you also have other cosmopolitans, most notably David Held[7] and Phillip van Parijs,[8] who had a kind of revelation about statism which turned them towards cosmopolitans. But other notable cosmopolitans include Thomas Pogge who takes the Rawlsian social contract and extends it across many societies and entire human species.[9] In essence, he says we can still stick with the social contract, but it is not our society first and then everybody else. We are just going to put all human beings situated within their societies into one social contract, and then let us see what we get from there.

What ended up happening is that the debate between the statists/social contractarians versus cosmopolitans died because the participating philosophers came to an agreement of sorts that it is neither "justice only exists within our country" nor "everybody is equal and we live in one big community and, therefore, everyone has equal moral rights and duties across any borders that may exist". Instead of these two extremes, there is an in-between place that we need to find and negotiate. Different philosophers landed in different places. However, it is worth noting that despite the flurry of publications and grand debates that took place in the early 2000s, it is unclear what this settlement among global justice philosophers offered as solutions or guidance to addressing some of the pressing issues of our times.

What is interesting about the global justice literature from the 2000s to around 2015 is that philosophers often started with the health example as a motivation for talking about global justice – like "consider those poor people dying or starving over there", and so the question was what we owe those people in those kinds of situations. Different philosophers produced different arguments, whether it be for increasing access to medicines in poor countries or addressing neglected diseases affecting poor people in poor countries. There were others who moved from that initial problem of poor health or low life expectancy to proposals for changing economic conditions and institutions. However, if we pay attention to the causation and distribution of disease and death and regard these as central to justice, then proposals for more medicines or changing economic institutions seem off-target. The idea that people in resource-poor settings are dying and suffering because they do not have access to medicines or healthcare more broadly is true. But to argue that justice demands that the concern for health deprivations and preventable deaths be addressed primarily through providing more access to medicines lacks both an understanding of nature of the problem and takes minimal advantage of what the concept of justice can offer in terms of scope and scale.

Nevertheless, one school of global justice philosophy that has really resonated and really progressed over the last 15 years is utilitarianism, particularly the group known as Effective Altruists. But another kind of utilitarianism that has been enormously effective in the practical policy world is one making use of the DALY (Disability Adjusted Life Years). Like the classic metric of utility in utilitarianism, a DALY is essentially a unit that combines mortality and morbidity into one measure. Before DALYs, we only had life expectancy and no disease-specific calculations of harm. DALYs help make comparisons of harm across different diseases and impairments. DALYS are also used to measure the impact of medical interventions. When combined with cost-efficiency calculations, they help identify which interventions will reduce the most harms or put "the most life years" back into populations.

This line of reasoning about maximising health life years in a population has profoundly influenced the way we think about and address global and domestic health policy. This is not only because of the intuitive attractiveness of the idea, but also because Bill Gates/The Gates Foundation has given the Institute of Health Metrics – which is centred around the DALY – over six hundred million dollars over the last 15 years in order to develop and apply that particular kind of approach.[10] Effective altruists, following Peter Singer, also started with the idea of cost efficiency and sought to identify which disease interventions should global donations support. As utilitarian justice demands maximising the valued outcome, the quest was to identify which disease intervention will have the most impact anywhere in the world. A group of them have now moved on and are thinking about the long-term future horizon. The idea is that if we care about maximising wellbeing of human beings around the world now, then we should also think about human beings in the future. This then leads to thinking about the millions and billions of people of the future under threat by our present actions, and how we should identify and address those threats. This line of reasoning asserts that future people have equal value as the present living people. Therefore, we should focus on the threats we are posing to future people rather than on the threats that current human beings are facing now. This is because justice demands that we act to have the greatest good impact, and the health and wellbeing of billions of human beings in the future is at stake. Addressing the deaths and suffering affecting those alive in the present would be doing less good, and less justice.

In contrast to the profound impact that utilitarians have had not only on global justice philosophy but also on global health justice philosophy, the other philosophical option available is Norman Daniels' approach.[11] Daniels is a Rawlsian who has argued that a just society would distribute healthcare fairly because it is an important commodity that supports people to have equality of opportunity to pursue their life plans (among a possible standard range in a given society). Daniels writes that the original formulation of the theory proved to be impracticable because when we actually distribute healthcare with equality of opportunity in mind there is no one formula or principle to make decisions. In fact, there are many valid and incommensurate competing distribution principles. For example, some people may believe those who are most in need should get healthcare. Others might believe that healthcare should be given to those who will benefit the most. Yet others may believe that more people should receive healthcare than few. In the face of multiple incommensurate values at play in decision making, Daniels revised this theory. He argued for a fair decision-making process which entailed certain criteria (transparency, relevant reasons, and revisability).[12] The idea is that if the process is fair, then the outcome is legitimate and fair.

In addition to that revision, there was another major one. Daniels had a revelation in the years after putting out his initial theory that while health is important for equality of opportunity, health is not primarily about healthcare: health, disease, and mortality are actually more significantly determined by something called "social determinants of health". And, significantly, the second part to this revelation was that despite being incorrectly focused on just healthcare in his initial theory, serendipitously, under John Rawls's theory of justice the social determinants of health get distributed fairly. So, according to Daniels, he does not have to change anything because of the new awareness about social determinants of health because the theoretical framework he was using, already addressed them. But Daniels does not solve a third problem that was visible to him given the global justice debates that flourished in the early 2000s. In the revised theory presented in the 2007 book, Daniels does not have a solution to the question of what we owe to people regarding their health outside one's own country, whether in ideal Rawlsian theory or real world. Curiously, he states openly that it is up to us, the future generations, to figure out that philosophical solution.

I have discussed Daniels's theory in depth elsewhere.[13] Briefly, I believe Daniels is wrong at least in two ways: one is that what are called the "social determinants of health" are actually bad things, not good things to be distributed fairly. These are bad socially created conditions that cause and distribute disabilities, disease, and premature mortality. So, if and when we say that social determinants are distributed fairly, what we are saying is that we are distributing bad things across society fairly. In Rawls's theory, primary goods are "all purpose means" or good things that help people pursue diverse kinds of lives they value. Everyone would want more of them. As a result, they cannot be bad or harmful things. In his original theory, Daniels considers healthcare as a possible primary good, but for various reasons chooses to give it ethical value for being a supportive means for equality of opportunity, which is a primary good. So, when Daniels says Rawls's theory distributes the social determinants of health fairly, it is unclear where or how. Is it through primary goods, or through other aspects of the Rawlsian architecture?

Indeed, it is possible to disconnect from the social epidemiological literature and reimagine social determinants of health as good things. Let's imagine that we are able to and/or should identify good social determinants of health. Then we would identify claims to such goods and want to distribute them fairly. While it may be interesting and productive to do so for philosophical discussions, disconnecting from the epidemiological literature we mean losing the ability to speak across relevant and quite important disciplines. Imagine philosophers disconnecting from economics literature and redefining some basic economic concepts in novel ways that are interesting to philosophers (only). While it is not an either or choice, redefining influential scientific concepts would likely diminish our ability to be relevant, engage in reciprocal learning, and have impact on real-world injustices. In any case, the main point was whether Daniels handles social determinants of health appropriately in saying they are distributed fairly in a Rawlsian just society, and if that provides guidance for real-world action.

The second concern has to do with Daniels's argument for accountability for reasonableness criteria. As he and others have stated, the criteria have been implemented in various hospitals and even health policymaking decisions of various countries. However, there is something that does not sit right regarding implementing a fair healthcare resource allocation process that does not take account of a surrounding social context of injustice. As we saw early in the Covid-19 pandemic, many hospitals tried to implement a fair allocation process/principles for distributing limited healthcare during various waves of infections. But it became clear that such implementing fairness procedures can do injustice to people twice: within the hospital, someone who has multi-morbidities is told that "we don't think you are going to benefit very much from this healthcare, and because we have a limited amount of resources we are going to give it to someone who will benefits more". Benefit, as we know, may not be the only principle to use. At the same time, that person with multi-morbidities is in the hospital because of a lifetime of social disadvantage. The Black Lives Matter public demonstrations in the United States and worldwide made clear how people's lives are under persistent threat on a daily basis. People became sick with Covid-19 and different kinds of multi-morbidities, not primarily because of their individual choices but because of a lifetime of disadvantages and harmful social conditions. So, many people experience injustice by being exposed to social causes of various diseases over a lifetime, and when they go to the hospital, they are told that according to a fair procedure, "unfortunately, we are going to help someone else rather than you because they need it more, can benefit more, is more urgent" and so forth. As can be imagined, in places like urban Chicago, the person who is not likely to be helped is usually Black while the person who will benefit a lot more and helped is usually White. So, Daniels's accountability for reasonableness principles, as well as other such frameworks being proposed and used, do not adequately address the lifetime of disadvantages in a de facto context of social injustice. The fair process inside the hospital or committee room has to be connected to doing more justice outside. The reality of social and health injustices being made more visible during the pandemic has led to some novel solutions. In the United States, these included using geographical data of deprivations and developing "equity weights" in the distribution of health-care and Covid-19 vaccines.[14]

In contrast to the utilitarians, or Daniels's approach where we muddle through what we do in our unjust society as well as about our duties in other places, we also have Amartya Sen (and Martha Nussbaum)[15] proposing a cosmopolitan approach to global health justice, called the "capabilities approach". While not expressly focused on health, health is considered to be a basic concern that motivated the approach. Two aspects which they were clear from the beginning of the development of the approach are that we should think about human wellbeing in terms of what individuals are able to be and do in their daily lives, and that social justice is about developing, protecting, expanding, and recovering the capabilities of individuals, wherever we find them. And when we do look at the space of human capabilities, within and across countries, we should be looking to identify and address the greatest capability deprivations. This aspect implicates various kinds of philosophical discussions. For example, Sen writes that people with diverse ethical commitments are more likely to agree on the worst scenario of injustice than on the perfect or ideal conception of justice. Addressing the worst cases of injustices in the real world helps us make progress on justice, despite profound disagreements. Second, one of the main motivations of thinking about wellbeing in terms of capabilities is that it allows for making comparisons across individuals and groups. This, then allows us to "grade" either ordinally or cardinally the severity of capability constraints, as well as the level of injustice implicate in such constraints.

There is a third, and important dimension worth noting. On the one hand, Sen states that we should not think of our own capabilities or that of others as just forms of social advantage. Capabilities are not like Rawlsian primary goods of social advantage but also produce responsibilities. Having the capabilities to be and do things such as alleviating someone else's deprivations produces at least an ethical duty to consider to do so. Such duties arising from capabilities have implications for realising health justice within our own societies as well as elsewhere in the world. On the other hand, when we look more closely as the causation and distribution of capability constraints and failures, including of health capability, we will quickly be able to identify who or what is morally responsible. By focusing on capabilities, we are more likely to identify the causes in the socio-structural policies, processes and neglect rather than in the lack of finite commodities such as medicines, food, or water. It is here that social epidemiology and causation and distribution of capabilities have a great overlap.[16] These two approaches to identifying injustice in capability failures are distinct from that of Nussbaum's approach.[17] She asserts that every individual has a claim to ten basic capabilities, and each to a threshold that constitutes a minimally decent life. There is less emphasis on the injustice in the causes and distribution patterns of capabilities constraints, and more on every individual's claim to basic capabilities akin to basic rights identified in national constitutions.

The above is a rough and ready sketch of my understanding of the state of the field of global health justice – and it is possible that this understanding needs correction. As someone who has been following global justice and global health justice literature since the mid-1990s, in Anglo-American philosophy, we have the utilitarians, the Rawlsians, and the capabilitarians all wanting to reason about and guide public action to realise real-world global health justice. There are many other approaches to global health that are not grounded in justice but rather, in charity, self-interest, power, and so forth. The idea is that just like a concept of social justice might manage the diverse factors working within a society setting, a concept of global health justice might do the same in global health. However, in 2023 and moving forward, we cannot easily take as a given the theories and discussions that have been prominent in the literature, particularly in Anglo-American and rich country academia. To decide which of the available options is a good theory for global health justice, or if some other one is needed, we need some criteria for what we want from or in such a theory.

There has been much discussion on what constitutes a theory of social justice, what purpose it serves, and so forth. Perhaps of all the different discussions, Elizabeth Anderson's description that any theory of social justice has a metric (what is valued) and a distribution rule is quite helpful.[18] But in light of many discussions on justice that have happened since, we can say that Anderson was talking specifically about distributive justice. It may be that a global health justice theory should do more work than just distribution; we may want it to also do relational justice, corrective justice, or reparative justice. This is why I started this chapter saying that I am presenting rough sketches. I would value being partially right in sketches than totally wrong with a full argument. In any case, I would argue that a theory of global health justice should at least satisfy or reflect four criteria. I have provided the above discussion to show how the weakness and blind spots in other approaches inform these criteria. And these criteria, I believe, are specifically relevant to global health, and are not generic to what would be needed of a global justice theory.

13.3 The Three Criteria

The first might seem very obvious: relevance. There is a valid concern that global justice philosophy debates and literature, and similarly global health justice philosophy literature is very "ideal" – and I am not against ideal theory or abstract theory or idealised theory. But I have found it hard to see the real-world relevance of ideal theorising such as "in a perfect society under Rawlsian conditions" what would this or that look like? Ideal theory does have some use, but it may be far removed from the reality of the situation and there may be much disagreement on this one ideal conception of justice. Starting from a real-world health injustice is an understandable and laudable way to begin theorising of global health justice. But not circling back after theorising to solve the problem can be seen as weakness of such theorising. Now, utilitarians may absolutely say that their theory has direct relevance because they are looking at what people are dying from now, and they are focusing on maximising the benefit for that issue. And underneath the criterion of relevance, I think that not only must a theory be relevant to the current situation in the world, but the proposed theory must provide both theoretical guidance and practical guidance. Perhaps, this should be seen as being responsive. Being relevant to the real-world suffering and deaths of people, and being responsive to new problems and old ones long ignored are not the same thing, but inter-related. A good global health justice theory cannot just be a beautiful theoretical discussion or philosophical architecture; it must be able to guide our actions; to actually do the things that we want justice to do in the real world.

The second criterion that I believe is important to a theory of global health justice is perseverance; more precisely our concepts of justice and global health justice must be stable and persevere over time. This ability to persist requires the theory to be at a certain level of abstraction – but not ideal theory – that provides theoretical power to guide action beyond the immediate situation. This feature is really important because many people who are using the words "health justice" or "global health justice" in the last few years have been using these words to make very contextually specific claims: "we want access to *this* vaccine" or "we want access to *this* medicine". To put it another way, imagine me saying "justice demands that I get this piece of cake in front of me". There is something valuable about the concept of justice that makes us step back from the immediate and reason at a higher level of generality. Moreover, in light of the potential scope of global health justice, the coherence of "justice means access to *this* particular healthcare treatment available now" is not going to last very long. By that, I mean only relevant for a few years till new treatments come along. It is a very time-bound and epidemiologically-bound situation. The idea that a theory of global health justice should persevere over time helps us step back from the immediate political and social conflicts over biomedical or healthcare resources, and reason at much higher or more general level of causation and distribution of health within and across countries, state of global institutions and world order, and means and ends of global health.

The third important criterion is inter-theoretical coherence. Recall that in *Justice as Fairness* Rawls shows a fairly deep engagement with macro-economics.[19] He spends a significant amount of time discussing how his theory aligns with basic economic principles, and how this provides more external justification; that it has inter-theoretical coherence. Despite it being a hugely important contribution, one of the big blind spots with Rawls's theory is that he does not engage very much with public health, or the underlying sciences of epidemiology and biostatistics. He does recognise the value of healthcare, and lets people choose their level of healthcare consumption up to them. But, given that so much of the theory is about the rules of social cooperation, it seems odd that there is very little consideration of the spread of harmful diseases among a group of human beings precisely because they are choosing to live together. While other philosophers have also recognised the health blind spot in Rawls's reasoning, they have chosen to address the issue within philosophical terms and concepts rather than reach across relevant disciplines. That is, philosophers have worked on how would luck-egalitarian, care ethics, libertarian, or other ethical approaches deal with health and healthcare.

That is what my work is about; I try to bring a theory of justice in line with our latest understandings of causation and distribution of disease, and also what is possible in terms of prevention mitigation and care. What I have found is that there are different kinds and levels or intensity of engagement with relevant disciplines. There is also a real question about what are the most relevant disciplines and spheres that need to be involved in a theory of global health justice. For example, Rawls's theory brings together political philosophy with economics, law and later, international relations. Norman Daniels tries to integrate social epidemiology, which I don't think he does correctly, but he still does use that further justification for his approach ("reflective equilibrium"). Utilitarians also bring in epidemiology, cost-effectiveness, and economics together. These kinds of inter-disciplinary informed efforts are great, but it is not and has not been enough. There must be some more relevant disciplines included for a global health justice theory to be inter-theoretically coherent, practice guiding, relevant, and persevere over time.

This is why I am an advocate of the capabilities approach. Such approach brings political philosophy, economics, social epidemiology, and what it still needs – and this is what I'm looking to do in my work – is the integration of history. The inspiration is Paul Farmer, who worked for a long time on this. He initially brought the history of colonialism into the modern-day understanding of the causation and distribution of disease in Haiti and other countries.[20] He and others have applied that to many other global health contexts. We have a much better understanding of the causal determinants of the current situations (capability constraints and failures) from a historical perspective, which then raises good questions about reparations, corrections, and equity. Such questions are more difficult to perceive even if one is working with social epidemiology. And they are impossible to see if we just look at individual-level risk factors and access to medicines. Epidemiology is one of the most pernicious sites of epistemic domination and exclusion in global health. But that is another story. The main point was that the capabilities approach is inter-disciplinary, reaching into the discipline of history may help provide more insight and explanatory power, as well as guidance.

Aside from public health sciences and history disciplines, there is also a need for a better understanding of how health policymaking works, not only at a national level but also at a global level. Because we want our conceptions of global health justice to be able to be practical and guide actions and conversations, we need to understand where theories of justice or concepts can influence policy. This might not satisfy philosophers who are purely interested in philosophical questions. But for those who are interested in a theory of global health justice, and want it to persevere, guide action, and do justice in the world, we need to be able to talk about and to health policy-makers. A theory of global health justice that speaks across disciplinary theories and paradigms is also more plausible and more justifiable.

13.4 Conclusion

My initial work focused on the idea of health justice being about a capability-centred approach to not only health justice but social justice as well. The argument that I presented in the *Health Justice* book is about how to think about health justice at an individual level, in terms of capabilities rather than utilities or resources.[21] I recognised at that time that there were significant intellectual challenges in applying this argument to groups (public health) and to global health. The three criteria I have proposed for global health justice theory reflect the weakness of other approaches as well as to further develop my own argument into a global health justice theory. It should surprise no one when I say that according to the three proposed criteria, I think the capability approach fares much better than its rival approaches to global health justice. It is indeed suspect that someone is choosing and presenting the criteria by which their effort should be judged. But, putting the capabilities approach aside, the proposed criteria are worth discussing regarding any theory or approach to global health justice.

In my own case, I would argue that a global health justice theory would be or should be a capability approach theory. In *Health Justice*, I argue that any justice theory that is interested in taking health seriously would be a health capabilities theory. This is because, correctly understood, health is a meta-capability (a cluster of capabilities) not absence of disease, or normal functioning, or something else. So doing justice regarding health means addressing health capabilities.[22] This is also how I would think about global health justice: we need to think of a global theory of health justice as an argument for not only more justice in global health but for more global justice. This would entail reforming the present global architecture to centre more on individual capabilities. The aim of global justice is to protect, expand, manage, and recover health capabilities.

I can give some practical examples. During the first two years of the Covid-19 pandemic, when different countries, particularly rich countries, implemented lockdowns, they were engendering and protecting health capabilities. They were saying, you stay home in order to protect yourself from exposure to a harmful virus, at the same time we as a society are going to provide you the conditions in order to be able to have at least some basic or minimal flourishing. You should be at home, there will be electricity, water, and food in the stores, the post will be delivered, the trash will still get picked up, and so forth. We will make sure that your internet is working, and we will also pay you while you are not able to work. This shows that we were engendering and protecting a (minimum set of) capabilities while preventing people from getting harmed, while also trying to find lasting solutions for this crisis. We can think of vaccines as also engendering or protecting capabilities.

For a number of weeks and months, almost all governments of all societies were expressly focused on protecting the life and health of their people against a harmful threat and implemented policies that sought to support people's basic capabilities. They did not primarily seek to maximise something, or provide a ration of basic goods, or try to identify who was morally responsible for the harm they were experiencing. It was more clearly an approach of protecting and ensuring a sufficient or basic level of capabilities, or quality of life. Such experience during an acute crisis reveals what is the standard situation during non-crisis times. Conditions support the health and wellbeing of some, often the majority of people. Others suffer greatly. A capabilities approach to global health justice would emphasise the importance of social conditions (shaped by forces from the global to the local) that engender and support basic capabilities of people and protect them from acute health threats. Identifying and addressing the situation of people with the most constrained capabilities would likely receive global support. It would also likely contribute to protecting the capabilities of people in far-away places, most directly in preventing or slowing down future pandemics.

Notes

1 Chatterjee DK (ed), *The Ethics of Assistance: Morality and the Distant Needy* (Cambridge University Press 2004).
2 Rawls J, *A Theory of Justice* (Harvard University Press 1971).
3 See Sen A, *The Idea of Justice* (Belknap Press 2011).
4 Rawls J, *The Law of Peoples: With, the Idea of Public Reason Revisited* (Harvard University Press 1999).
5 Miller D, *Justice for Earthlings: Essays in Political Philosophy* (Cambridge University Press 2013).
6 Singer P, 'Famine, Affluence, and Morality' (1972) 1 Philosophy & Public Affairs 229.
7 Held D, 'Cosmopolitan Democracy and the Global Order: Reflections on the 200th Anniversary of Kant's "Perpetual Peace"' (1995) 20 Alternatives: Global, Local, Political 415.
8 van Parijs P, 'Demos-Cracy for the European Union: Why and How' in Luis Cabrera (ed.), *Institutional cosmopolitanism* (Oxford University Press 2018).
9 Pogge TW, 'An Egalitarian Law of Peoples' (1994) 23 Philosophy & Public Affairs 195.

10 Schwab T, 'Are Bill Gates's Billions Distorting Public Health Data?' <https://www.thenation.com/article/society/gates-covid-data-ihme/> accessed 30 March 2023.

11 Daniels N, *Just Health Care* (Cambridge University Press 1985); Daniels N, *Just Health: Meeting Health Needs Fairly* (Cambridge University Press 2007).

12 Daniels, *Just Health* (n 11).

13 Venkatapuram S, 'Health and Justice: The Capability to Be Healthy.' (Thesis, University of Cambridge 2008) <https://www.repository.cam.ac.uk/handle/1810/224951>.

14 Mikell IM, Hoggard CLS and Schmidt H, 'What Should Be Roles of Federal Clinician Governors in Motivating Equity in Locally Coordinated Triage Protocols?' (2023) 25 AMA Journal of Ethics E179.

15 Sen A, 'Capability and Well-Being' in Nussbaum MC and Sen A (eds.), *The Quality of Life* (Oxford University Press 1993); Nussbaum MC, *Creating Capabilities: The Human Development Approach* (Belknap Press 2013).

16 Marmot M and others, 'Closing the Gap in a Generation: Health Equity through Action on the Social Determinants of Health' (2008) 372 The Lancet 1661.

17 Nussbaum MC, *Frontiers of Justice: Disability, Nationality, Species Membership* (Harvard University Press 2006).

18 Anderson E, 'Justifying the Capabilities Approach to Justice' in Brighouse H and Robeyns I (eds.), *Measuring Justice: Primary Goods and Capabilities* (Cambridge University Press 2010).

19 Rawls J, *Justice as Fairness: A Restatement* (Harvard University Press 2001).

20 Farmer P, *AIDS and Accusation: Haiti and the Geography of Blame* (2nd edn, University of California Press 2006).

21 Venkatapuram S, *Health Justice: An Argument From the Capabilities Approach* (Polity Press 2011).

22 ibid.

Bibliography

Anderson E, 'Justifying the Capabilities Approach to Justice' in H. Brighouse and I. Robeyns (eds), *Measuring Justice: Primary Goods and Capabilities* (Cambridge University Press 2010).

Chatterjee DK (ed), *The Ethics of Assistance: Morality and the Distant Needy* (Cambridge University Press 2004).

Daniels N, *Just Health Care* (Cambridge University Press 1985).

Daniels N, *Just Health: Meeting Health Needs Fairly* (Cambridge University Press 2007).

Farmer P, *AIDS and Accusation: Haiti and the Geography of Blame* (2nd edn, University of California Press 2006).

Held D, 'Cosmopolitan Democracy and the Global Order: Reflections on the 200th Anniversary of Kant's "Perpetual Peace"' [1995] 20 Alternatives: Global, Local, Political 415.

Marmot M and others, 'Closing the Gap in a Generation: Health Equity through Action on the Social Determinants of Health' [2008] 372 The Lancet 1661.

Mikell IM, Savage Hoggard CL and Schmidt H, 'What Should Be Roles of Federal Clinician Governors in Motivating Equity in Locally Coordinated Triage Protocols?' [2023] 25 AMA Journal of Ethics E179.

Miller D, *Justice for Earthlings: Essays in Political Philosophy* (Cambridge University Press 2013).

Nussbaum MC, *Frontiers of Justice: Disability, Nationality, Species Membership* (Harvard University Press 2006).

Nussbaum MC, *Creating Capabilities: The Human Development Approach* (Belknap Press 2013).

Parijs P van, 'Demos-Cracy for the European Union: Why and How' in L. Cabrera (ed), *Institutional cosmopolitanism* (Oxford University Press 2018).

Pogge TW, 'An Egalitarian Law of Peoples' [1994] 23 Philosophy & Public Affairs 195.

Rawls J, *A Theory of Justice* (Harvard University Press 1971).

Rawls J, *The Law of Peoples: With, the Idea of Public Reason Revisited* (Harvard University Press 1999).

Rawls J, *Justice as Fairness: A Restatement* (Harvard University Press 2001).

Schwab T, 'Are Bill Gates's Billions Distorting Public Health Data?' <https://www.thenation.com/article/society/gates-covid-data-ihme/> accessed 30 March 2023.

Sen A, 'Capability and Well-Being' in M. Nussbaum and A. Sen (eds), *The Quality of Life* (Oxford University Press 1993).

Sen A, *The Idea of Justice* (Belknap Press 2011).

Singer P, 'Famine, Affluence, and Morality' [1972] 1 Philosophy & Public Affairs 229.

Venkatapuram S, 'Health and Justice: The Capability to Be Healthy.' (Thesis, University of Cambridge 2008) <https://www.repository.cam.ac.uk/handle/1810/224951>

Venkatapuram S, *Health Justice: An Argument From the Capabilities Approach* (Polity Press 2011).

INDEX

Note: Page numbers followed by "n" refer to notes

Printed in the United States
by Baker & Taylor Publisher Services